J. Haddad
D. Christmann J. Messer (Eds.)

Imaging Techniques of the CNS of the Neonates

With Contributions by

D. I. Altmann, B. Brunot, G. M. Bydder, E. B. Cady, A. Calame, D. Christmann, A. Constantinesco, D. T. Delpy, C. L. Fawer, J. Haddad, J. Hennig, E. Martin, J. Messer, J. J. Volpe, J. S. Wyatt

With 251 Figures

Springer-Verlag
Berlin Heidelberg New York
London Paris Tokyo
Hong Kong Barcelona
Budapest

JOSEPH HADDAD, M. D.

Service de Médecine et Réanimation du Nouveau-Né
Centre Hospitalier Universitaire de Hautepierre – Strasbourg
Avenue Molière

67098 Strasbourg Cedex, France

DOMINIQUE CHRISTMANN, M. D.

Radiopédiatrie – Service de Radiologie II
Centre Hospitalier Universitaire de Hautepierre – Strasbourg
Avenue Molière

67098 Strasbourg Cedex, France

JEAN MESSER, Prof.

Service de Néonatologie
Service de Médecine et Réanimation du Nouveau-Né
Centre Hospitalier Universitaire de Hautepierre – Strasbourg
Avenue Molière

67098 Strasbourg Cedex, France

Library of Congress Cataloging-in-Publication Data. Imaging techniques of the CNS of the neonates / J. Haddad, D. Christmann, J. Messer (eds.). p. cm. Includes bibliographical references and index.

ISBN-13: 978-3-642-76490-5 e-ISBN-13: 978-3-642-76488-2

DOI: 10.1007/ 978-3-642-76488-2

1. Central nervous system-Imaging. 2. Infants (Newborn)-Diseases-Diagnosis. 3. Central Nervous System-Diseases-Diagnosis. I. Haddad, J. (Joseph) II. Christmann, D. III. Messer, J.
RJ290.I42 1991 618.92′80754-dc20 91-20738

Reproduction of the figures: Gustav Dreher GmbH, D-7000 Stuttgart
Typesetting: Konrad Triltsch, Graphischer Betrieb, Würzburg
21/3130-543210 – Printed on acid-free paper

Preface

There has been increasing interest in neonatal neurology, especially since imaging techniques were introduced in the neonatal ward. Looking at the natural history of imaging techniques, we can identify three main axes of its development.

Logically, it was first essential to image the brain morphologically. For this purpose, computed tomography was initially used, followed by ultrasound. However, to improve the quality of the images, magnetic resonance imaging was introduced. Major features of ultrasound and magnetic resonance imaging are their safety and lack of ionization.

Morphological imaging techniques have proved to be insufficient to explain the mechanisms underlying CNS injuries. Thus, it was essential to develop functional techniques to assess cerebral hemodynamics and oxygenation. The use of Doppler ultrasound, PET scanning, SPECT scanning and, more recently, NIRS have widened our knowledge of general neurological problems.

Finally, to achieve our goal of attaining a better understanding of CNS injuries, it is important to assess cerebral cellular metabolism. Magnetic resonance spectroscopy was introduced to achieve this goal.

We hope that this book links these different techniques in order to widen our horizon. The future is promising and bound to provide further developments, which however can only be understood if we grasp the present level of development.

JOSEPH HADDAD

Contents

List of Contributors

D. I. Altman, M. B., B. Ch.,
Assistant Professor, Washington
University School of Medicine
St. Louis Children's Hospital
400 S. Kingshighway Blvd.
St. Louis, MO 63110, USA

B. Brunot, M. D.
Service de Médecine Nucléaire
Hospital University of Strasbourg
Hopital de Hautepierre
67098 Strasbourg Cedex, France

G. M. Bydder, Prof.
N.M.R. Department
Hammersmith Hospital
Du Cane Road
London W12 OHS,
United Kingdom

E. B. Cady, Ph. D.
Department of Medical Physics
and Bio-Engineering
University College London
1st Floor Shropshire House
11-20 Capper Street
London WC1E 6AJ,
United Kingdom

A. Calame, M. D., Prof.
Division de Néonatologie
Service de Pédiatrie
Centre Hospitalier Universitaire
Vaudois
1011 Lausanne, Switzerland

D. Christmann, M. D.
Hospices Civils de Strasbourg
Radiopédiatrie – Service de
Radiologie II
Centre Hospitalier Universitaire de
Hautepierre – Strasbourg
67098 Strasbourg Cedex, France

A. Constantinesco, M. D., Ph. D.,
Prof.
Service de Médicine Nucléaire
Hospital University of Strasbourg
Hopital de Hautepierre
67098 Strasbourg Cedex, France

D. T. Delpy, Ph. D.
Departments of Paediatrics
and Medical Physics
and Bioengineering
University College & Middlesex
School of Medicine
Rayne Institute
University Street
London WC1E 6JJ,
United Kingdom

C. L. Fawer, M. D., Ph. D.
Division de Néonatologie
Service de Pédiatrie
Centre Hospitalier Universitaire
Vaudois
1011 Lausanne, Switzerland

J. Haddad, M. D.
Hospices Civils de Strasbourg
Service de Pédiatrie II
Médecine et Réanimation du
Nouveau-Né
Avenue Molière
67098 Strasbourg Cedex, France

J. Hennig, Ph. D.
Radiologische Universitätsklinik
Chirurgie/Kernspintomographie
Hugstetter Str. 55
W-7800 Freiburg i.Br., FRG

E. Martin, M. D.
Magnetresonanz
Kinderspital Zürich
Steinwiesstr. 75
8032 Zürich, Switzerland

J. MESSER, M.D., Prof.
Service de Néonatologie, Medecine et Réanimation du Nouveau-Né
Pédiatrie II
Centre Hospitalier Universitaire de Hautepierre – Strasbourg
Avenue Molière
67098 Strasbourg Cedex, France

J. J. VOLPE, M.D.
Bronson Crothers Professor of Neurology
Harvard Medical School
Neurologist-in-Chief
Children's Hospital
Boston, MA 02115, USA

J. S. WYATT, M.D.
Departments of Paediatrics and Medical Physics and Bioengineering
University College & Middlesex School of Medicine
Rayne Institute
University Street
London WC1E 6JJ,
United Kingdom

1 Principles of Magnetic Resonance Imaging

G. M. Bydder

CONTENTS

1.1 Introduction

Magnetic resonance imaging (MRI) is a new noninvasive method of mapping the internal structure of the body which completely avoids the use of ionizing radiation and appears to be without hazard. It employs radiofrequency (rf) radiation in the presence of carefully controlled magnetic fields in order to produce high quality images of the body in any plane. It usually displays the distribution of hydrogen nuclei and parameters relating to their motion in water and lipids.

The phenomenon of MR was described independently by Bloch and Purcell in 1946 and for their discovery they were jointly awarded the nobel prize for physics in 1952. Since its discovery, MR has been used extensively as a laboratory method for studying the properties of matter at the molecular level.

The use of MR for imaging required a method for spatial localization. In 1973 Lauterbur showed that this could be done by applying a linearly varying magnetic field to the body. Clinical images were first published in 1980 by Hawkes et al. The subject has evolved rapidly and there is now a large text devoted solely to MRI in children (Cohen and Edwards 1990).

1.2 Principles of MRI

1.2.1 Basic Physics

MR describes the phenomenon whereby the nuclei of certain atoms, when placed in a magnetic field, absorb and emit rf energy of a specific frequency. The spectrum of absorbed or emitted rf energy depends upon the nucleus under observation and its chemical environment.

Nuclei suitable for MRI are those which have an odd number of protons or neutrons and therefore possess a net charge and have angular momentum. As a result of the combination of charge and angular momentum, these nuclei behave as magnetic dipoles. Almost all images produced to date have been of the nuclear magnetism of the hydrogen nucleus (or proton), which is a particularly favourable nucleus from the MRI standpoint and is present in virtually all biological materials. Other naturally occurring magnetic nuclei which are of interest include phosphorus (^{31}P), sodium (^{23}Na), carbon (^{13}C) and potassium (^{39}K).

The proton can be regarded as a small, freely suspended bar magnet spinning rapidly about its magnetic axis. When a group of protons are placed in a uniform magnetic field, their magnetic moments experience a couple tending to turn them parallel to the direction of the field. In a

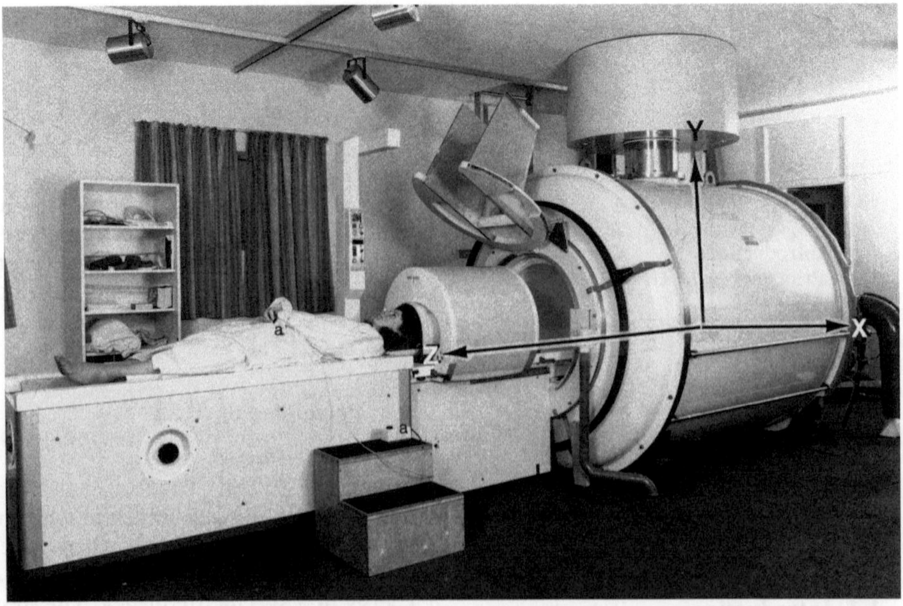

Fig. 1.1. MRI scanner based on a cryogenic magnet. The x, y and z axes are labelled

strong magnetic field, many more of these nuclear magnetic dipoles align with the applied static magnetic field in the direction of the field rather than against it. This produces a net magnetization in the direction of the field and conventionally defines the z axis, which is generally along the longitudinal axis of the patient in an MRI machine (Fig. 1.1).

The strong magnetic field, which must be homogeneous over a volume large enough to contain the human body in an MRI machine, is provided by a resistive, permanent or superconducting magnet. Magnetic field strengths used for clinical imaging currently range from 0.02 to 4 T.

Since the nuclei are spinning, they respond to the magnetic couple like a gyroscope and their axes are tilted so that they come to rotate at exactly the same frequency about the magnetic field direction in a movement known as precession. The frequency of precession is directly proportional to the applied magnetic field; for protons in a field of 1 T, it is 42.6 MHz. This relationship is expressed as the Larmor equation:

$$f = \gamma B \qquad (1.1)$$

where f is the resonant frequency, γ is the gyromagnetic ratio and B is the applied field.

If a pulse of oscillating rf from a coil is imposed on a group of protons in a magnetic field, there is a strong interaction or resonant effect, providing that the frequency of the oscillator is equal to the precession frequency of the protons. This is called magnetic resonance and manifests itself in the following way: rf energy is absorbed from the transmitter coil which causes the motion of the elementary magnets to be disturbed and the direction of the total nuclear magnetization to be altered. The net magnetization along the z axis is deviated through an angle which depends upon the strength and duration of the pulse of the rf magnetic field. So-called 90° and 180° pulses are commonly used. These rotate the magnetization in the z direction through 90° and 180°, respectively. After the disturbance induced by the applied pulse or pulses, the magnetization returns to its equilibrium position along the *z* axis in an exponential manner, and, as it does so, the changing magnetization induces a small voltage in a receiver coil which surrounds the patient.

The electrical signal picked up following an rf pulse is known as the free induction decay (FID). The magnitude and length of the FID is determined by the nuclear relaxation times, which reflect molecular motion.

The first of these relaxation times, T_1, or the longitudinal relaxation time, is the time taken by the system of nuclei to return to thermal equilibrium after the rf pulse. The second relaxation time, T_2, or the transverse relaxation time, is the characteristic decay time of the FID and is due to the irreversible dephasing of the initially coherent precession of individual protons which follows the rf pulse. In liquids or systems containing mobile protons, T_2/T_1 is approximately 1, whereas in solids T_2/T_1 is very small. Unlike computerized tomography (CT) images in which contrast is determined by differences in one parameter (the linear X-ray attenuation coefficiency μ), multiple parameters influence the MRI signal including proton density, T_1 and T_2. In addition, flowing material within the image plane alters contrast. T_1 and T_2 variations between tissues are usually very much greater than variations in proton density; thus, images with greater dependence on T_1 or T_2 have greater contrast. The principal pulse sequences are:

1. Partial saturation (PS) or saturation recovery (SR) which typically utilizes a 90° rf pulse but can use a greater or smaller pulse.
2. Spin echo (SE) which utilizes a 90° pulse followed at time TE/2 by an 180° pulse. At a further time, *TE*/2, an echo of the original signal is detected.
3. Inversion recovery (IR) which utilizes a 180° pulse followed at time *TI* by a 90° pulse.

Variations in the timing of the rf pulses in these pulse sequences may produce marked differences in image contrast.

1.2.2 Localization of the MRI Signal

In addition to information at the molecular level, the MRI signal can also be used to provide macroscopic spatial information. The resonant frequency is proportional to the strength of the magnetic field. If a linearly increasing gradient is applied in one direction, then the frequencies of the components of the body being studied will increase with distance. Each volume element in the body is therefore labelled by having a different resonant frequency for the protons within it. The resulting complicated FID signal is digitized and frequency analysed in a computer using a mathematical technique known as Fourier analysis.

If an additional gradient magnetic field is applied prior to the detection of the signal, differences in the phase of the local nuclear signals are produced. By using a series of phase encoding gradients of different strengths, the spatial distribution of signals along a perpendicular gradient direction can also be obtained. This is the basis of the widely employed two-dimensional Fourier transform method of imaging.

The rf radiation from the transmitter coil cannot be collimated into a narrow beam as can X-rays. There is, therefore, a fundamental difference in the method of selecting the slice to be imaged. A gradient field is applied during excitation by an rf pulse which contains a predetermined narrow band of frequencies. Only those regions in which the local resonant frequency falls within the range of frequencies determined by the gradient field and corresponding to that of the rf pulse are excited. In this way imaging can be restricted to a particular slice of the desired thickness.

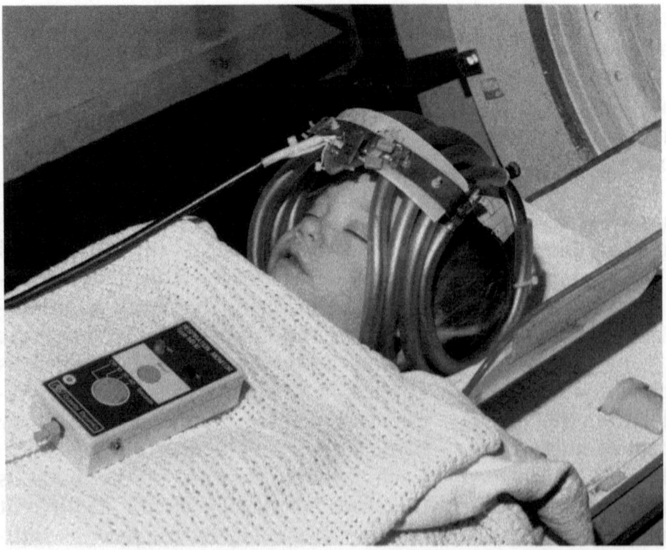

Fig. 1.2. Child in a quasispherical receiver coil

1.2.3 Instrumentation

All MRI scanners are constructed around a large magnet. Within this are situated gradient coils. In MR systems which have separate transmitter and receiver coils, appropriately configured coils can be placed in close apposition to the region of interest in order to receive the signal (Fig. 1.2) (Dubowitz et al. 1986).

Gradient amplifiers are required to generate the magnetic field necessary to spatially encode the detected signal and select a slice. A large computer is required to control the system, reconstruct the images and display them.

MRI scanners present the data obtained as an analogue display of the pixel values of the signal in a given anatomical cross section. Since the dynamic range of the MRI signals exceeds what can be partitioned into a grey scale that can be appreciated by the visual system, the data is viewed at different window widths around a chosen central level. The numerical data underlying the images can be stored on magnetic tape or floppy discs and can be manipulated in various ways before being displayed. High frequency filtration gives a smoothed image with a reduced noise content at the expense of resolution; low frequency filtration gives edge enhancement at the boundaries of high contrast structures. Colour may provide a valuable method of presenting the multivariable information provided by MRI.

1.2.4 Image Parameters

The problem of interpretation facing the clinician can be illustrated in Fig. 1.3, in which on one side the tissue within the voxel is represented and on the other side is the signal intensity within that voxel.

For unenhanced CT, the physics connecting the two can be represented as in Fig. 1.3. There is an essentially linear relationship between pixel signal intensity (image brightness) and the X-ray linear attenuation coefficient μ, which is scaled relative to air and water and converted to an integer. This is expressed in Hounsfield units (H) with air having a value of

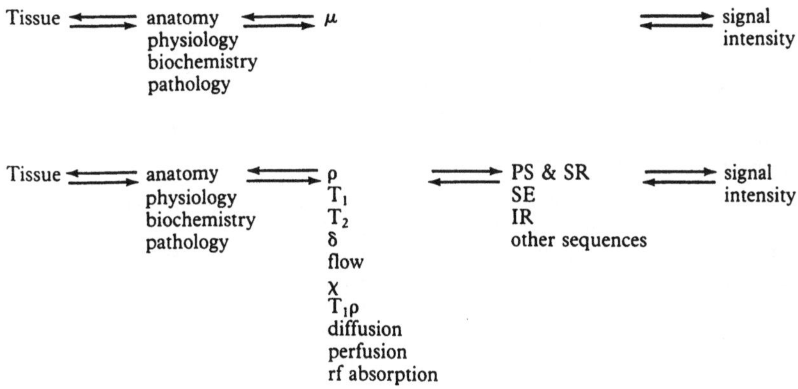

Fig. 1.3. Models for CT (*upper*) and MRI (*lower*) image interpretation. The CT image can be interpreted with knowledge of the X-ray attenuation coefficient μ. The MR image requires a knowledge of 10 image parameters, P, T_1, T_2, δ, flow, χ, T_1 P, D, perfusion, RF absorption and the pulse sequences, partial saturation or saturation recovery (*PS* or *SR*), spin echo (*SE*), and inversion recovery (*IR*)

-1000, water a value of 0 and most soft tissues (except fat) about 20–60 H. On the patient side of this model, it is necessary to consider the anatomy, physiology, biochemistry and pathology of various tissues and how this changes μ. For example, calcification usually increases μ, whereas oedema in the brain decreases it. From the change in tissue μ, it is possible to make inferences about the tissue including particularly whether it is normal or abnormal. Other anatomical information contributes to the diagnosis but the physics necessary for image interpretation of the unenhanced CT image can very largely be understood in terms of changes in the single parameter, μ.

The situation with MRI is much more complex (Fig. 1.3). Instead of a single parameter there are at least ten potential image parameters. These include proton density (P), T_1, T_2, chemical shift (δ), flow, susceptibility (χ), $T_1 P$ (T_1 in the rotating frame), diffusion (D), perfusion and rf absorption. It is necessary on the patient side (Fig. 1.3, left) of this model to 'think through' the MR properties of tissues in terms of these image parameters for both healthy and pathological tissues. On the machine side (Fig. 1.3, right) it is necessary to relate differences in the image parameters to the observed signal intensity via the pulse sequence. The pulse sequence defines the dependence of the MR image signal intensity on the ten image parameters. The pulse sequence has no equivalent in CT in which there is only one image parameter and only a single pattern of dependence of the image on this parameter. Some other factors affect signal intensity on the machine side of this model including the choice of receiver coil and magnetic field strength. Planar surface coils tend to be nonlinear and produce a decrease in signal intensity with distance from the coil, whereas solenoidal, spherical and saddle coils display a more uniform signal intensity.

A systematic approach to image interpretation involves further consideration of the left (patient) and right (machine) sides of Fig. 1.3. This will form the subject matter for the remainder of this section beginning with the left side of the model.

1.2.4.1 Proton Density

Only protons are considered here, but the same concepts are applicable to all MR sensitive species. The dominant role of protons in MRI is a consequence of both their abundance and their high sensitivity. It is useful to rank fluids and tissues according to their relative proton density. Highest is CSF, urine and other fluids; these are followed, in order, by various soft tissues such as liver, kidney and spleen, grey matter, white matter, articular cartilage, fibrocartilage, membranes, cortical bone and air. It is important to recognize that it is only mobile protons which give a MR signal with conventional techniques. When the protons are in large molecules or immobilised in solids they give no detectable signal with most MRI techniques. Thus cortical bone contains protons but these do not give a detectable signal.

There is a variety of pathological circumstances in which proton density is increased. These include oedema, infection, inflammation, acute demyelination, acute haemorrhage, some tumours, cysts and other conditions. Since the formation of oedema is a common response to a wide variety of insults, an increase in *P* is a frequent occurrence. A decrease in proton density may be seen in scar formation, fibrosis, some tumours, capsule and membrane formation and calcification. The changes in proton density are often relatively small (5% – 10%) in comparison to the changes seen in T_1 and T_2, which may be 20% – 200%.

1.2.4.2 Relaxation Times

T_1 and T_2 are very important determinants of image contrast. There is a wide range of normal values of T_1 and T_2 for different tissues. A general knowledge of these values is a necessary prerequisite for understanding differences in signal intensity on images. Table 1.1 lists values of T_1 and T_2 at 0.15 T for some common tissues. The information is obtained from a collation of values of T_1 and T_2 published by Bottomley et al. (1984, 1987). The values of T_1 and T_2 depend on many factors, but in general terms there is a relationship between the viscosity of a tissue and its T_1 and T_2. Thus liquids have a very long T_1 and T_2, soft tissues have shorter values of T_1 and T_2 and solids have very long T_1s and very short T_2s. Within the imaging range, T_2 changes relatively little with field, whereas T_1 increases with field. It approximately doubles between 0.15 T and 1.5 T for many tissues, although the change in fat is rather less (1.5 times) and CSF changes relatively little. The ratio of T_1 values for different tissues at different fields is shown in Table 1.2. For the tissues of principal interest an increase in water content will generally result in an increase in T_1 and T_2. Fluid accumulates in many pathological conditions (e.g. oedema, inflammation and infection) so

Table 1.1. Values of T_1, T_2 and the ratio of T_1/T_2 at 0.15 *T* for various tissues

Tissue	T_1 (ms)	T_2 (ms)	T_1/T_2
Grey matter	453 ± 77	101 ± 13	4.5
White matter	353 ± 60	92 ± 22	3.8
Cardiac muscle	377 ± 60	57 ± 16	6.6
Liver	206 ± 45	43 ± 14	4.8
Spleen	364 ± 69	62 ± 37	5.9
Kidney	368 ± 99	58 ± 24	6.3
Skeletal muscle	330 ± 59	47 ± 13	7.0
Fat	173 ± 49	84 ± 36	2.1

Table 1.2. Ratio of T_1 at different fields to that at 0.15 T for various tissues

Tissue	Field strength (T)				
	0.15	0.3	0.5	1	1.5
Grey matter	1	1.24	1.45	1.79	2.03
White matter	1	1.27	1.52	1.93	2.23
Cardiac muscle	1	1.28	1.55	1.99	2.30
Liver	1	1.30	1.58	2.05	2.39
Spleen	1	1.24	1.49	1.88	2.15
Kidney	1	1.19	1.35	1.60	1.77
Skeletal muscle	1	1.34	1.66	2.22	2.63
Fat	1	1.13	1.24	1.39	1.50

that an increase in T_1 and T_2 is a common observation in many diseases.

Another major determinant of T_1 and T_2 is the presence of paramagnetic species. These may be endogenous including organic iron compounds such as the breakdown products of haemoglobin. They may also be exogenous in the form of paramagnetic contrast agents such as intravenous gadolinium-DTPA (Gd-DTPA). Paramagnetic species tend to decrease T_1 and T_2. The observed values of T_1 and T_2 for liver are not as high as might be expected from its generally 'wet' nature. This is probably a consequence of the presence of organic iron within the liver. In pathological circumstances, effects due to paramagnetic species are seen in haematomas in which deoxyhaemoglobin, methaemoglobin, haemosiderin and free Fe^{3+} may all play a role in decreasing T_1 and T_2.

The changes in T_1 and T_2 may be very large. For example, the neonatal brain contains about 92% water. During the first 2 years of life this drops to 83%–85%. The T_1 of the brain (at 0.15 T) typically decreases from 1300–1500 ms at birth to 300–500 ms during the second year of life. Thus there is about a 300% decrease in T_1 for a 7%–9% decrease in water content. Similarly, in disease a small increase in water content may be associated with a 50%–100% increase in T_1 and T_2. From an imaging point of view, the large changes in T_1 and T_2 are of more value in diagnosis than the relatively small changes in proton density.

1.2.4.3 Chemical Shift

Although this parameter has been of major importance in spectroscopy it has a smaller role in imaging. The proton spectrum of many tissues contains two large peaks – one from protons in water and the other from protons in $-CH_2$ (lipid) bonds. There are many other resonances but these two peaks are generally much greater than those of other species. The peaks are typically separated by about 3.5 parts per million (ppm). From an imaging point of view it is useful to consider the phase of the signal from a voxel after a 90° pulse. As a result of the difference in resonant frequency between these two main proton species, their signals will alternatively be in and out of phase. The detected signals tend to cancel out when they are 180° out of phase and add when they come back into phase. The phenomenon is like the beating effect from two musical notes which are slightly out of tune. The time TE_0 for the signals to become 180° out of phase after a 90° pulse is given by:

$$TE_0 = \frac{1}{2f\delta} \qquad (1.2)$$

where f is the resonant frequency and δ is the chemical shift between them. For protons using $\delta = 3.5$ ppm for fat and water

$$TE_0\,(\mathrm{ms}) = \frac{3.3}{B_0\,(\mathrm{tesla})} \qquad (1.3)$$

where B_0 is the static magnetic field. Note that TE_0 decreases with increasing field. Thus 22 ms is the time for cancellation at 0.15 T, whereas 2.2 ms is the corresponding time at 1.5 T.

For the cancellation effect to be obvious, a voxel must contain at least roughly equal proportions of protons in water and lipid. This occurs normally in voxels at interfaces between subcutaneous fat and other tissues as a result of partial volume effects and produces a dark 'india ink' line surrounding many organs and marking certain tissue planes. In red bone marrow there are roughly equal proportions of protons in lipid and water and cancellation effects are normally seen.

1.2.4.4 Flow Effects

The movement of fluids produces important changes in signal intensity. The situations of interest include both blood and

CSF flow and fluid collections such as urine in the bladder, joint fluid, cysts and ascites. Flow phenomena are dealt with in detail by Bradley and Waluch (1985) and only a brief outline is included here.

The method of analysis takes a slice and considers: (a) the behaviour of the fluid remaining in the slice between excitations, (b) the fluid that is washed into the slice between excitations, (c) the fluid that is washed out of the slice between excitations and (d) phase changes in the presence of a magnetic field gradient.

The fluid remaining in the slice is stationary or moving very slowly and, to a first approximation, behaves like the stationary tissue outside the fluid filled region in the slice, although with thick slices and rapid repetition rates it is possible to have significant movement of fluid which is still within the slice. From a practical point of view it is still useful to consider a greater or smaller fraction of the fluid as 'stationary' within the slice.

The fluid washing into the slice may not have been excited by an rf pulse previously. Alternatively, it may have experienced an rf pulse as part of a non-slice selected excitation or as a slice selected excication when it was within another slice of a multislice set. When the fluid flowing into the slice is unsaturated (i.e. it has no recent experience of an rf pulse), a 90° pulse will give a high signal; if the blood has not fully recovered from a previous excitation, the signal will be lower. Some of the options and the various appearances that result are discussed by Axel (1984). The appearance of the inflowing fluid depends both on the type of flow (laminar or turbulent) and on its velocity. The appearances may also vary depending on whether the image is gated to the heartbeat or not and, if it is gated, on what phase of the cardiac cycle. Cardiac gating and respiration also affects the pattern of CSF flow. With pulse sequences involving two or more rf excitations, it is possible for blood flowing into the slice to only experience the second or a subsequent excitation. Thus the blood in effect experiences a different pulse sequence than the surrounding tissue.

The signal from outflowing blood depends on a number of factors. With very rapid rates of flow it is possible for the excited blood to disappear from the vicinity of the receiver coil before the data is collected, resulting in loss of the signal. More common is for some of the fluid in the slice to experience only part of the pulse sequence since it has moved out of the slice before the second or subsequent rf pulse is applied. Thus moving blood may experience a 90°–180° pulse sequence with an SE sequence, whereas faster moving blood may only experience a 90° pulse sequence. Incomplete exposure to a pulse sequence occurs with both inflowing and outflowing fluid.

A phase change in the presence of a gradient is an important cause for both a loss and a relative increase in signal. When fluid elements within a voxel move with different velocities along a magnetic field gradient, they experience different changes in phase. When the signal is received from this voxel, the phase shifts may produce a net cancellation with a reduction in signal intensity. This is a common mechanism for the reduction in signal frequently seen with flowing blood. Another phenomenon, even echo rephasing, is seen with SE sequences with multiple echoes (Waluch and Bradley 1984). The signal received from the even echoes is higher than that from the preceding odd echoes. Thus the signal intensity from venous blood in the sagittal sinus often gives a higher signal from the second echo than it does for the first echo.

The effects of flow vary with the angle of incidence of the vessel to the slice. The principles are the same for in-plane flow, in which the blood is entirely within the slice. In this situation, wash-in and wash-out effects are much less important and the effects of magnetic field gradients dominate. The position of the flowing blood on the image may be displaced since it moves in the time between receiving its phase-encoding pulse and when its signal is received.

In order to predict the appearance of blood flow it is necessary to know the type of flow, the rate of flow, its direction, whether gating has been used or not and the full details of the pulse sequence. Care is necessary in recognising flow effects, for it is relatively easy to diagnose a solid lesion when all that is being seen is an unusual flow effect within a fluid filled space.

1.2.4.5 Susceptibility Effects

It is possible to divide tissues into three categories according to the way they effect the static magnetic field B_0. Diamagnetic materials produce a slight reduction in the field, paramagnetic materials produce a slight increase and ferromagnetic materials produce a large and persistent increase. These changes in magnetic field produce a corresponding change in the phase and frequency of the resonant nuclei. If there is a difference in field within a voxel this will lead to dephasing of any excited signal with a loss of intensity. The effect increases with magnetic field strength and with echo time. This mechanism is more important at high fields than at low fields and accounts for some of the changes seen in paramagnetic lesions such as haematomas. Susceptibility effects may also be seen at air-tissue interfaces as a result of differences in susceptibility between air and tissue. On transverse images this can result in artefacts in the temporal lobes above the mastoid sinuses.

1.2.4.6 Other Image Parameters

While considerable clinical experience has accumulated with the use of the parameters listed above (P, T_1, T_2, δ, flow and χ). Use of other parameters is still the subject of further research. $T_1 P$ (T_1 in the rotating frame) provides information analogous to T_1 and T_2 but the methods required to obtain this information may involve high rf power deposition. It may provide information about large molecules but the number of patients examined to date is quite small.

Assessment of diffusion (D) has formed a part of MR spectroscopy since the 1950s. It is usually assessed as part of tissue perfusion which also involves elements of flow. The application is to ischaemia, arteriovenous malformations and other disturbances of blood supply (Le Bihan et al. 1986). Its importance in infancy derives from the fact that the diffusion of water in nerve fibres is highly restricted by myelin. Assessment of diffusion has been proven to be more sensitive than highly T_1 weighted imaging in detecting the presence of myelin and has shown areas of abnormality not detected with other sequences (Rutherford et al. 1991).

This section covered tissues and their MR properties in order to understand how the image parameters change in health and disease. In the next sections pulse sequences are considered. Pulse sequences determine the dependence of the signal intensity of the image voxel on the ten basic image parameters.

In order to describe each pulse sequence it is necessary to consider another set of parameters – the pulse sequence parameters. A list of these is shown opposite the first six image parameters in Table 1.3 for a PS sequence. TR is the repetition time, i.e. the time between cycles; TE is the time from the rf pulse to the middle of the data collection, and α is the flip angle, i.e. the angle of the excitation pulse. Other factors include the use of spoiler pulses, the number of averages, the spatial resolution and motion suppression techniques. The essential task is to analyse each sequence and determine how changes in each of the pulse sequence parameters affects the dependence of the signal intensity on the image parameters. An approach to this problem is described below for the PS sequence.

Table 1.3. Image parameters and pulse sequence parameters for the PS sequence

Image parameters	Pulse sequence parameters
P	TR
T_1	TE
T_2	α
δ	Spoiler pulses
Flow	Bandwidth and data collection time
χ	Spatial resolution
	Projection reconstruction or two-dimensional Fourier transform
	Motion artefact suppression
	Single slice, multislice or volume

1.2.5 Principal Pulse Sequences

1.2.5.1 The PS Pulse Sequence

Proton density (P) is an easy parameter to model. For each of the common sequences, PS, SE and IR (with a minor exception), signal intensity is proportional to proton density. This rule applies to the PS sequence, in which for example, cortical bone ($P=0$) gives no signal.

In order to follow the effects of T_1 and T_2 it is useful to construct composite graphs of the recovery of the longitudinal magnetization (M_z) during the time TR followed by the decay (after a 90° pulse) of the transverse magnetization M_{xy} (Fig. 1.4). The signal intensity on the image is proportional to the height of M_{xy} at the time of the data collection. These figures can be drawn for tissues with short and long values of T_1 and T_2. A tissue with a short T_1 is likely to have a short T_2 and vice versa. If a curve is plotted for a tissue with a short T_1 and T_2 and another for a tissue with a long T_1 and T_2, then it is easy to see that at a certain value of TE there will be a 'crossover' in which the signal intensity of the two tissues is equal in spite of the fact that the tissues differ in their values of T_1 and T_2 (Fig. 1.5). The crossover

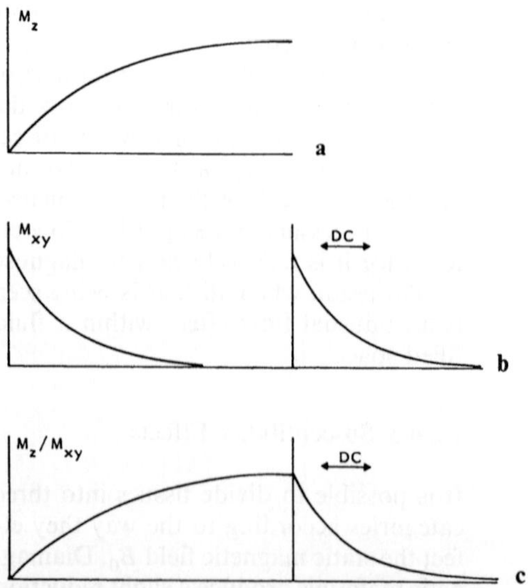

Fig. 1.4a–c. PS sequence. **a** Plot of M_z against time after a 90° pulse, and **b** M_{xy} against time with the data collection (DC) shown. **c** A composite of M_z/M_{xy} against time for two 90° pulses

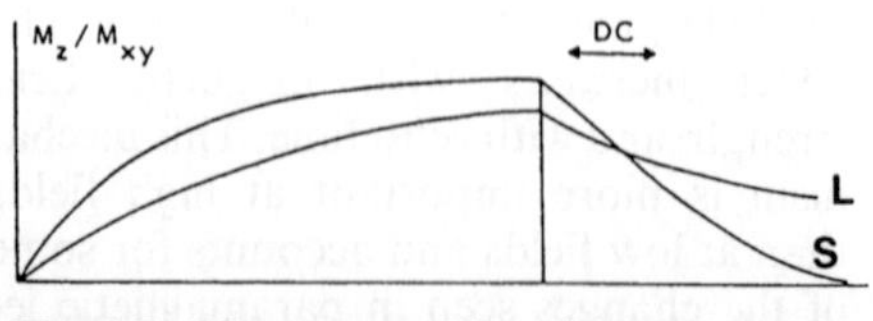

Fig. 1.5. PS sequence. Plot of M_z/M_{xy} against time for a tissue (S) with a short T_1 and T_2 and a tissue (L) with a long T_1 and T_2. The data collection (DC) is shown. The curves cross at which time there is a loss of contrast between L and S

point should be avoided in clinical practice.

In general, it is most useful to maximise either T_1 or T_2 dependent contrast with a pulse sequence. To maximise T_1 dependent contrast, TR is chosen about equal to the anticipated mean T_1 of the tissues of interest and TE is kept as short as possible to minimise the T_2 dependent

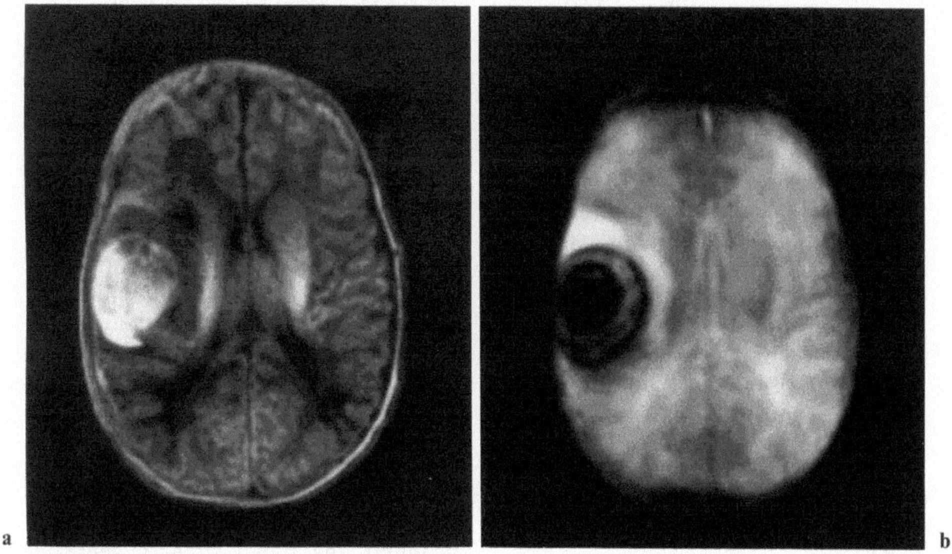

Fig. 1.6 a, b. Intracerebral haematoma. IR 1500/500/44 (**a**) and PS 1660/193 (**b**) images. The haematoma has a high signal intensity in **a** and a mixed pattern with low signal intensity areas in **b** due to susceptibility effects

contrast. In order to maximise T_2 dependent contrast, TE is lengthened to the likely mean value of T_2 and TR is made as long as practical to reduce the T_1 dependence.

Optimisation of the signal to noise ratio, by using an appropriate value of the flip angle α is well known in spectroscopy. Reducing α reduces the T_1 dependence of the PS sequence. This may be used in situations in which low T_1 dependence and high T_2 dependence is being sought, such as with rapid T_2 dependent sequences. Typical values of α for low T_1 dependence are in the range of 10°–30°.

In addition to affecting the T_2 dependent contrast, *TE* also controls phase dependent chemical shift changes. The key concept here is the time, TE_0, which will produce a cancellation effect in voxels containing roughly equal proportions of protons in water and lipid. At a time equal to 2 TE_0 the signals add again and so on. *TE* also controls susceptibility effects; these increase as B_0 is increased and as TE is lengthened (Fig. 1.6).

1.2.5.2 The SE Pulse Sequence

Much of the reasoning used in the previous section also applies to the SE sequence. The additional 180° pulse creates new options and these vary depending on whether the 180° pulse is slice selected or not. In general the SE sequence is used in three forms: (1) the T_1 dependent form, (2) the T_2 dependent form, and (3) the asymmetrical SE form in which chemical shift phase effects are apparent. Frequently, multiple echoes are produced with different values of TE. This affects the T_2 dependence, flow effects (including phenomena such as even echo rephasing) and susceptibility effects. The sequence tolerates field inhomogeneity well and has become the most commonly used approach in clinical MRI.

In the first step of a SE pulsing sequence, a 90° rf pulse flips the existing longitudinal magnetization from the *z* axis 90° into the transverse *xy* plane. Whenever transverse magnetization is present, it rotates at the Larmor frequency and induces an oscillating MR signal in a receiving coil. The magnitude of the transverse magnetization after the 90° pulse is approximately equal to the magnitude of the longitudinal magnetization which had recovered during the interval allowed between repetitions. This interval is called the repetition time (TR) and is one of the programmable sequence parameters.

In the process of rotating the magnetization 90° into the transverse orientation, the longitudinal component of magnetization is totally lost and must be allowed to recover before another signal can be generated. The amount of longitudinal magnetization which is recovered depends on the rate of recovery (T_1) and the time allowed for recovery to occur (TR).

The magnitude of the signal detected depends not only on longitudinal recovery between repetitions, but also on how slowly the transverse magnetization decays from its initial maximum value. This decay depends on the T_2 of the tissue. The amount of time allowed for decay to occur – the time between the initial 90° rf pulse and the detection of the SE – is called the echo delay time (TE) and is another programmable sequence parameter.

When considered in the most simplistic terms, the SE is a two step process. The first step (longitudinal recovery) determines the starting intensity for the second step (transverse decay). The starting intensity reflects the relationship between T_1 and TR, modified by the proton density. The subsequent decay from this starting intensity reflects differences in T_2 and TE.

The difference in T_1 values between brain parenchyma (shorter T_1) and CSF (longer T_1) can be used to enhance contrast between the two. This is important when seeking abnormalities at the brain-CSF interface. A short TR time allows a shorter T_1 tissue (such as brain) to recover between repetitions to a much greater extent than a longer T_1 fluid (such as CSF). The contrast in short TR, short TE sequences is based primarily on differences in T_1; they are called 'T_1-weighted' sequences. Note that tissues with low values of T_1 have the highest signal intensity on T_1-weighted images.

As the *TR* is prolonged, all tissues fully recover their longitudinal magnetization between repetitions and the pixel intensity becomes more independent of T_1. At short TE values the effect of T_2 decay is minimised and one is left with an image with little T_1 or T_2 dependence. This is called a 'proton density-weighted' image.

Tissues with longer T_2 times generate stronger signals than those with shorter T_2 times, if both are acquired at the same TE and if proton density and T_1 are comparable. When multiple spin echoes are acquired, the signal strength generally decreases as TE is lengthened due to T_2 decay.

Increasing the TE generally increases T_2 weighting of sequences. Images with a long TR and TE are regarded as 'heavily T_2 weighted'.

A typical oedematous or cystic lesion has a longer T_1 and T_2 than brain. On T_1-weighted images such a lesion will appear dark, i.e. it will have negative contrast. On heavily T_2-weighted images it will appear bright and will thus have positive contrast. If a short TR, long TE sequence is inadvertently chosen, the tendencies towards positive and negative lesion contrast will cancel and the lesion may not be detected.

The SE signal is greatest when the T_1 is short and the T_2 and proton density are high; it is decreased if the T_1 is long and the T_2 and proton density are small. The differentiation of lesions from normal tissues can be enhanced if one is aware of the differences in the proton density and magnetic relaxation times and selects the sequence times accordingly.

Flow effects are complex. Blood may appear of high, medium or low signal intensity depending on its rate and direction of flow.

1.2.5.3 The Inversion Recovery Pulse Sequence

If a 180° pulse is placed in front of either the PS sequence or the SE sequence an IR sequence results. In principle all the options available with both of the previous sequences are available with the IR sequence as well as those introduced by the additional 180°.

The effect of the 180° pulse depends on whether it is slice selected or not and the inversion time (TI) between the 180° pulse and the subsequent 90° pulse. The IR pulse sequence is generally used in a highly T_1 dependent form although there is interest in the short TI T_2 dependent form.

The proton magnetization induced in the patient by the static magnetic field can be represented by a vector M. The component of the magnetization in the transverse plane at any given time is then represented by M_{xy} and that in the longitudinal direction at the same time by M_z. The effect of a 90° pulse is to rotate M_z into the transverse plane to become M_{xy} (Fig. 1.4).

Following a 90° pulse, M_z increases exponentially from zero with time constant T_1, and M_{xy} decays exponentially with time constant T_2. At the following 180° pulse, M_z is inverted to become $-M_z$ and recovers with a time constant T_1, but at twice the rate of the earlier longitudinal recovery after the 90° pulse. At the next 90° pulse, M_z is rotated to become M_{xy}, which then decays exponentially with time constant T_2. Using a SE or FID data collection, signal is collected at a mean time, TE, after the 90° pulse and the cycle is repeated.

A composite diagram is shown (Fig. 1.7) which first follows M_z then M_{xy} after the second 90° pulse. This can be used to represent the 'potential signal intensity' at various stages in the sequence in order to understand how this may be varied.

The size of the received signal and ultimately the signal intensity or pixel value in the image is proportional to the value of M_{xy} at the time of the data collection. M_{xy} is also proportional to tissue proton density.

Using Fig. 1.8 as a model of the IR sequence, we can compare the signal intensities of white matter (a tissue with a relatively short T_1), grey matter (a tissue with a longer T_1) and CSF (which has a very long T_1). The signal intensity observed is proportional to the height of M_{xy} and it can be seen that the shorter T_1 of white matter results in a higher signal intensity than for grey matter. The very long T_1 of CSF gives a low signal intensity which may be negative. The last segment of the decay converges towards zero for both grey and white matter with their positive signal intensities and for CSF with its negative signal intensity. Display of the resultant image after phase-corrected processing gives white

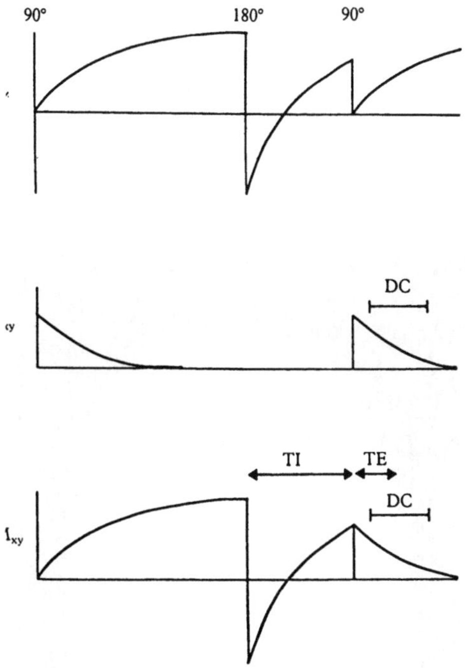

Fig. 1.7 a–c. IR sequence. M_z plotted against time (**a**), and M_{xy} plotted against time (**b**) and M_z/M_{xy} (**c**). The 90° and 180° pulses are shown with the data collection (*DC*), *TI* and *TE*

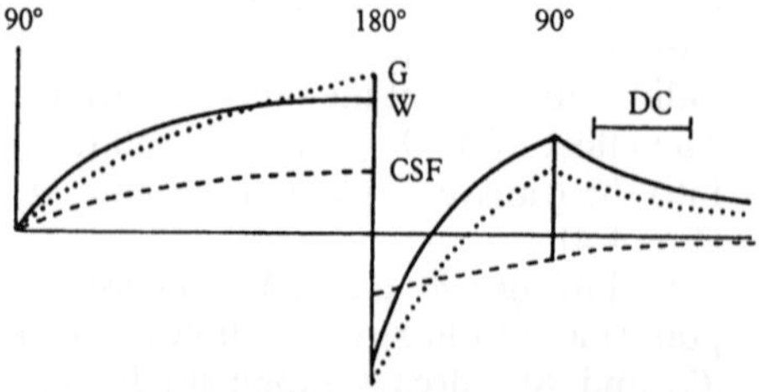

Fig. 1.8. IR sequence. Comparison of potential signal intensity for grey matter (*G*), white mater (*W*) and *CSF.* The signal intensity is proportional to the height of M_z/M_{xy} at the midpoint of the data collection (*DC*)

for white matter, grey for grey matter, and black for CSF (Fig. 1.9). The signal for grey matter is slightly greater than that for white matter at the time of the 180° pulse because of its greater proton density.

1.2.5.4 Fast Pulse Sequences

Conventional MRI techniques typically require several minutes to acquire each image set. An examination requiring the use of several pulse sequences and imaging in several planes may take as long as an hour to complete. The requirement to eliminate obtrusive movement derived artefacts in abdominal imaging and also improve patient throughput have stimulated the development of faster imaging methods. One of the simplest approaches has been to reduce the pulse TR, thus increasing the frequency per unit time that each pulse cycle is applied. Most commercial MR systems employ standard SE sequences and there is a limit below which TR can be shortened without seriously impairing the available signal to noise ratio and contrast; furthermore, the minimum achievable TR is constrained by power deposition, particularly at high field.

A second approach to fast imaging is to use fast PS sequences. These differ from SE sequences in using only a single rf pulse (which may be less than 90°) and a signal is generated by gradient reversal instead of a 180° refocussing pulse. With very rapid pulsing TR may be much less

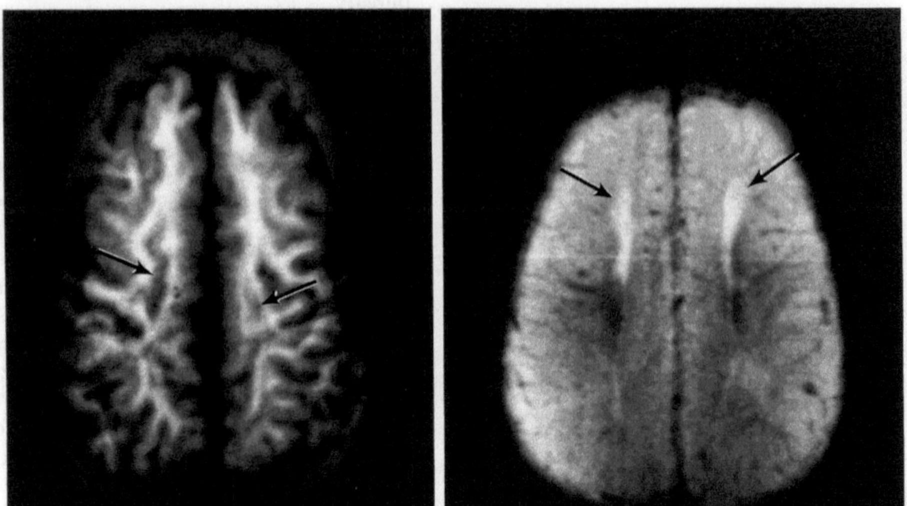

a b

Fig. 1.9 a, b. Periventricular leucomalacia. Comparison of IR 1800/33/600 (**a**) and SE 1500/130 (**b**) scans. There is high grey to white matter contrast in (**a**). The cystic areas are low signal in (**a**) and high signal in (**b**) (*arrows*) than T_1 and so there is insufficient time for full recovery of longitudinal magnification between pulses which leads to a reduced signal. More signal can be preserved if the pulse angle is reduced below 90°. A number of pulse sequences have been devised which use gradient echoes for signal generation and allow images to be obtained in a few seconds; for example, the "fast low angle shot" or FLASH sequence (Frahm et al. 1986).

The relatively long imaging times using conventional pulse sequences frustrated early attempts to exploit the potential for the three-dimensional data acquisition by MRI.

An alternative approach to fast imaging is echo planar imaging (EPI) (Stehling et al. 1990). In this distinctive variant of MRI, a train of gradient echoes is generated from a single excitation of the protons in the imaging plane in such a way that a complete image reconstruction can be achieved.

Ultra high-speed EPI allows acquisition of complete two-dimensional images in 64–128 ms, eliminating the need for any gating techniques in studying the heart, liver or foetus. A range of spin sequences is available and these permit the introduction of differing degrees of T_1 and T_2 weighting whilst retaining the inherent high-speed capability. The method provides an opportunity to study, in real time, dynamic events such as flow phenomena in the vascular and CSF compartments of the brain and the kinetics of administered contrast agents.

1.3 Contrast Agents

Following extensive pharmacological and animal studies, volunteer studies with intravenous Gd-DTPA (Schering) were begun at the end of 1983. The compound is now widely used in MRI of the central nervous system and is marketed under the name of Magnevist.

In general terms, the clinical results with Gd-DTPA parallel those seen with the iodinated contrast agents used in X-ray CT, but there are important differences, particularly in relation to the choice of pulse sequences and the effect of increased concentrations of Gd-DTPA.

More recently, variants of Gd-DTPA, such as Gd-DOTA and the non-ionic compounds Gd-HP-DO3A and Gd-DTPA *bis*-methylamide have been used in phase II and III trials. All produce results very similar to those of Gd-DTPA.

Gd-DTPA is the first parenteral agent to be used in clinical practice but many other possibilities exist. Another agent, magnetic iron oxide particles (MIOPs), has undergone clinical trials in Boston and in Europe.

1.4 Hazards and Safety

The safety of MRI is an important consideration and, as yet, no basic hazard has been identified provided the machine is used sensibly. The National Radiological Protection Board in the UK and the Food and Drug Administration (FDA) in the USA have published guidelines for the medical use of MRI and these have recently been revised. Three possible adverse effects have been considered, including the static magnetic field, induced currents due to changing magnetic fields, and heating effects on vulnerable tissues, such as the lens of the eye, due to the rf pulses. Guidelines for exposure limits have been suggested. As the possibility exists that ferromagnetic aneurysm clips may become dislodged by magnetic fields, patients with these in place should not be examined. Patients with cardiac pacemakers should also be excluded. Other hazards to be considered include the effect of the magnetic field on external ferromagnetic objects such as scissors and scalpels, which can become dangerous missiles if accidentally released near the magnet.

References

Axel L (1984) Blood flow effects in magnetic resonance imaging. Am J Radiol 143:1157–1206

Bottomley PA, Foster TH, Argersinger RE, Pfeifer LM (1984) A review of normal tissue hydrogen NMR relaxation times and relaxation mechanisms from 1–100 MHz. Med Phys 11:425–448

Bottomley PA, Hardy CJ, Argersinger RE, Allen-Moore G (1987) A review of ^1H nuclear magnetic resonance relaxation in pathology. Med Phys 14:1–37

Bradley WG, Waluch V (1985) Blood flow: magnetic resonance imaging. Radiology 154:443–450

Cohen MD, Edwards MK (eds) (1990) Magnetic resonance imaging in children. Becker, Philadelphia

Dubowitz LMS, Pennock JM, Johnson MA, Bydder GM (1986) High-resolution magnetic resonance imaging of the brain in children. Clin Radiol 37:113–117

Frahm J, Haase A, Matthaei D (1986) Rapid NMR imaging of dynamic processes using the FLASH technique. Magn Reson Med 3:321–327

Hawkes RC, Holland GN, Moore WS, Worthington BS (1980) NMR tomography of the brain: a preliminary clinical assessment with demonstration of pathology. J Comput Assist Tomogr 4:577–586

Lauterbur PC (1973) Image formation by induced local interactions: examples employing NMR. Nature 242:190–191

Le Bihan D, Breton E, Lallemand D, Grenier P, Cabanis E, Laval-Jeantet M (1986) MR imaging of intravoxel incoherent motions: application to perfusion and diffusion in neurological disorders. Radiology 161:401–408

Rutherford MA, Cowan FM, Mansur A, Pennock JM, Hajnal JV, Young IR, Bydder GM (1991) Magnetic resonance imaging of anisotropically restricted diffusion in infants. J Comput Assist Tomogr 15(2):188–198

Stehling MK, Mansfield P, Ordidge RJ, Coxon R, Chapman B, Blamire A, Gibbs P, Johnson IR, Symonds EM, Worthington BS, Coupland RE (1990) Echo-planar imaging of the human fetus in utero. J Magn Reson Med 13:314–318

Waluch V, Bradley WG (1984) NMR even echo rephasing in slow laminar flow. J Comput Assist Tomogr 8:594–598

2 Magnetic Resonance Imaging: Application to the Neonatal Period

D. CHRISTMANN and J. HADDAD

CONTENTS

2.1 Introduction

The application of magnetic resonance imaging (MRI) has recently been extended to include neonates. We feel that it is necessary to elaborate on the application of this technique to the exploration of the neonatal CNS. In Chap. 1, Bydder has provided an overview of the principles of MR and has explained the different terms used. We will try, based on our own experience since 1986, to show to what extent MRI may be useful in the diagnosis of brain disorders in the neonatal period. In some sections, interest will be focussed on the pathophysiology of cerebral injury, clinical data and neurodevelopmental outcome in order to provide the reader with extensive knowledge of the cerebral injury diagnosed. In some instances, comparisons between MRI, CT and US will be made. The purpose is not to prove the superiority of MRI, but to locate its appropriate place in the choice of brain imaging techniques in the neonatal period. We will give, at the end of this chapter, several references which will complete your knowledge of MRI. Only some of these will be mentioned in the text.

2.2 Materials and Methods

A total of 102 neonates, ranging in postconceptional age (PCA) from 30 to 44 weeks at the time of the study were imaged. MRI was repeated in several neonates in the first year of life. Thus, a total of 167 examinations were per-

Table 2.1. Indications for cerebral MRI examination in the neonatal period ($n = 102$)

Birth asphyxia (mild to severe)	15
Malformations	25
Central nervous system infection	10
Ischemia and hemorrhage	40
Miscellaneous	17

formed on this population, which constitutes the patient sample in this study. The indications for cerebral MRI are summarized in Table 2.1. Informed consent was obtained from the parents.

2.2.1 Sedation and Patient Handling

Satisfactory sedation is essential for a proper examination and for improving the quality of the images. The sedation protocol used in this study depended on the age of the infant:

- In premature babies, the examinations were performed after feeding.
- In full-term babies, chloral hydrate was given via a nasogastric tube (50 mg/kg) 30 min before the exam.
- In early infancy, 50–100 mg/kg of chloral hydrate was required.

Neonates were wrapped on a special nonmagnetic bed and were moved to and from the MR facility. Older infants did not require this type of handling. In addition to direct monitoring by touching, seeing and hearing the patient, we monitored vital parameters (electrocardiogram monitor, pulse oximeter and blood pressure monitoring). Infants needing ventilation were ventilated by hand with a breathing circuit devoid of ferromagnetic material or by a Monal ventilator. Sources of oxygen and suction were available. A neonatologist was always present in the magnet room. After careful monitoring of the patients, no adverse effects were noted.

2.2.2 MR System and Pulse Sequences

All examinations were performed on a Compagnie Generale Radiologie-General Electric (CGR-GE) MR system of 0.5 T with the conventional 28 cm headcoil. We used the following pulse sequences:

1. Spin echo T1 weighted images (SET1) with a repetition time (TR) of 400–600 ms and an echo time (TE) of 20–32 ms
2. Spin echo T2 weighted images (SET2); multiple echoes with a repetition time of 2000 or 2200 ms and an echo time of 40–120 ms
3. Gradient echo (GE) with a repetition time of 400–520 ms and an echo time of 12 or 13 ms and 90° flip angle; images similar to SET1 images

The matrix element used was 256 × 256. The duration of an exam did not exceed 45 min.

2.2.3 Additional Brain Imaging Techniques

In addition to MRI, cerebral ultrasound (US) with a 5 MHz probe and computed tomography (CT) scans were performed. In some cases these images were compared to MRI images.

2.2.4 Neurodevelopmental Outcome

Short-term (at 2 years of age) neurological follow-up was available for most infants. Assessment of neurodevelopmental outcome was based upon the results of a neuromotor exam. A developmental quotient (DQ), when available, was assigned according to a Brunet-Lezine test. Electrophysiological measurements (visual and auditory evoked responses) were performed, in most cases, in early infancy.

2.3 Normal Appearance of the Neonatal Brain

2.3.1 Patients

A total of 19 MR examinations from 19 neonates whose PCA ranged from 33 to 43 weeks were studied. The main indication for MRI was mild birth asphyxia or abnormal neurological exam. We followed 13 of these neonates, none of whom exhibited an abnormal neurological outcome at 2 years of age. The classification of these infants is shown in Table 2.2.

This series will be used to illustrate, by MRI, the normal appearance of the neonatal CNS. We were not able to examine a normal premature baby less than 33 weeks PCA, since it was rather difficult to scan such a baby safely. However, a few premature babies were examined for several of the pathologies in the following sections. The imaging features of these infants can be used to illustrate the more immature brain. The characteristics of immature brains will be discussed later.

2.3.2 Results

In full-term babies cerebral sulci and gyri appear well developed, whereas in the premature baby a smooth cortex was noted. This is particularly obvious on MRI scan, especially on sagittal view (SV).

The neonatal brain is characterized by a high brain water content and poor myelination. Thus, the appearance of white matter is different from that of the adult on MRI. On SET1, white matter exhibits a low signal intensity (hyposignal) compared to gray matter; on SET2, a high signal intensity (hypersignal) is noted. The white to gray matter differentiation pattern in the neonate is strictly the opposite of that of adults.

Table 2.2. Classification of neonates based on post-conceptional age ($n = 13$)

PCA (weeks)	*n*
33	1
34	1
35	2
40	6
43	3

PCA, post-conceptional age

Depending on whether SET1 or SET2 is used, myelinated fibers exhibit a different signal, hyper- or hyposignal, respectively (see Sect. 2.3.3), than does gray matter.

In premature babies, myelinated fibers are located mainly at the level of the brain stem, cerebral peduncles, in part at the posterior limb of the internal capsule and to a lesser degree at the ventral posterior nuclei of the thalami (Fig. 2.6). At term, myelinated fibers progress more cephalad and reach the centrum semiovale at its central portion (Figs. 2.1 and 2.2). Myelin is also seen in a portion of the cerebral parietal cortex (sensorimotor) (Fig. 2.11). Cerebral spinal fluid (CSF) appears hypointense on SET1 and hyperintense on SET2.

2.3.3 Discussion

Pulse sequences used in the neonatal period are mainly SET1 or GE, with a flip angle of 90°, and SET2. The former show good anatomic details and are mostly used in the evaluation of brain malformations. The latter appears to be more indicative of cerebral maturation. Thus, MRI provides more information on both anatomy and cerebral maturation than US or CT.

2.3.3.1 Anatomy

SET1 or GE allows good recognition of the anatomy of the CNS, especially when

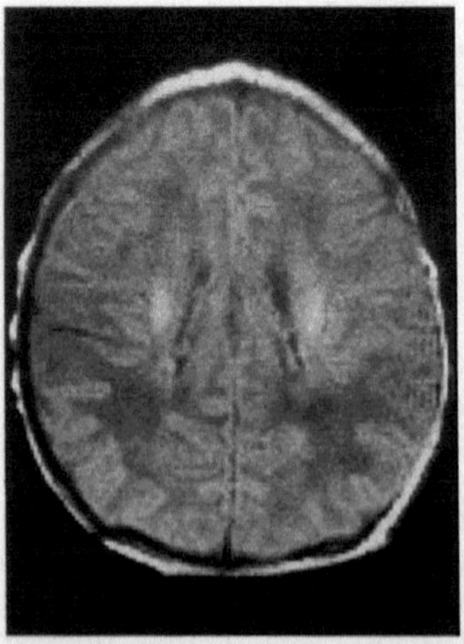

2.1

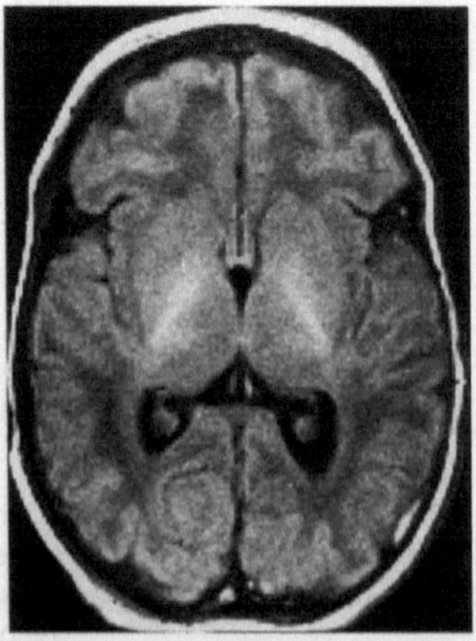

2.2

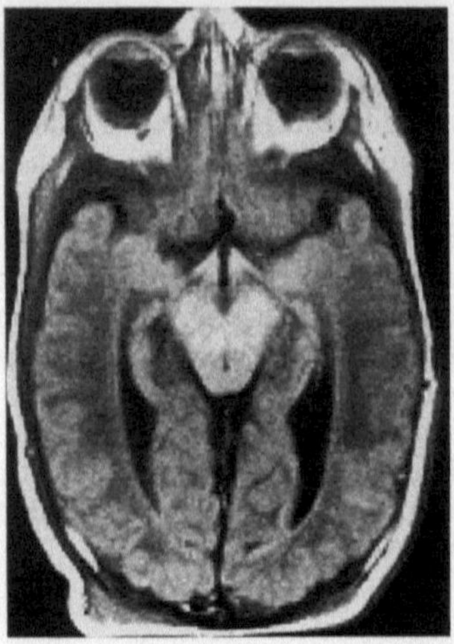

2.3

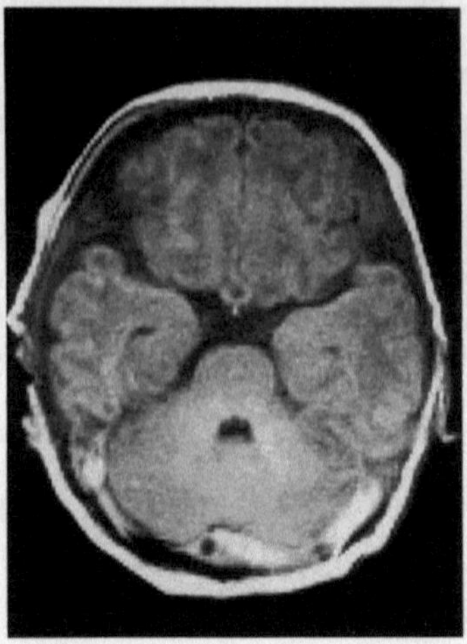

2.4

Fig. 2.1. SET 1, 600/32 ms, AV at the level of the centrum semiovale; full-term baby. Note that the convolutions and gyri are well developed. There is a hypersignal at the level of the corona radiata at its central part. Note the hyposignal of the white matter and the white to gray matter differentiation pattern

Fig. 2.2. SET 1, 600/32 ms. AV at the level of the basal ganglia; full-term baby. Note the hypersignal of the posterior limb of the internal capsule; the hyposignal of the white matter is still obvious

Fig. 2.3. SET 1, 600/32 ms. AV at the level of the cerebral peduncles; full-term baby. Note the hypersignal of the cerebral peduncles

Fig. 2.4. SET 1, 600/32 ms, AV at the level of the cerebellar peduncle; full-term baby. Note the hypersignal of the cerebellar peduncles

multiplanar images are used. We can easily separate on MRI the different cerebral lobes (frontal, parietal, occipital and temporal), whereas this seems to be difficult with US and CT. The corpus callosum is well visualized as is the pituitary gland, the pituitary gland stalk and the chiasma on sagittal view (Fig. 2.5). The ventricular system and extracerebral space are well defined and one can differ-

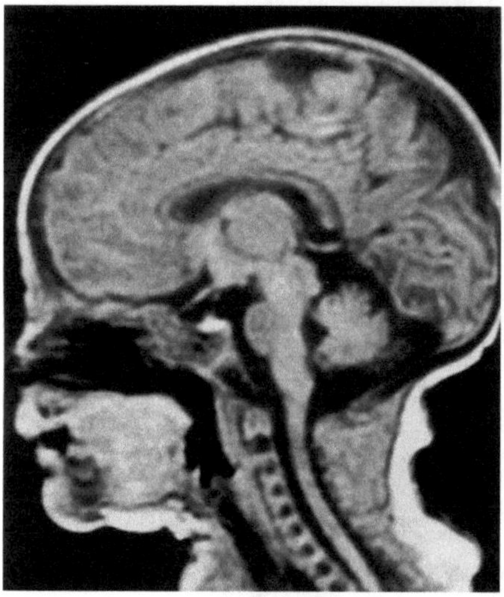

Fig. 2.5. GE, 450/12 ms/90°, SV; full-term baby. Note the normal aspect of the corpus callosum; the aqueduct of sylvius is obvious but narrow; the extracerebral space is clearly visible (subarachnoidal space is crossed by vascular component); the posterior fossa cisterna, the vermis, the pituitary gland, the pituitary gland stalk and the chiasma are also clearly visible; the sulci and gyri are well developed

entiate a subdural from a subarachnoidal collection by MRI. It is well known that ventricular size and extracerebral spaces change with advanced gestational age. McArdel et al. (1987b) documented the normal range of widths of the extracerebral space and lateral ventricles in this population. In premature babies they can be summarized as follows: the lateral ventricles are prominent, the extracerebral space and the posterior fossa cisterna may both be wide. The cavity of the septum pellucidum is mainly present in all prematures, decreases in size with progression of gestational age and disappears in early infancy. The developing changes, from smooth cortex with few convolutions and sulci in the premature baby to compactly infolded cortex in the normal-term infant, can also be seen.

2.3.3.2 Cerebral Maturation

One of the major criterion for judging cerebral maturation is myelination of the CNS. Myelination is characterized by acquisition of myelin membranes around axons. Myelination begins in utero at the fifth fetal month and progresses rapidly after birth. Moreover, myelination occurs simultaneously with the development of functional activity in the CNS, as evidenced by positron emission tomography (PET). The ability of MRI to depict myelin tracts is certain. Thus, it allows an "in vivo" approach to studying cerebral maturation.

Myelin exhibits a different signal on MRI, depending on whether SET1 or SET2 is used. On SET1, myelin gives a hypersignal, whereas on SET2 it gives a hyposignal. When myelin appearances on SET1 and SET2 in the same baby are compared, myelination seems to be less developed when seen on SET2 than on SET1 (Figs. 2.2, 2.9); this discrepancy is not seen in the adult. A possible explanation could be that SET1 is more sensitive to promyelin formation (deposit of lipids around the axon) and SET2 more sensitive to mature myelin. As depicted by MRI, myelination progresses cephalad. With the progression of gestational age, fibers become myelinated infratentorially (inferior cerebral peduncle) and at term supratentorially: thalamus, posterior limb of the internal capsule, centrum semiovale, and parietal cortex (sensorimotor). Those imaging features are in agreement with myelogenetic cycles in the human brain as described by Yakoulev and Lecours. Moreover, cerebral maturation, as evidenced by myelination, correlates well with neuromotor behavior. Indeed, neonatal behavior is dominated by subcortical brain structure activity. Intrinsic brain stem reflexes are prominent and cortical function is mostly limited to the sensorimotor cortex. The other aspect of cerebral maturation was seen by MRI, is the ratio of the signal between white and gray matter. As noted

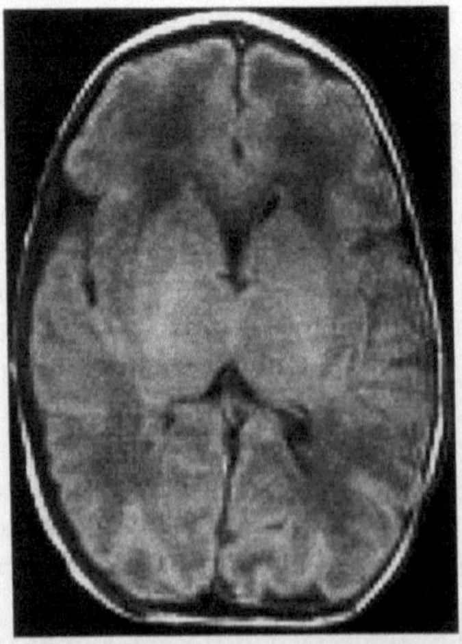
2.6

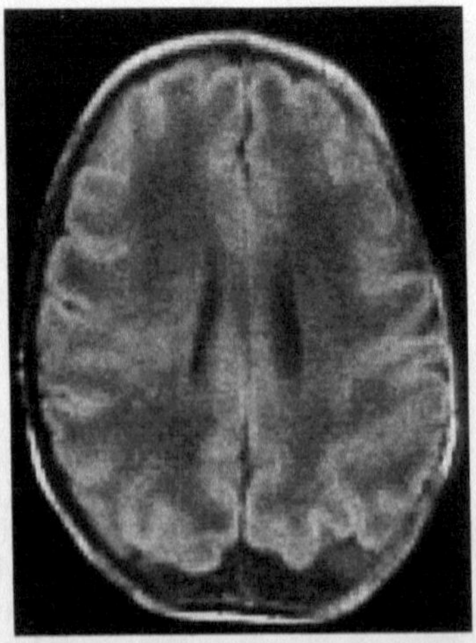
2.7

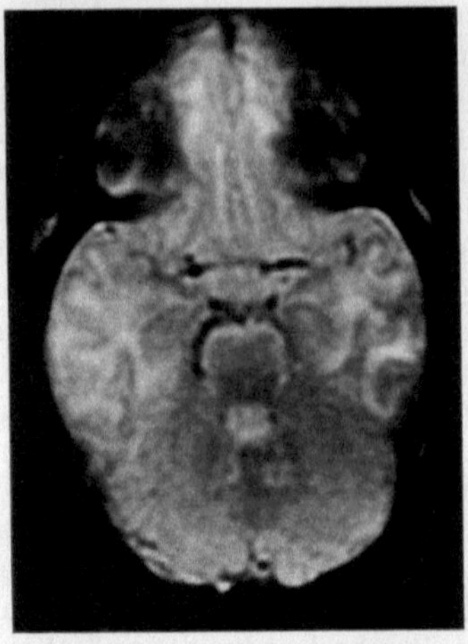
2.8

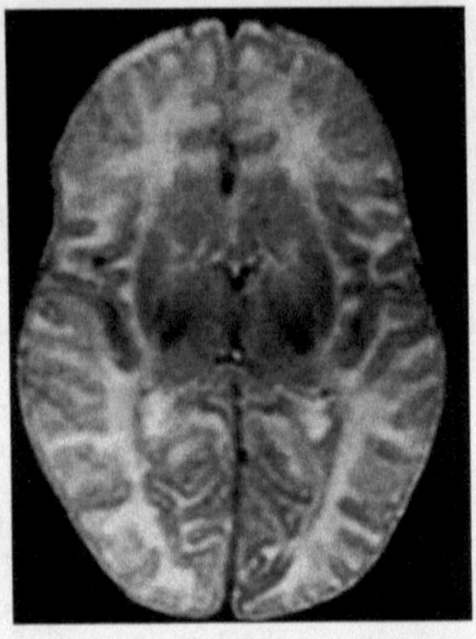
2.9

Fig. 2.6. SET1, 600/32 ms AV at the level of the basal ganglia; premature baby (34 weeks GA). Note the slight hypersignal of the posterior limb of the internal capsule. The hyposignal of the white matter and the white to gray matter differentiation pattern are more accentuated than in a full-term baby

Fig. 2.7. SET1, 600/32 ms, AV at the level of the centrum semiovale; premature baby (34 weeks GA). Note the hyposignal of the white matter. The sulci and gyri are less developed than in a full-term baby and there is no hypersignal at the corona radiata

Fig. 2.8. SET2, 2000/120 ms, at the level of the cerebellar peduncle; full-term baby. Note the hyposignal of the cerebellar peduncles

Fig. 2.9. SET2, 2000/120 ms, level of the basal ganglia; full-term baby. Note the hyposignal of the posterior limb of the internal capsule and of the posterior ventral nuclei of the thalamus. White matter appears as a hypersignal and white to gray matter differentiation is obvious

above, the white to gray matter differentiation pattern is related to both the high water content and poor myelination. Since brain water exhibits a hyposignal (long T1) and a hypersignal (long T2), this differentiation pattern may be easily displayed. As seen on MRI, the thickness of the cerebral cortex is reduced in the

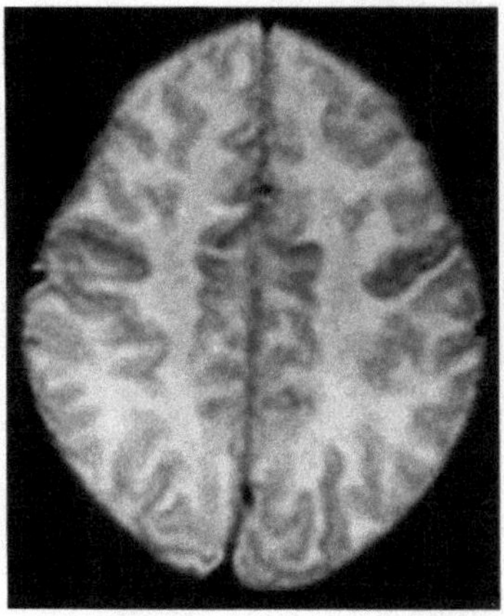

2.10

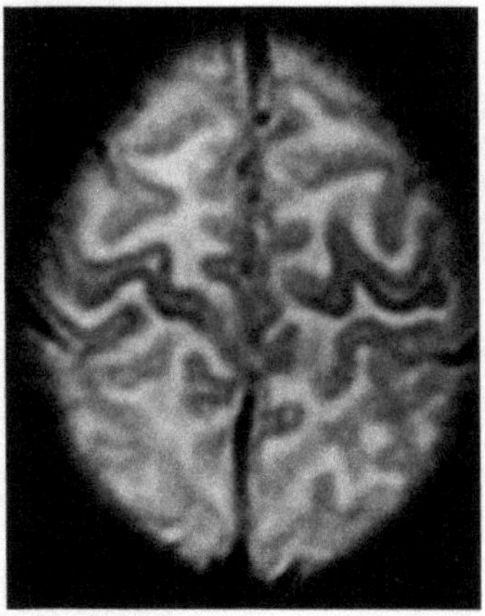

2.11

Fig. 2.10. SET2, 2000/120 ms, level of the centrum semiovale; full-term baby. A mild hyposignal in the central portion of the centrum semiovale is noted

Fig. 2.11. SET2, 2000/120 ms, at the vertex; full-term baby. Note hyposignal in the parietal cortex (sensorimotor); convolutions and gyri are well visualized

premature baby as are the number of convolutions and gyri. Thus, one should be cautious in evaluating the very immature brain, since the high brain water content can lead to difficulties in interpreting ischemic lesions.

We can conclude that MRI provides good visualization of both the anatomy and cerebral maturation of the neonatal CNS. It thus constitutes a useful tool for assessing perinatal brain disorders. The following sections are devoted to studies of brain anomalies in the premature baby and the neonate.

2.4 Malformations

Twenty five cerebral malformations were collected. Neonatal brain malformations are not uncommon. Diagnosis is often suspected by ultrasound (US) during pregnancy and confirmed by transfontanellar US during the first days of life. Nevertheless, this method has anatomical limits. Instead, MRI is the method of choice for a thorough evaluation of brain malformations since it allows evaluation of multiplanar slices. The more frequent malformations are:

- Cystic malformations
- Occlusion anomalies
- Diverticulation anomalies
- Posterior fossa anomalies
- Anomalies of neuronal growth and migration and of myelination
- Vascular anomalies

2.4.1 Cystic Anomalies

Some cysts are normal manifestations in newborns or prematures, for example, cysts of the septum pellucidum, cavum vergae, cavum of the velum interpositum. Normally, these cysts resolve by themselves and are only pathologic when they persist. Clinical manifestations of cystic malformations include macrocephaly or asymmetric cranial deformation.

A relatively frequent cystic malformation is the *medial cerebral fossa cyst*. This is generally associated with temporal lobe agenesis, which can be easily seen by MRI.

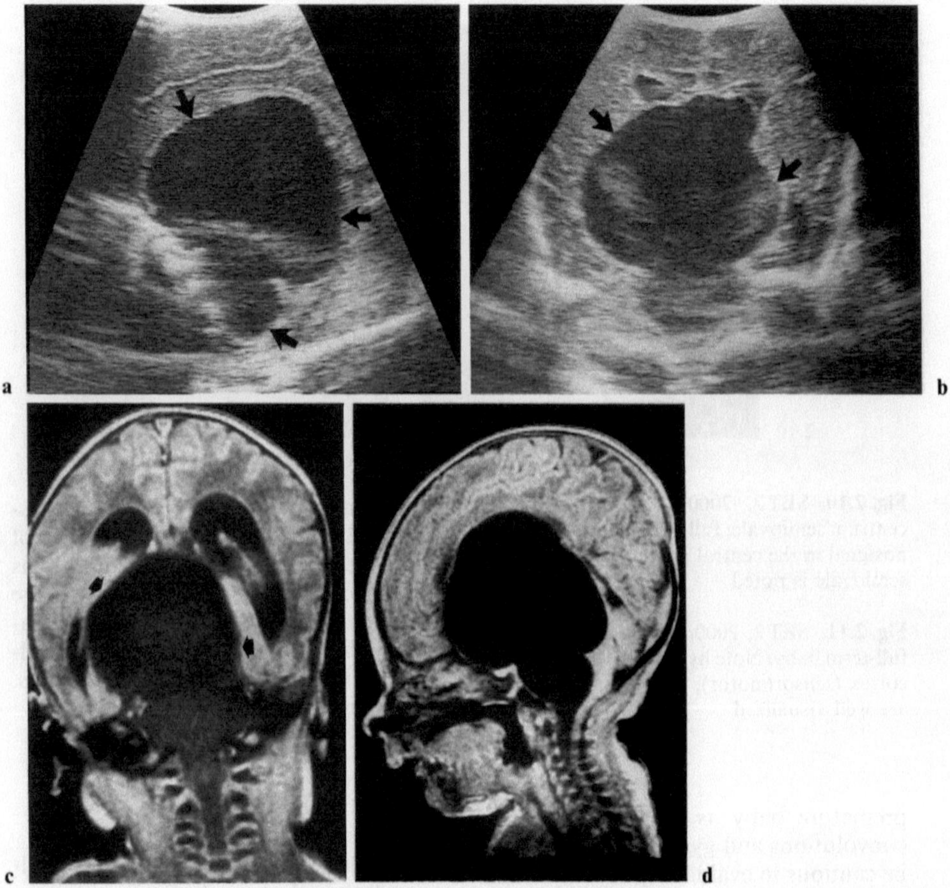

Fig. 2.12 a–d. Suspicion of a brain cyst during pregnancy. Postnatal US, FV (**a**) and SV (**b**). Corpus callosum is present. Very large suprasellar cyst with posterior extension (*arrows*). Posterior fossa not easily seen. GE, FV (**c**) and SV (**d**) 560/12 ms: Suprasellar cyst with posterior and superior extensions compressing the third ventricle and the brain stem. Very small posterior fossa. Moderate hydrocephalus without modification of the fourth ventricle. Corpus callosum is easily seen and normal

Suprasellar cysts often cause hydrocephalus due to obstruction of Monro's foramina. They can extend superiorly, laterally or posteriorly. These cysts are better demonstrated by multiplanar sequences using MRI (Fig. 2.12). Furthermore, MRI is the best method to look for other frequently associated brain malformations, such as corpus callosum agenesis (Fig. 2.12) or temporal cysts.

Interhemispheric cysts are seen especially together with corpus callosum agenesis, but they may also be isolated (Fig. 2.13). MRI delineates such cysts better than CT and excludes the diagnosis cystic anterior expansion of the third ventricle.

2.4.2 Occlusion Anomalies

2.4.2.1 Cephaloceles

These brain malformations appear very early during pregnancy. A cephalocele is a herniation of intracranial structures through an osseous defect and can appear as either a meningocele (Fig. 2.14) or a meningoencephalocele (Fig. 2.15). Prognosis is based on the nature of the herniated intracranial structures and on associated brain malformations.

After transfontanellar US, MRI is the method of choice for the evaluation of these brain malformations, especially when they are of significant size. Multiplanar images are possible without mobilization of the baby's head or of the mass and are thus without risk of complications such as infection, rupture or volvulus.

MRI allows determination of the cephalocele contents, the width of the osseous defect, the presence or absence of associated brain malformations and the estimation of brain maturation. In addition, MRI allows identification of other extracranial tumoral pathologies, such as hemangiopericytomas (Fig. 2.16) or dermoid cysts, either of which could clinically simulate meningoceles.

Three differents types of cephaloceles can be differentiated:

1. Sphenoidal: This type is frequently associated with facial malformations; the chiasma and pituitary gland are easily identified by MRI.

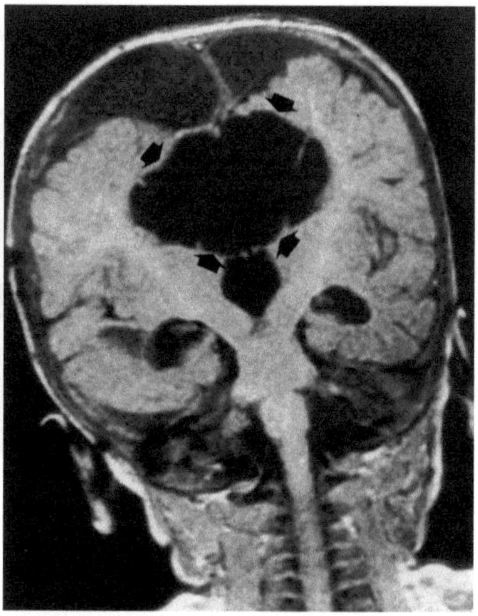

Fig. 2.13. GE, FV, 550/12 ms. Infected external hydrocephalus. Interhemispheric cyst (*arrows*) with corpus callosum agenesis well differentiated from the pericerebral collection by its different signal

2. Ethmoidal: This type may be associated with nasal obstruction.
3. Occipital (Fig. 2.15): MRI allows determination of the exact location of associated malformations, such as Arnold-Chiari malformations or Dandy-Walker syndrome, and of deformations of the posterior fossa. Injection of contrast media is useful for seeing the topography of vascular structures.

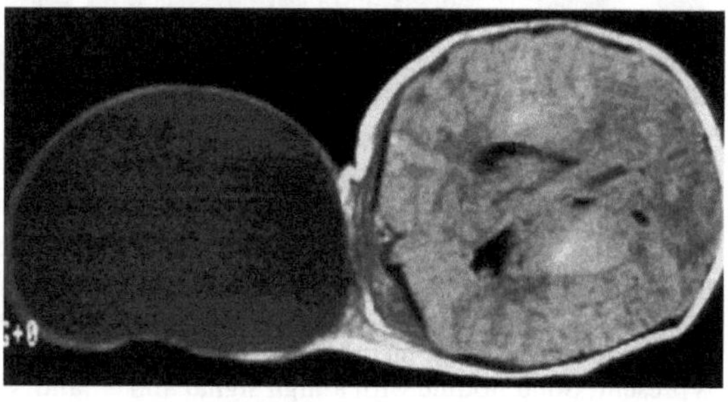

Fig. 2.14. SET 1, AV, 600/32 ms. Parieto-occipital meningocele seen in utero and without complication after resection. No other brain malformation

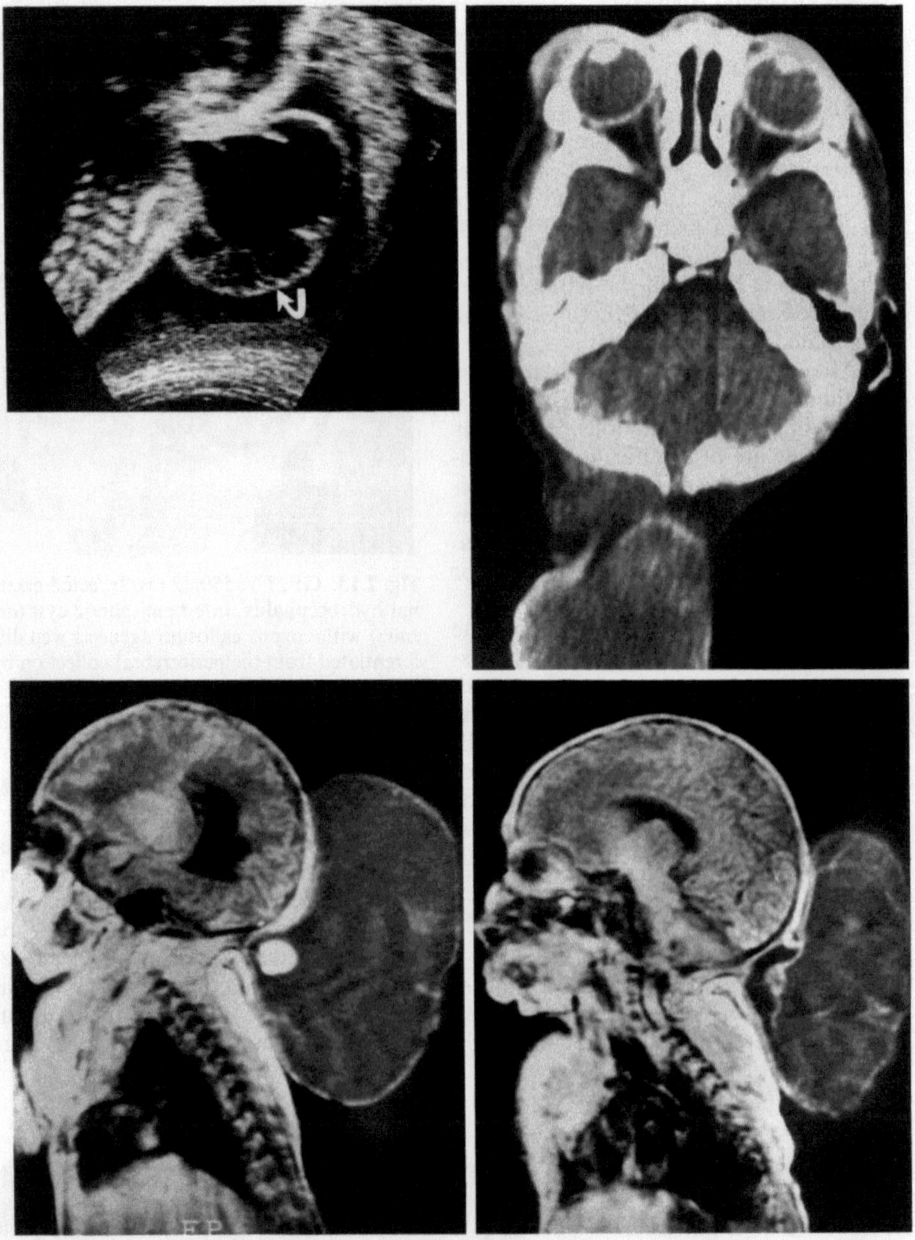

a b c d

Fig. 2.15. **a** In utero US, SV. Suspicion of cervical cystic lymphangioma (*arrow*). **b** CT without contrast media; occipital meningoencephalocele. Posterior fossa seems to be normal; solid nodule near the osseous defect. – **c, d** GE, SV, 460/12 ms. **c, d** The baby is lying on its side. A very large meningoencephalocele is present. Solid nodule with a high signal and a high and heterogeneous signal from the vermis. Based on pathological data, it was determined to be a necrosed cerebellum. Osseous defect is very well delineated and without associated vascular dysplasia. Moderate ventricular dilatation with normal brain maturation. Hydrocephalus after resection of the meningoencephalocele. (US provided by Drs. Nisand and Weil)

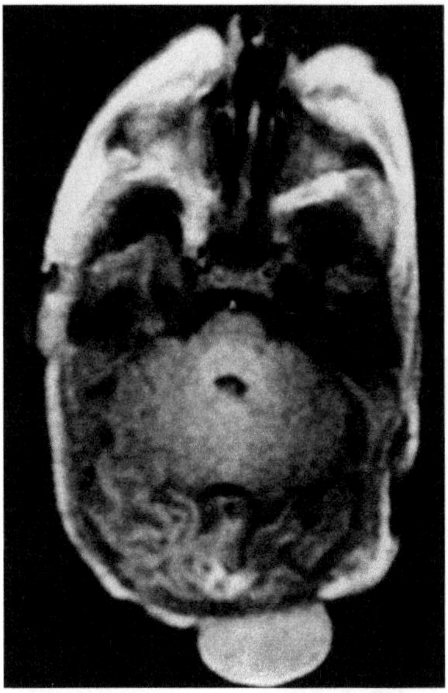

Fig. 2.16. GE, AV, 450/12 ms. Occipital mass, which appears liquid, detected in a neonate. Mass was originally suspected following US. Extracranial mass gives a increased slightly signal and is a hemangiopericytoma

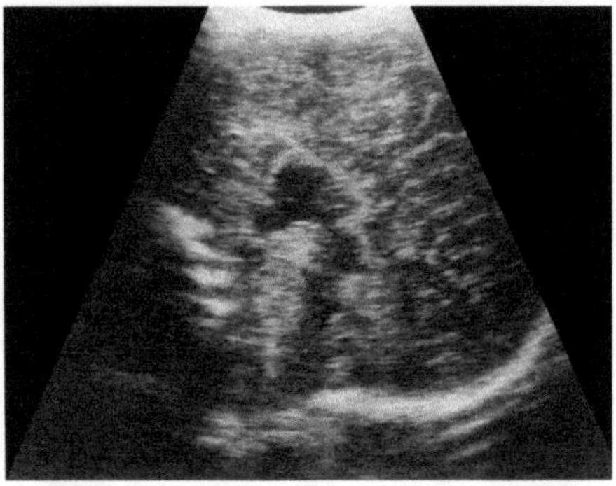

Fig. 2.17. US, SV. Total corpus callosum agenesis

2.4.2.2 Corpus Callosum Malformations

Corpus callosum agenesis is the most frequent malformation of the corpus callosum. This abnormality can be recognized during pregnancy. The etiopathogenesis is not clear, and the newborn is usually asymptomatic. Developmental delay and epilepsy may appear in early infancy. Agenesis can be total (Figs. 2.17 and 2.18) or partial and is most often posterior (Fig. 2.19).

After birth, cerebral US allows visualization of the corpus callosum (Fig. 2.17); however, visualization is sometimes limited by the small size of the anterior fontanelle. Thus, evaluation of possible associated anomalies is difficult. By contrast, MRI shows the cortical interhemispheric sulci radially disposed (Fig. 2.18 a), the steerhorn shape of the frontal horns (Fig. 2.18 b), the lateral ventricle separation (Fig. 2.18 d) and colpocephaly (Fig. 2.18 c). MRI also shows corpus callosum agenesis. In fact, in normal newborns, the corpus callosum is easily recognized as a thin line isosignal. Growth and maturation of the corpus callosum occurs during the first year of life.

Corpus callosum agenesis may either be isolated or various cerebral anomalies may be present. Such associated anomalies include:

1. An interhemispheric cyst (possibly multiple), when very large and parasagittal, may cause unilateral ventricular dilatation. In this case, SET2 is useful to distinguish between an isolated arachnoid cyst (Fig. 2.20) and a cystic anterior dilatation of the third ventricle. The cyst may appear as a communicating porencephaly. When it is near the anterior fontanelle, the cyst may cause compression of the third ventricle or ipsilateral Monro's foramina. In these instances, the cyst must be treated by puncture. Follow-up survey is made by regular US and sometimes MRI.

2. Lipoma of the corpus callsoum is seen in partial posterior corpus callosum age-

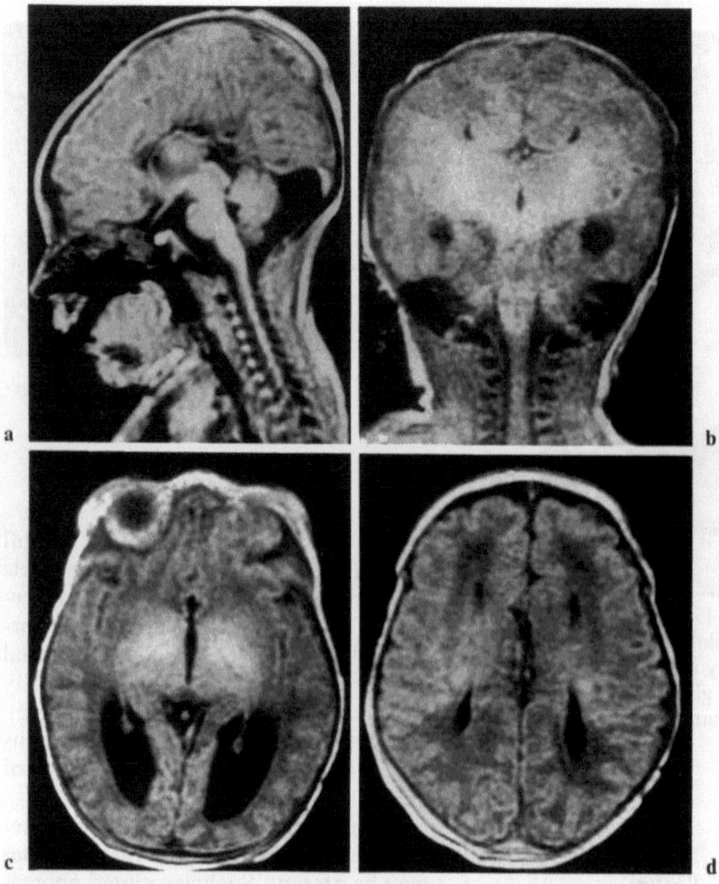

Fig. 2.18. GE, SV (**a**). FV (**b**) and AV (**c, d**), 450/12 ms. Total isolated corpus callosum agenesis with radially disposed interhemispheric sulci (**a**). Diagnosis suspected in utero. No corpus callosum is seen; mega cisterna magna. Steerhorn shape of frontal horns (**b**). Dilatation of the occipital horns (**c**). Separation of the lateral ventricles, which have lost their normal inner convexity (**d**)

nesis and is located just above the anterior part of the corpus callosum. It is easily detectable by MRI in sagittal view because of high signal doubling due to the high signal coming also from the anterior part of the corpus callosum.

3. *Other associated anomalies* include: *posterior fossa malformations* (Fig. 2.19a); *gray nuclei malformations* (Fig. 2.21d); and *ischemia*. We have seen two patients with corpus callosum agenesis associated with ischemic lesions, perhaps suggesting a common vascular etiopathogenesis. In one patient there was a subcortical ischemia of vascular topography (Fig. 2.21) and in the other there were cystic lesions (Fig. 2.22).

2.4.2.3 Arnold-Chiari Malformations

These malformations are usually type II and associated with a lombar myelomeningocele with osseous, meningeal, cerebellar and ventricular anomalies. MRI clearly demonstrates all the anomalies suspected by US (Figs. 2.23 and 2.24).

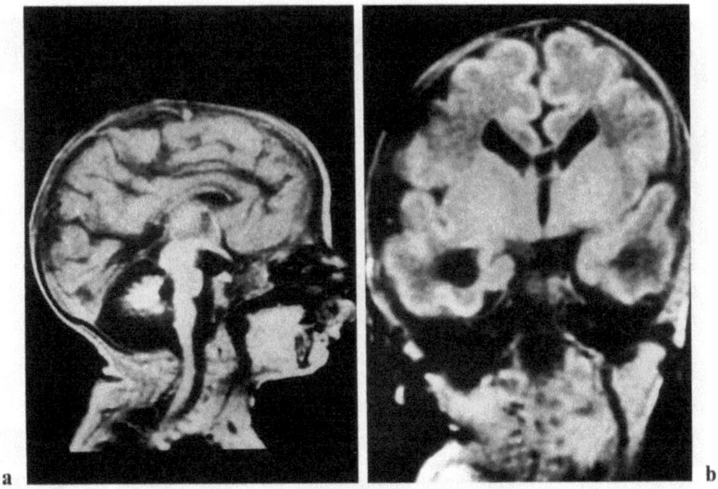

Fig. 2.19. GE, SV (a) and FV (b), 450/12 ms. Posterior corpus callosum agenesis (a) without deformation of the frontal horns (b) in a patient with Pierre Robin syndrome with posterior fossa anomaly

2.4.3 Diverticulation Anomalies

2.4.3.1 Septum Agenesis

This entity can be acquired to the newborn when there is severe hydrocephalus during pregnancy. Septo-optic dysplasia occurs in a newborn with neonatal hypoglycemia, micropenis and a small sella turcica. MRI demonstrates optic nerve atrophy, a thickened pituitary stalk, septum pellucidum agenesis and sometimes

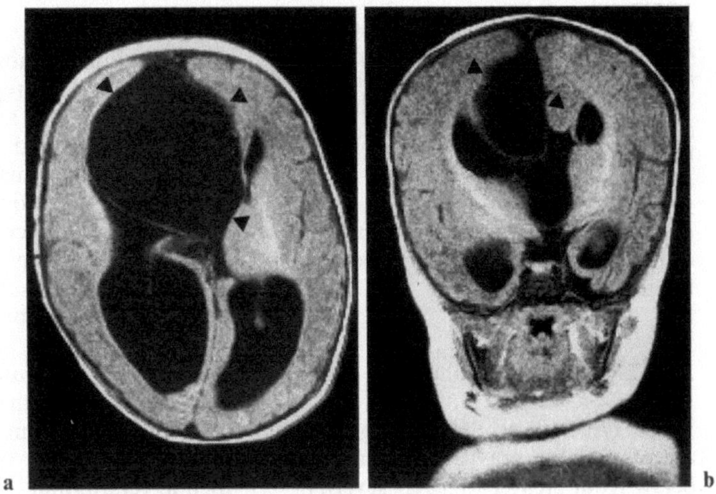

Fig. 2.20 a, b. SET1, AV (a) and FV (b), 450/14 ms. Corpus callosum agenesis associated with an interhemispheric cyst (*arrows*). Large cyst with dilatation and deformation of the third and right lateral ventricles

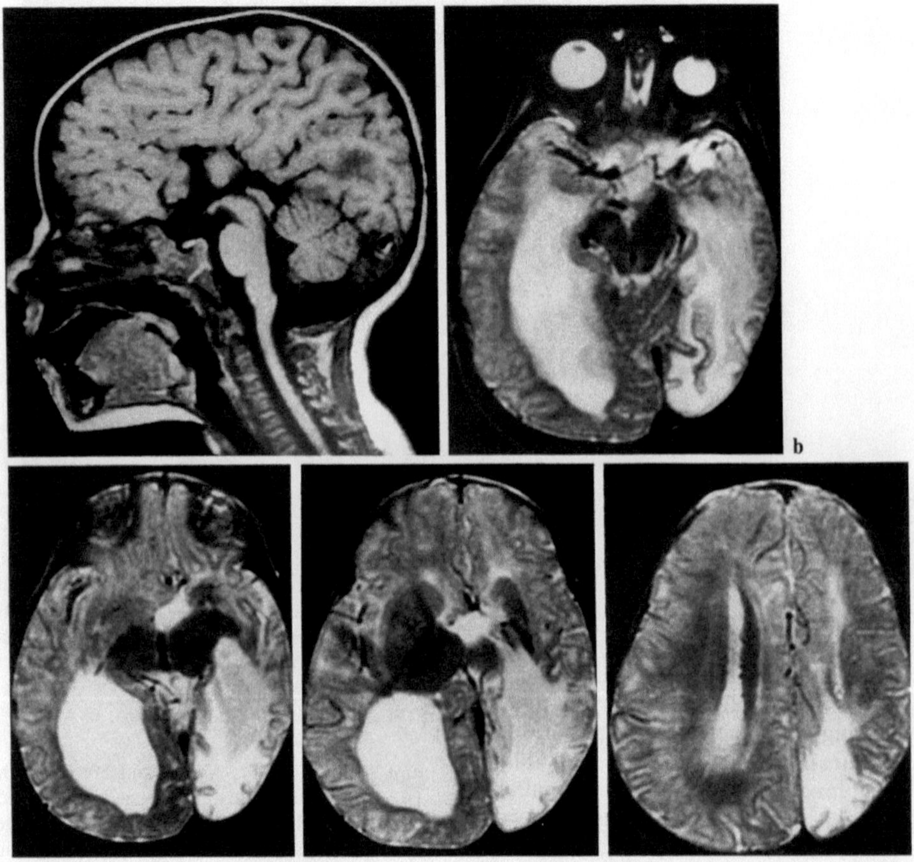

Fig. 2.21. SET2. SV (**a**) and AV (**b–e**), 1990/40–120 ms. Total corpus callosum agenesis (**a**). Occipital left ischemia (**b, c**) with malrotation of the left thalamus (**c**) and colpocephaly (**d, e**) occipital ischemia and atrophic left hemisphere

associated malformations such as corpus callosum agenesis or gyral developmental abnormalities.

2.4.3.2 Holoprosencephalies

These types of cerebral malformations are of variable gravity. They are listed below from greater to lesser severity:

1. Alobar holoprosencephaly is a severe malformation diagnosed in utero leading to interruption of pregnancy. If the baby is born, there are always severe facial malformations and the prognosis is death. This malformation consists of an absence of separation of the cerebral hemispheres, absence of interhemispheric fissure and fusion of the thalami. The corpus callosum is always absent; the posterior fossa is normal.

2. Semilobar holoprosencephaly is a partial separation of the two hemispheres. The corpus callosum may be present or absent. Clinically, there is significant mental retardation.

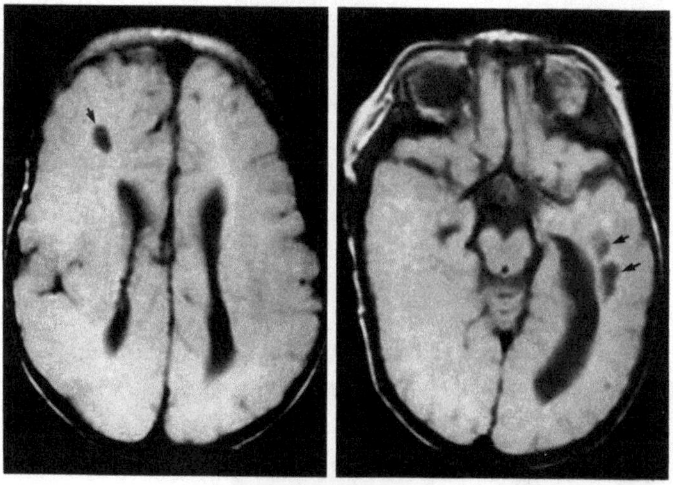

2.22 a b

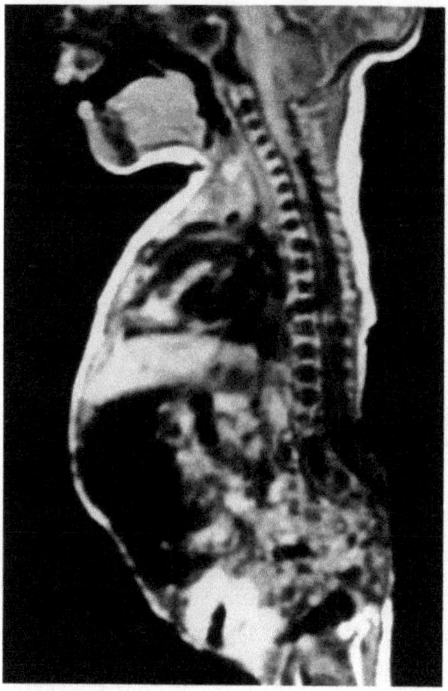

2.23

3. *In lobar holoprosencephaly,* only the frontal lobes are not separated. The anterior part of the interhemispheric fissure and septum pellucidum are absent. Mental retardation is mild.

It is useful to confirm the diagnosis of holoprosencephaly especially when it leads to interruption of the pregnancy. These anomalies may be suspected based on US results; CT is usually demonstrative. Nonetheless, MRI is very informative because of its multiplanar sequence ability and its evaluation of the entire brain (Fig. 2.25). MRI easily demonstrates the different anomalies: thalamic fusion, dorsal pouches of various dimensions, gyral developmental anomalies or corpus callosum agenesis. Furthermore, MRI excludes hydranencephaly or severe hydrocephalus.

2.4.4 Posterior Fossa Abnormalities

Diagnosis of posterior fossa abnormalities is difficult by US and CT but easier by MRI in SV. It should be noted that a large cisterna magna is a normal feature of many newborns.

Fig. 2.22 a, b. SET2, AV, 1990/40–120 ms. Total corpus callosum agenesis. Some right frontal (**a**) and left temporal (**b**), periventricular, small cystic formations (*arrows*) with left subcortical atrophy

Fig. 2.23. GE, SV, 450/12 ms. Lombar myelomeningocele with Arnold-Chiari II malformation; small posterior fossa, fourth ventricle not easily seen; inferior cerebellar ectopia

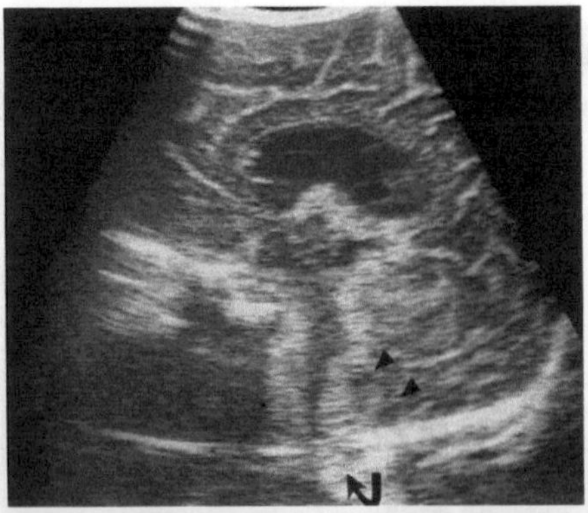

a

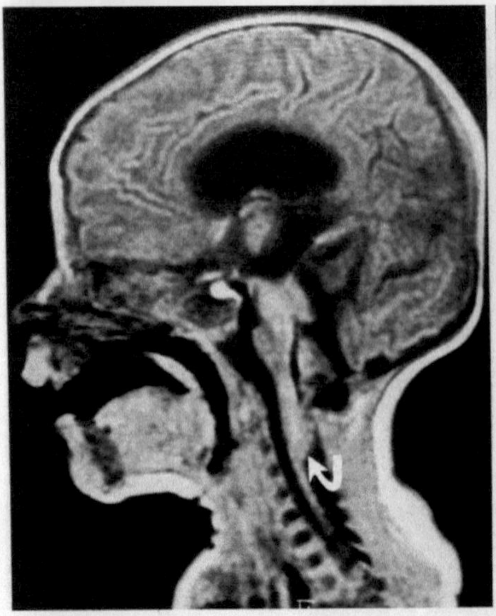

b

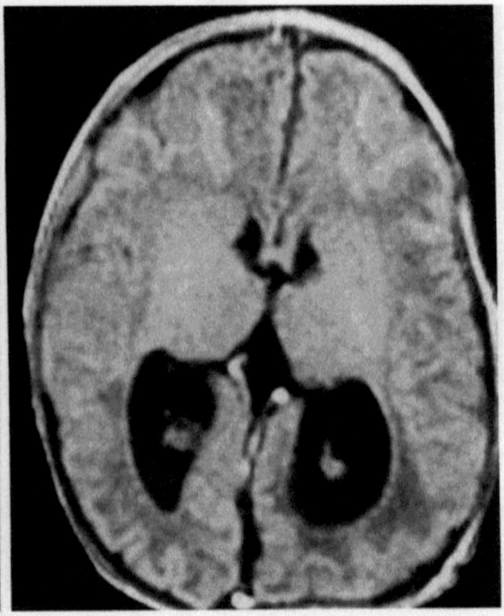

c

Fig. 2.24. (**a**) US, SV: Small posterior fossa but exact location of different cerebellar structures is difficult to determine. GE, SV (**b**) and AV (**c**), 450/12 ms. Arnold-Chiari II malformation associated with a myelomeningocele. Very small posterior fossa. Inferior ectopia of brain stem and cerebellum through occipital foramina (*black and white arrow*). No cisterna magna. Hypertrophy of gray commissure. Enlargement of the occipital foramina (**b**). Typical "USA eagle" shape of the dilated ventricles (**c**)

2.4.4.1 Dandy-Walker Syndrome

This deformity, whether in a variant form or not, is due to the obstruction of the foramina of Magendie and Luschka. It represents a malformation which is associated with cystic dilatation of the fourth ventricle, hypoplasia of the cerebellar hemispheres and vermis and a large posterior fossa with or without hydrocephalus. Diagnosis is made by US, but MRI demonstrates vermis rotation, the dimension of the aqueduct of Sylvius and associated malformations, such as heterotopic gray matter or corpus callosum agenesis (Fig. 2.26).

2.4.4.2 Cerebellar Hypoplasia

The vermis, cerebellar hemispheres or both are hypoplastic. The fourth ventricle and cisterna magna are enlarged (Fig. 2.27). In some patients, cerebellar hypoplasia is associated with corpus callosum agenesis, neuronal migration abnormalities or porencephalic cavities, which may suggest a vascular antenatal origin (Fig. 2.28).

Fig. 2.25 a–d. Semilobar holoprosencephaly without anterior cleft associated with a dorsal pouch. US (**a**); CT without contrast media (**b**); SET 2, FV (**c**) and AV (**d**), 1500/40–120 ms, E1. Thalamic fusion is easily seen as is the absence of an interhemispheric fissure in its anterior part and in the dorsal pouch

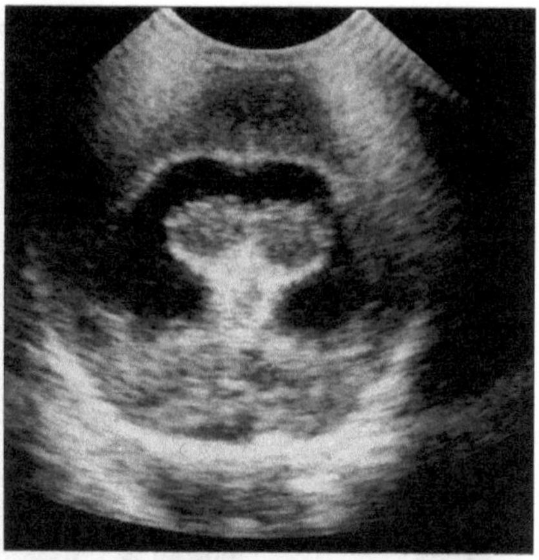

a

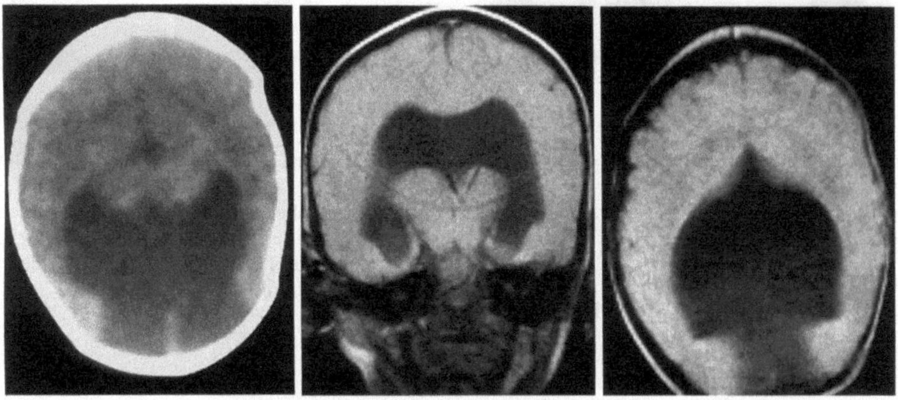

b c d

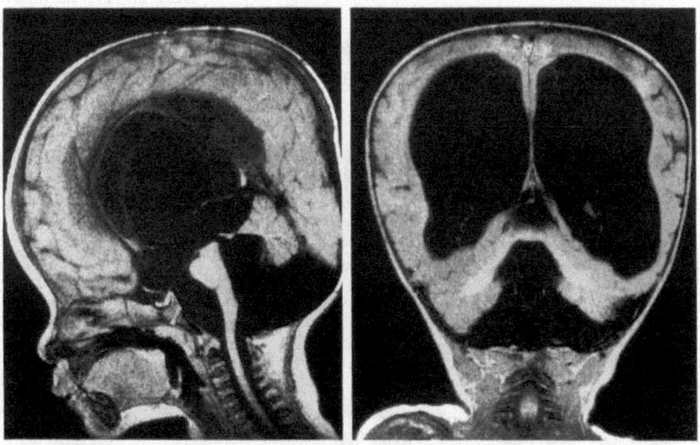

a b

Fig. 2.26 a, b. SET 1, FV (**a**) and FV (**b**), 500/14 ms. Dandy-Walker syndrome: macrocephaly, cystic dilatation of the fourth ventricle with rotation of the cerebellar vermis, large aqueduct of Sylvius, hypoplasia of cerebellar hemispheres more marked to the left; hydrocephalus and corpus callosum agenesis

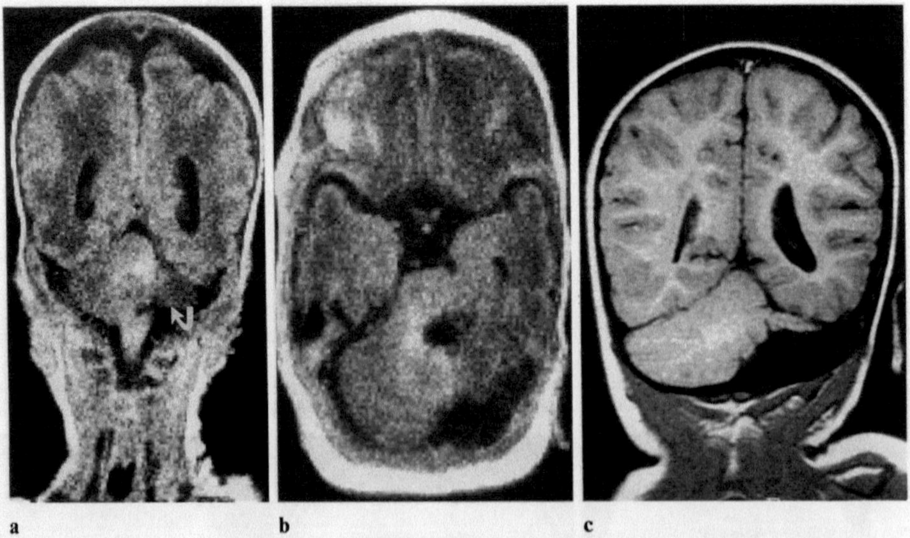

Fig. 2.27 a–c. SET 1, SV, FV and AV, 400/14 ms (**a, b**) and GE, FV, 450/10 ms (**c**). Left isolated cerebellar hypoplasia in the neonatal period (**a, b**) and at 2 years of age (**c**). Marked left cerebellar hemisphere hypoplasia clearly defined; moderate vermis hypoplasia

2.4.4.3 Obstructed Fourth Ventricle

There is no cerebellar hypoplasia or atrophy. Very often, dilatation of the fourth ventricle occurs secondary to a ventricular block-derived hydrocephalus, but it may also be isolated (Fig. 2.29).

2.4.5 Abnormalities of Neuronal Migration and Proliferation and of Myelination

In the neonatal period, diagnosis of these anomalies is difficult since neurologic

Fig. 2.28 a–c. GE, SV 450/12 ms (**a**) and SET 2, AV, 2040/50–120 ms (**b, c**). Left cerebellar hemisphere and moderate vermis hypoplasia associated with a right temporal porencephalic cavity, probably of vascular origin

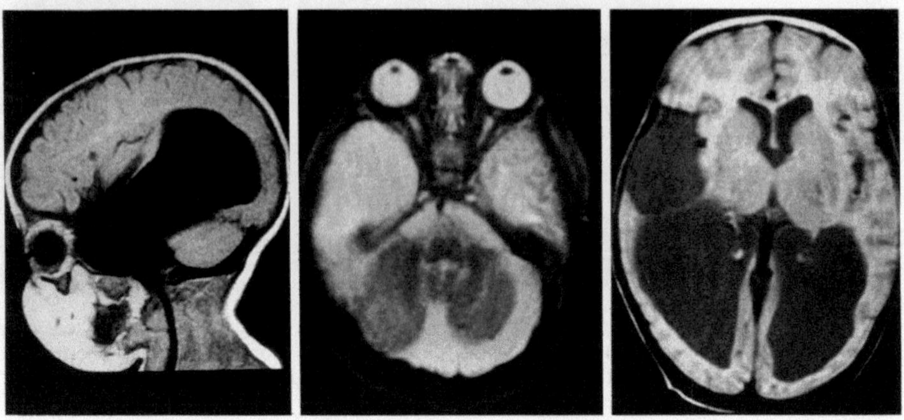

signs (mental retardation, epilepsy) appear only secondarily. Sometimes, US shows abnormalities of the cortical sulci. CT results are most often normal, especially in polymicrogyria. MRI is the examination method of choice because of its high gray and white matter contrast ability. Cerebral or extracerebral associated anomalies are frequent because of the duration of corticogenesis in utero.

2.4.5.1 Abnormalities of Neuronal Migration and Proliferation

Megaloencephaly is a rare anomaly characterized by macrocephaly with a significantly thickened cortex and corpus callosum. It resembles pachygyria but is not accompanied by a diminution of the brain volume (Fig. 2.30). Sometimes there is only a hemimegaloencephaly. In this case, MRI demonstrates an enlargement of all or part of the pathologic hemisphere, revealing a thickened cortex and ipsilateral ventricular dilatation.

Lissencephaly or agyria must be suspected when there is a microcephaly. There is hypoplasia of the brain, which appears to have a smooth surface and a thickened

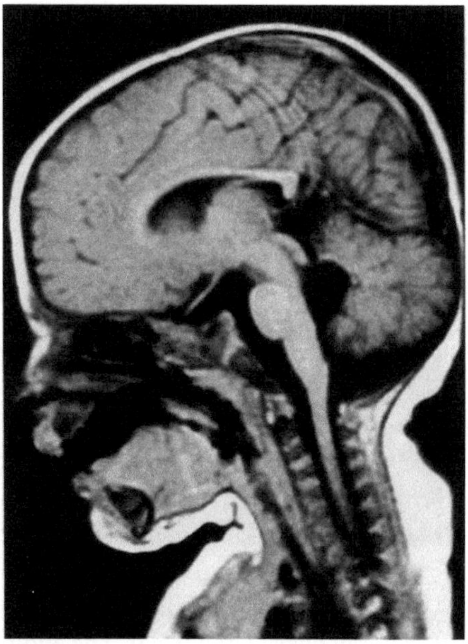

Fig. 2.29. GE, SV, 450/12 ms. Isolated dilatation of the fourth ventricle. There is no hypoplasia or atrophy of the cerebellar vermis or hemispheres and no hydrocephalus

Fig. 2.30 a, b. GE, SV (**a**), 450/12 ms and SET2, AV, 2050/120 ms (**b**). Megaloencephaly with increased cortex and corpus callosum (*arrowheads*) thickness; increased volume of white matter. *Abnormal myelination*

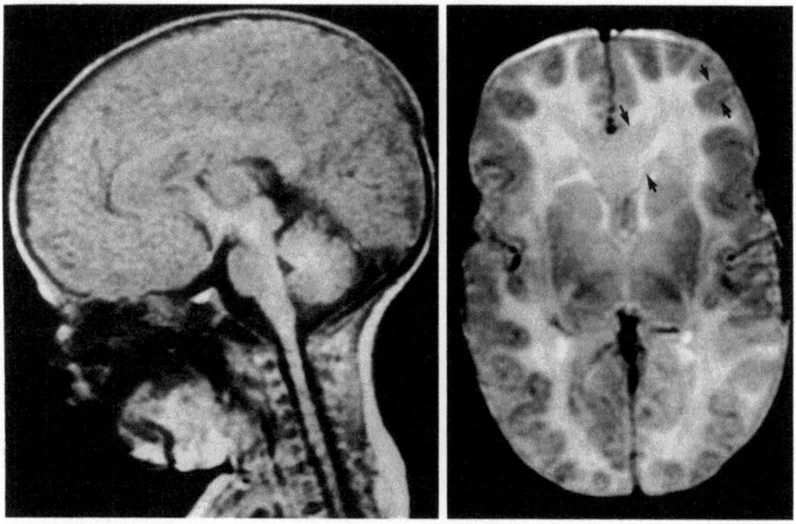

a b

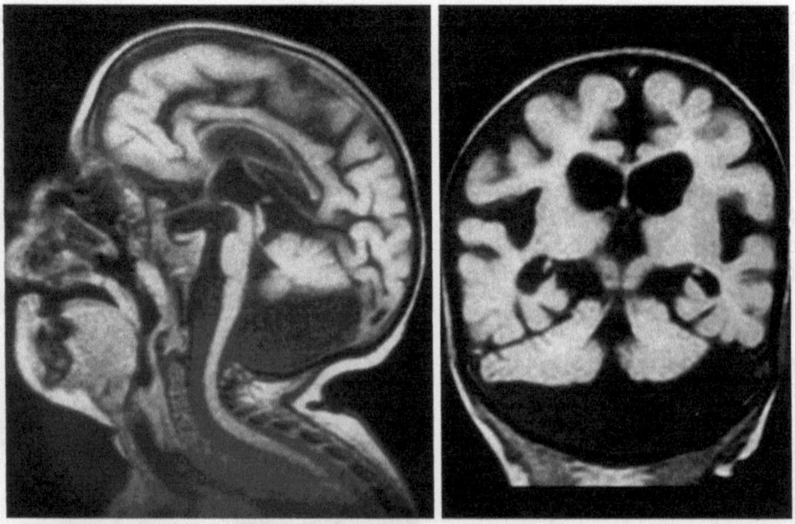

a b

Fig. 2.31. a, b. GE, SV (**a**) and FV (**b**), 450/12 ms. Microcephaly with significant mental retardation. MRI shows pachygyria, characterized by increased cortical thickness, shallow convolutions of the brain surface, some opercularisation and ventricular dilatation. There is also an arachnoid cyst of the posterior fossa associated with hypoplasia of the cerebellar vermis

cortex, and an absence of opercularisation. Gray nuclei are normal. The etiology of lissencephaly involves laminar necrosis impeding the migration of neuroblasts; however, vascular and genetic factors are probably also involved.

In pachygyria, sulci are rare but the cortex is more organized, less thick and there is some opercularisation (Figs. 2.31 and 2.32). This aspect differs from atrophy occurring in utero after infection (Fig. 2.33).

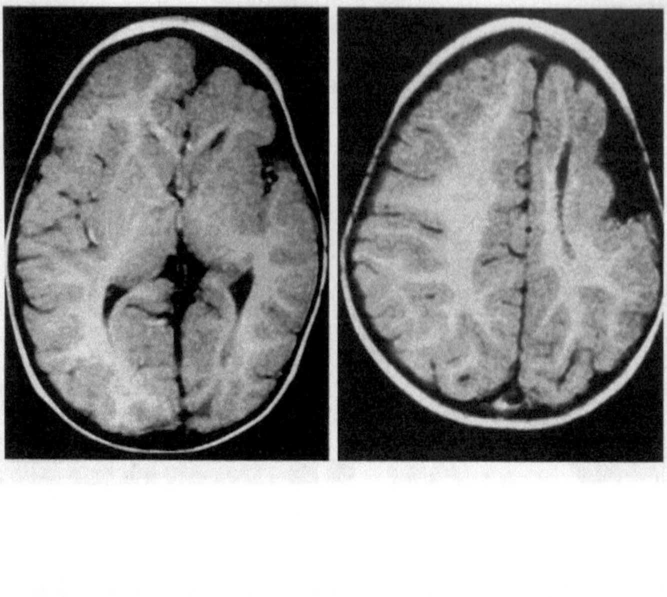

a b

Fig. 2.32. GE, SV (**a**) and FV (**b**), 450/13 ms. Left motor deficit; localized frontal left pachygyria with some opercularisation

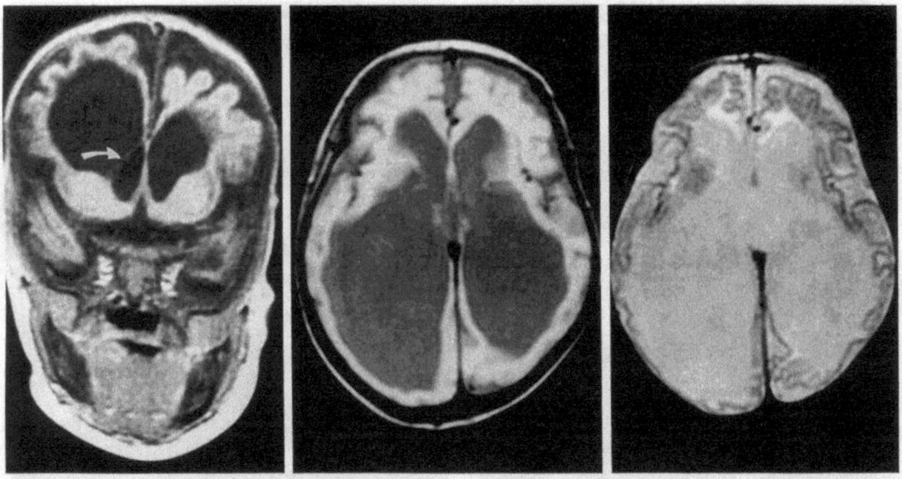

a b c

Fig. 2.33 a–c. GE, FV 450/12 ms (**a**) SET2, AV, 2020/40–120 ms (**b, c**). Microcephaly with significant ventricular dilatation and cortial atrophy. Normal cortical thickness, except for a right occipital cortical ischemic lesion, and normal opercularisation. Septa in the right frontal horn (**a**, *arrow*) suggest an infectious origin

Polymicrogyria is relatively more common. It is frequently localized in the insular area and associated with other cerebral malformations, such as schizencephaly (Fig. 2.34). There is an increased cortical thickness without the normal finger-like extensions of white into gray matter.

Schizencephaly is characterized by unilateral (Fig. 2.34) or bilateral (and then symmetrical) full thickness clefts within the cerebral hemispheres.

These neuronal migration anomalies may be diffuse or localized. In this latter case, a cortical migration anomaly is only suspected when a motor deficit or epilepsy appears. Even if they are total, many neuronal migration anomalies, i.e. pachygyria, polymicrogyria and heterotopic gray matter (Fig. 2.35), are difficult to diagnose in the neonatal period. This is because of the low contrast between gray and white matter, even in SET2.

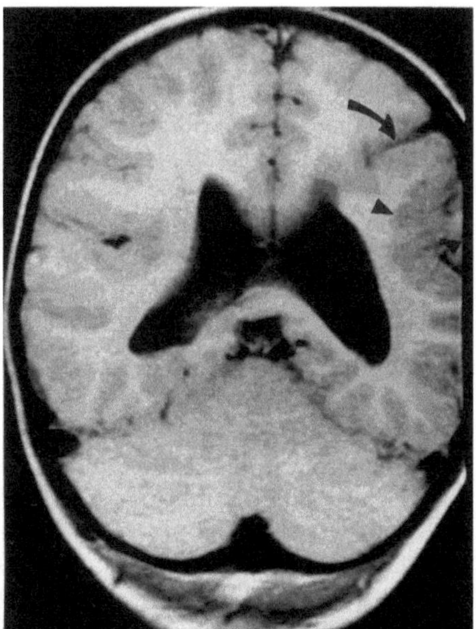

Fig. 2.34. GE, FV, 480/13 ms. Left motor deficit; localized pachygyria. Left cerebral cleft with agenesis of the septum pellucidum and polymicrogyria and the cleft's borders

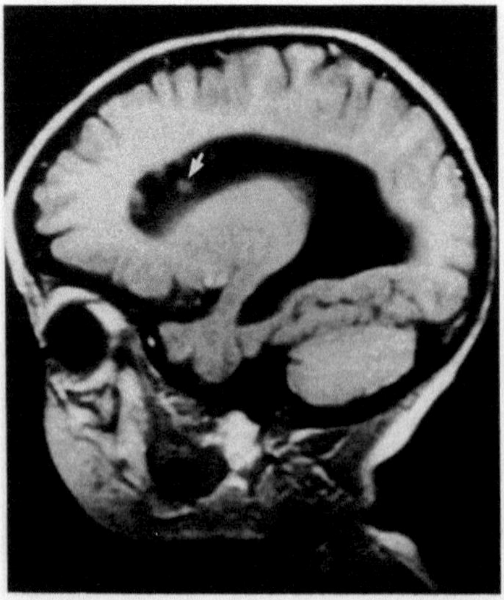

Fig. 2.35. GE, SV, 450/14 ms. Subependymal nodules (*arrow*) corresponding the heterotopic gray matter in a syndrome of hypomelanosis of Ito

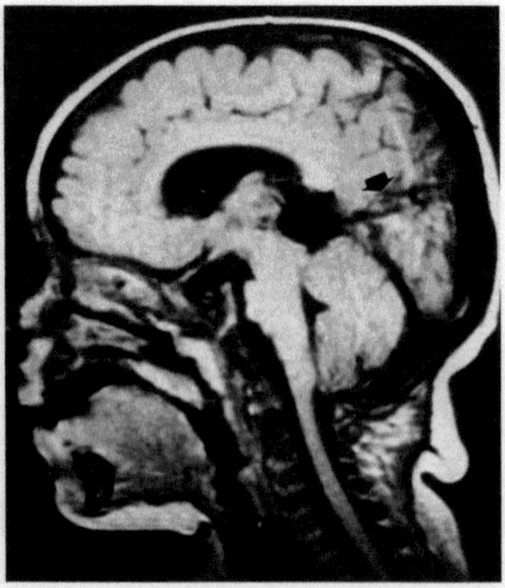

Fig. 2.36. GE, SV, 450/14 ms. Vein of Galen malformation (*arrow*) of little importance

2.4.5.2 Abnormalities of Myelination

Along with demyelinations due to ischemic lesions (described in Sect. 2.5), dysmyelinations are very difficult to diagnose in the neonate because there are no clinical signs and little information can be obtained using SET2 at this age.

2.4.6 Vascular Malformations

In utero diagnosis of arteriovenous malformation of Galen's vein is increasingly being detected using US. Cases without cardiac failure are more frequent. After Doppler US, MRI precisely identifies the extent of aneurysm (Fig. 2.36) and identifies the feeding arteries (Fig. 2.37a, c), dysplastic draining veins (Fig. 2.37b) and associated malformations. MRI contributes also to the follow-up. The efficacy of treatment, which consists of successive selective embolizations, is measured by the decrease in the dimensions of the aneurysm. MRI also detects possible ischemic lesions secondary to treatment which contraindicates new embolizations. Long-term, MRI estimates the significance of brain and corpus callosum atrophy (Fig. 2.38).

2.4.7 Phacomatosis

This diagnosis is rare in the neonatal period. If there is no familial data, it may be suspected in early infancy when there is a regression of neurologic development. This occurs in Recklinghausen's disease or tuberous sclerosis of Bourneville (Fig. 2.39b).

2.4.8 Conclusion

In the neonatal period, the presence of brain malformations is usually suspected following in utero and/or postnatal US. Nonetheless, MRI is necessary to confirm diagnosis and to look for associated brain malformations, especially neuronal migration or proliferation abnormalities, which are often not seen by US or CT.

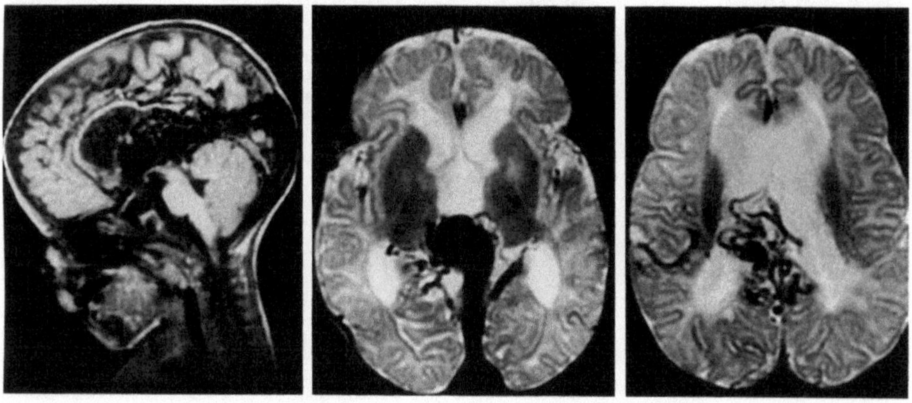

a b c

Fig. 2.37 a–c. GE, SV 450/12 ms (**a**) and SET 2, AV, 1990/120 ms (**b, c**). Vein of Galen malformation with cardiac failure. Small feeding vessels (**a, c**) and dysplastic venous sinus (**b**) well demonstrated. There is a slight ventricular dilatation and the splenium of the corpus callosum is deformed (**a**); brain maturation is normal

Fig. 2.38 a, b. GE, SV, 450/13 ms. Vein of Galen malformation with cardiac failure, diagnosed in utero. Three embolizations were performed. Significant cerebral and corpus callosum atrophy. Small round structures without signal correspond to the emboli; no ischemic lesion

2.5 Ischemia of the Neonate

2.5.1 Neuropathologic Features of Ischemia

Ischemia is one of the major neurologic problems of the perinatal period in both premature and full-term babies. It also constitutes a major determinant of neurologic impairment in infancy. Impaired autoregulation of cerebral blood flow (CBF) seems to be the most important factor in cerebral injury of the neonate (ischemia and hemorrhage). This impairment is mainly the result of perinatal asphyxia (hypoxia, hypercapnia). Other

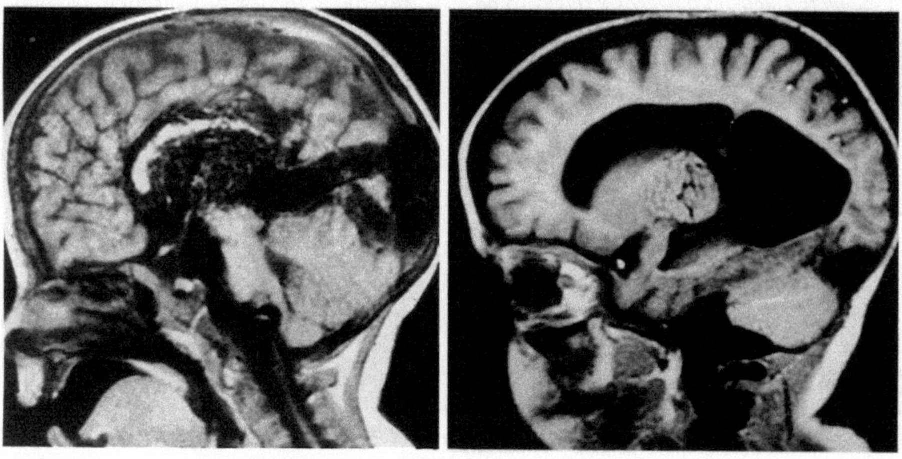

a b

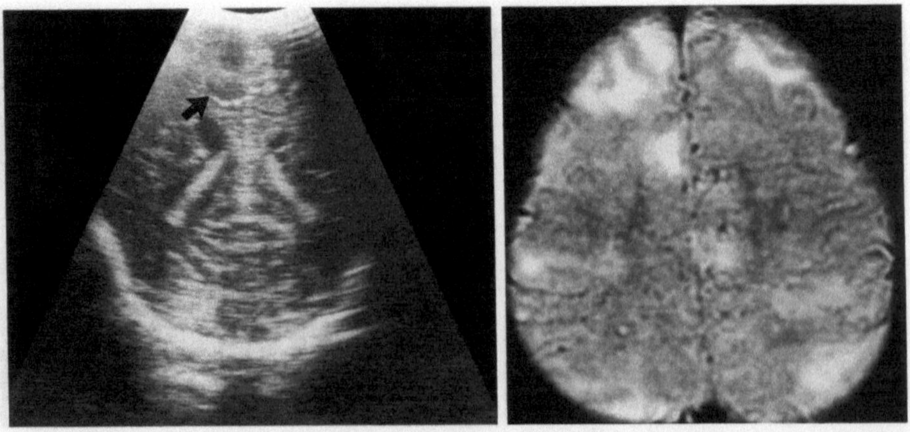

a b

Fig. 2.39 a, b. US, FV (**a**) and SET2, AV, 2000/120 ms (**b**). Regression of neurological development due to tuberous sclerosis of Bourneville. Multiple cortical tubers easily seen by MRI in SET2 because of their high signal but difficult to see by US because of their isoechogenicity

factors can lead to disturbance of CBF, especially in the premature baby: hypocapnia, patient handling and suctioning, and apnea and bradycardia.

In this section, we will review several patterns of ischemic injury in neonates with respect to Volpe's classification of neuropathologic features:

1. *Selective neuronal necrosis* refers to necrosis of neurons of the cerebral cortex, diencephalon, basal ganglia, midbrain, pons, medulla or cerebellum.
2. *Status marmoratus* of basal ganglia and thalami is characterized by hypermyelination; this disorder is the least common.
3. *Parasagittal cerebral injury* refers to a lesion of the cerebral cortex and subcortical white matter. The distribution of this injury is intimately related to the border zones and end fields of the anterior, posterior and middle cerebral arteries (parasagittal cerebral convexity).
4. *Cerebral leucomalacia* refers to a necrosis of white matter either adjacent to the external angle of the lateral ventricles (periventricular leucomalacia, PVL) or in the subcortical area at the depth of the sulcus (subcortical leucomalacia, SL). Abnormal vascular development appears to be the main predisposing factor leading to ischemia in these two particular regions. Indeed, in the premature baby, distal fields in the periventricular arterial border and end zones determine a watershed area vulnerable to systemic hypotension, hypoxemia, hypercapnia, etc. Lesions occurring within these areas are classified as PVL. With advanced gestational age and the development of convolutions and gyri, the depth of the sulcus reveals a relatively avascular triangular area vulnerable to the same factors mentioned above and predisposing to SL.
5. *Focal or multifocal ischemia* is related to necrosis that occurs within the distribution of the major cerebral vessels. Necrosis is associated with dissolution of the tissue and cavity formation. Thus, the terms porencephaly (single cavity), hydranencephaly (hemispheres reduced to cerebrospinal fluid filled sacs) or multicystic encephalomalacia (multiple cavities of necrosis) are used to describe those patterns of ischemia.

Even though the neuropathologic features are well classified, as mentioned above, distinction between these ischemic lesions is sometimes difficult and in some instances they seem to be interrelated. Other factors, such as gestational age, must be taken into consideration. With either advanced gestational age or in the full-term baby, selective neuronal necrosis, parasagittal cerebral injury, status marmoratus and focal or multifocal ischemia seem to be more frequent; in premature babies, cerebral leucomalacia is the most common lesion.

With the introduction of MRI, investigators have gained interest in the diagnosis and prognosis of cerebral injuries. We will see in this section to what extent MRI may be useful in diagnosing ischemia and providing a prognosis.

2.5.2 Patients

Since it was difficult to classify our patients according to the neuropathologic features described by Volpe (1987), we have adopted the following classification:

Group 1 includes neonates suffering from severe birth asphyxia, i.e. fetal distress as evidenced by abnormal cardiotocography; meconium staining; Apgar score ≤ 3 at 5 min; intubation and ventilation longer than 10 min; acidosis and neurologic impairment during the neonatal period.

Group 2 includes neonates admitted to the neonatal intensive care unit because of risk of cerebral leucomalacia.

Group 3 includes neonates suffering from focal ischemia, diagnosed by US or CT scan, with or without evident clinical signs.

All clinical data are summarized in Tables 2.3, 2.4 and 2.7.

2.5.3 Group 1: Cerebral Ischemia

2.5.3.1 Results

In this group several patterns of ischemia are noted (see Table 2.3 and Figs. 2.40–2.54).

In patient 1, ischemia was localized to the right occipital lobe with cortical necrosis (Fig. 2.40). The ischemia exhibited a low intensity signal more pronounced than that of white matter on SET1. By contrast, a high intensity signal was noted in the basal ganglia (lenticular nuclei) (Fig. 2.41). On SET1, a high signal intensity was related to hemorrhage. In this patient, we determined that ischemia was associated with basal ganglia injury.

In patient 2, several brain disorders could be noted and right temporal infarction was considered (Fig. 2.42). The infarct exhibited a low signal intensity more pronounced than that of the white matter on GE. We noted also a midline shift and compression of the lateral ventricle (Fig. 2.43). This seems to occur in

Table 2.3. Group 1: Perinatal data and patient outcome

Patient	GA (weeks)	Signs	MRI	Outcome
1	33	Coma seizures	D2	Died at D3
2	35	Coma seizures	D5	Died at D5
3	35	Seizures hypotonic	D28	Severely handicapped epilepsy
4	40	Hypotonia seizures	D15	Severely handicapped epilepsy
5	40	Seizures hypotonia	D16	Severely handicapped epilepsy
6	43	Seizures	D15	Severely handicapped epilepsy

GA, = gestational age at birth; MRI, day after birth of MRI study; D, day the early phase of cerebral infarction (see Sect. 2.5.5). It was also obvious that the signal of the white matter was abnormal based on the PCA. Thus, the cerebral parenchyma had undergone dissolution (multifocal ischemia?). Beside necrosis, hemorrhagic parenchymal involvement was identified in the left periventricular area and in the right subcortical parietal parenchyma. Hemorrhage was also seen in both the magna cisterna and the right subdural space. We determined that focal ischemia preceded multifocal ischemia and was associated with hemorrhage.

In patient 3, the pattern of ischemic lesion could be ascribed to parasagittal cerebral injury, more pronounced posteriorly (parietal lobes; Figs. 2.44–2.46).

In patients 4–6 (Figs. 2.47–2.54), several patterns of selective neuronal necrosis were observed. Cortical necrosis and cerebral white matter necrosis were noted in all patients to different degrees. However, the basal ganglia were spared in patients 4 and 5 and had necrosed in patient 6. In this latter patient, the basal ganglia exhibited a low intensity signal on SET1 and a high intensity signal on SET2. The brain stem was spared in all patients.

Fig. 2.40. SET1, 500/28 ms, AV; patient 1. Note cerebral ischemia (hyposignal) on the right occipital lobe with cortical necrosis associated with a hypersignal at the level of the lenticular nuclei

Fig. 2.41. SET1, 500/28 ms, AV at the level of basal ganglia; patient 1. Beside ischemia of the right occipital lobe, note the significant hypersignal on the lenticular nuclei (globus pallidus and putamen)

Fig. 2.42. GE, 450/12 ms/90°, medial SV; patient 2. Hemorrhage in the basal cisterna (hypersignal) and in the posterior fossa cisterna (hypersignal). Note the abnormal signal of the cerebral parenchyma

Fig. 2.43. GE, 450/12 ms/90°, FV; patient 2. Multiple parenchymal involvement associated with right temporal infarction and right subdural hemorrhagic collection. Note compression of the right lateral ventricle and the midline shift

Fig. 2.44. SET1, 600/28 ms, AV; patient 3. Note parasagittal ischemia (hyposignal) of the parietal lobe (posteriorly)

Fig. 2.45. SET1, 600/28 ms, FV; patient 3. Note cortical and subcortical parasagittal necrosis (hyposignal)

Fig. 2.46. AV; patient 3. Nonenhanced CT scan at day 28 after birth. Note parasagittal diffuse hypodensity

Fig. 2.47. SET1, 600/32 ms, AV; patient 4. Note diffuse ischemia (hyposignal) of frontal, parietal and occipital lobes. Basal ganglia are spared

Fig. 2.48. SET2, 2000/120 ms, AV at the same level as Fig. 2.36; patient 4. Ischemia exhibits high intensity signal; basal ganglia are spared

2.5.3.2 Discussion

Compared to other brain imaging techniques, MRI provides more information regarding the diagnosis, neuropathologic features and pathophysiological events of ischemia.

On MRI, cerebral ischemia exhibits a different signal depending on whether SET1 or SET2 is used. On SET1, a low intensity signal is found which seems to be more pronounced than the signal obtained from white matter. On SET2, ischemia exhibits a high intensity signal more marked than that of white matter. Although in our patients cerebral ischemia was easily identified by MRI, one ought to be cautious in interpreting these signals in the immature brain. Indeed, the large amount of brain water accounts for a large part of the signal. Thus, interpreting ischemia in immature brains requires careful attention.

In patient 1, ischemia was noted in the right temporal lobe. This was associated with hemorrhage within the basal ganglia and thalami. Basal ganglia injury in peri-

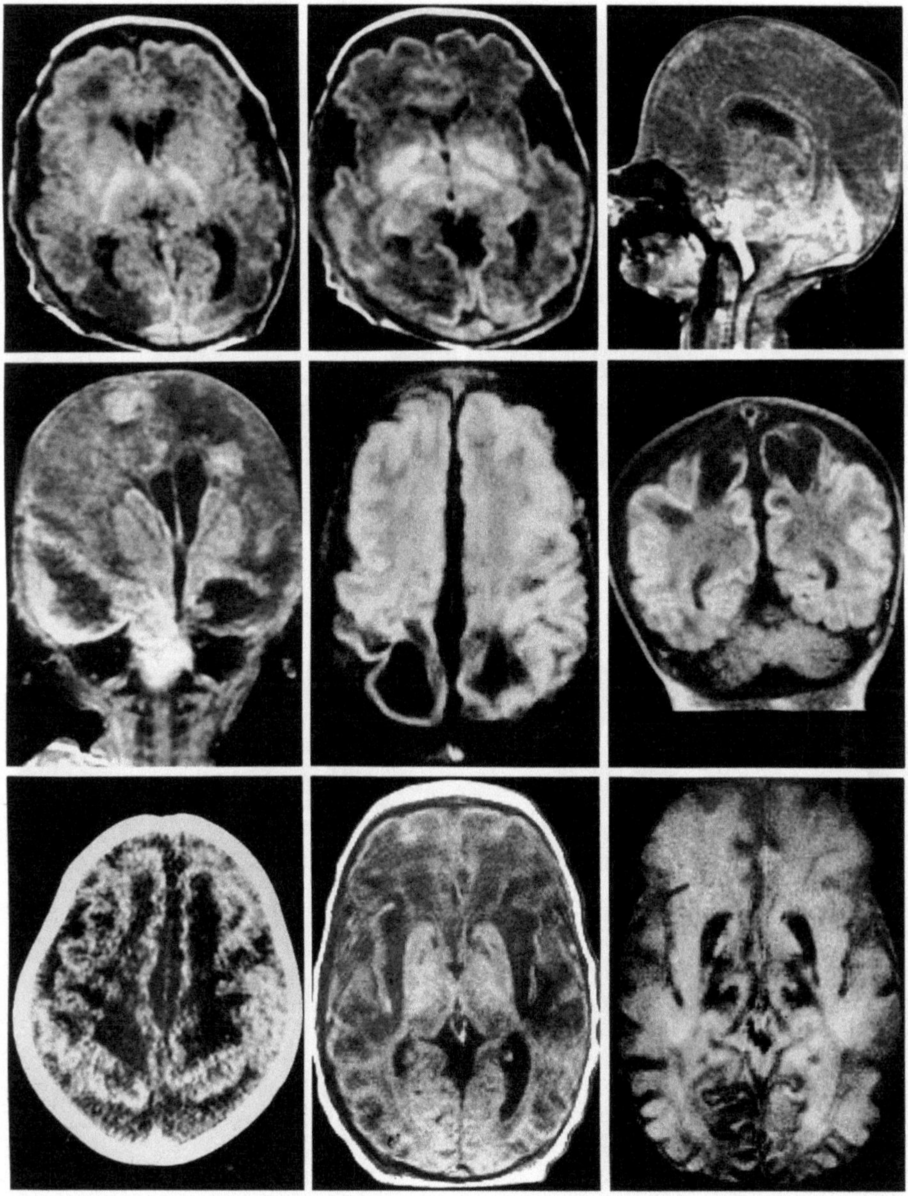

2.40 2.41, 42

2.43 2.44, 45

2.46 2.47, 48

natal asphyxia is related to status marmoratus. This lesion is apparently more common in term infants, the characteristic feature being hypermyelination. Although injury occurs in the perinatal period, the lesion itself (i.e. hypermyelination) is not seen until the end of the first year of life (*"état marbré"* or marbled appearance). However, after the acute period and during the following weeks, the affected area exhibits either capillary proliferation or hemorrhagic necrosis. These cellular changes were imaged by CT and US after the onset of the insult.

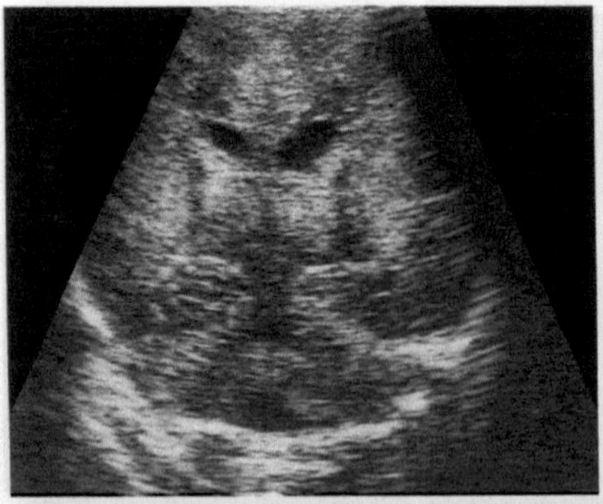
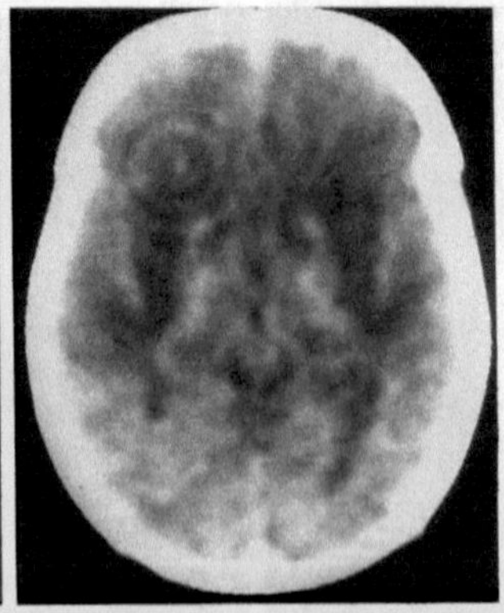

2.49, 50

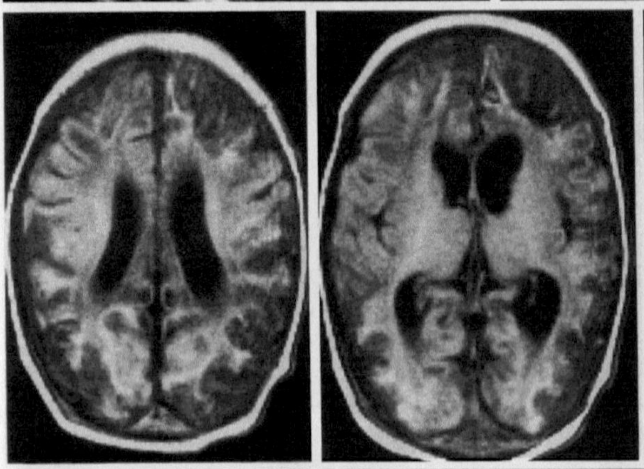

2.51 a, b

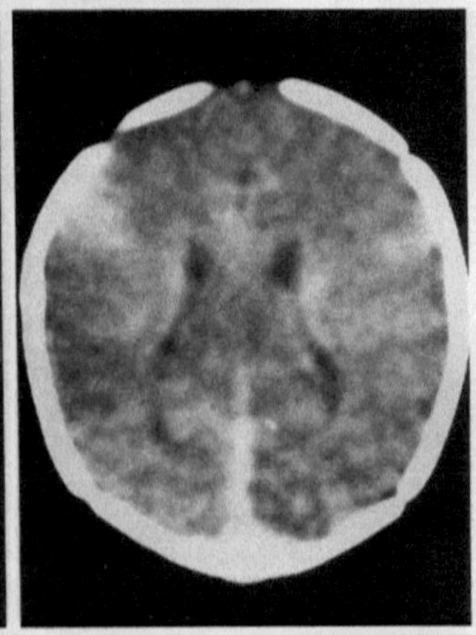

2.52

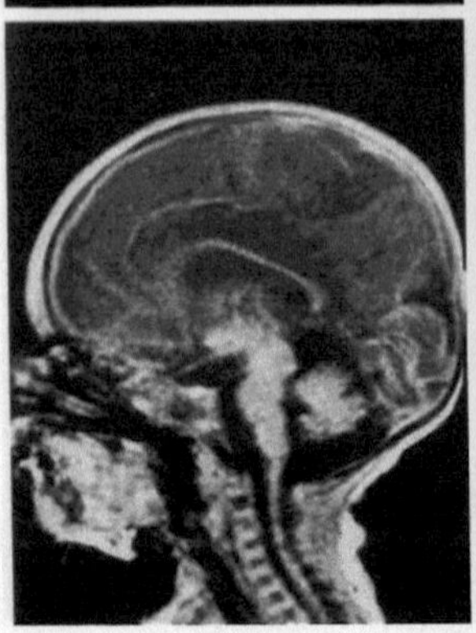

2.53

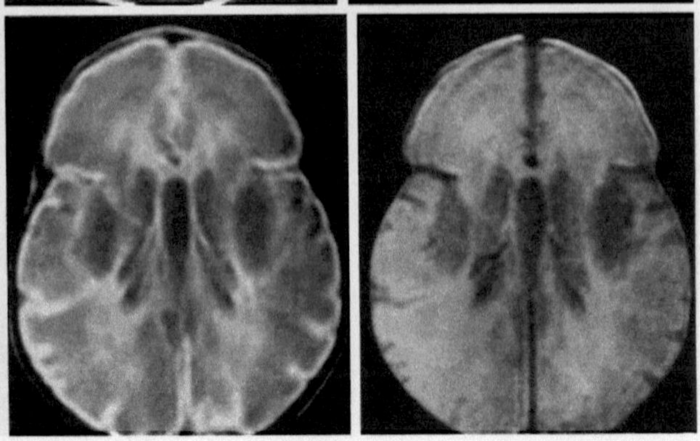

2.54 a,

On CT increased attenuation was found; on US, echo densities were shown. Whether these imaging features are related to hemorrhagic necrosis or exaggerated capillary proliferation is difficult to determine. In our patient, MRI applied earlier, at day 2, resulted in a high intensity signal in the affected area which could be related to hemorrhagic necrosis. Thus, MRI allowed us to distinguish between these two pathologic features.

In patient 2, several brain disorders were noted. This pattern of brain injury occurs particularly in the premature ba-

Fig. 2.49. US scan at day 14 day birth, FV; patient 4. Note dilated ventricules and bilateral altered echogenicity of cerebral parenchyma

Fig. 2.50. Nonenhanced CT scan, AV at the same level as Fig. 2.37 and 2.38; patient 4. Note diffuse hypodensity of the cerebral parenchyma; noninjured areas are difficult to identify

Fig. 2.51 a, b. SET1, 600/32 ms, AV; patient 5. Note ventricular dilatation, cortical and subcortical necrosis (hyposignal) of frontal, parietal and occipital lobes. Part of the parietal lobes (especially right) and basal ganglia are spared

Fig. 2.52. CT scan at day 10; AV; patient 5. Diffuse abnormal density in the cerebral parenchyma with mildly dilated ventricles. No evidence of normal parenchyma

Fig. 2.53. GE, 450/12 ms, SV; patient 6. Note diffuse hyposignal of cerebral parenchyma associated with a necrosis of the basal ganglia

Fig. 2.54 a, b. SET2, 2000/60 ms, first (**a**) and second (**b**) echo, AV; patient 6. Note diffuse cortical and subcortical necrosis and evolution from hypo- to hypersignal between the first (**a**) and second (**b**) echo

---

by. As demonstrated by MRI, focal ischemia and hemorrhage preceded multifocal ischemia. This diphasic pattern is mainly related to the severity of the hypoxic event. Indeed, following perinatal asphyxia, a redistribution of cardiac output occurs with an increase in CBF which could lead to hemorrhage. If hypoxemia persists a decrease in CBF occurs leading to ischemia. The more severe the hypoxic event, the more cerebral artery territory gained by ischemia. Here again, MRI was useful in determining the pathophysiological event occurring after perinatal asphyxia.

In patient 3, the pattern of ischemic lesion could be ascribed to parasagittal cerebral injury. This lesions is observed in the near-term infant. The areas affected are in the border zones between the end fields of the major cerebral arteries and thus a necrosis of the cortical and adjacent parenchyma, most marked in the posterior cerebrum, occurs. The reason why premature brains are spared is related to the presence of meningeal interarterial anastomoses between the three major cerebral arteries. Thus, cortical and subcortical perfusion is relatively spared in case of an hypoxic event. However, these anastomoses tend to regress toward term, mainly due to the increased surface area of the cortex and the development of convolutions and gyri. This leads to a parasagittal watershed area vulnerable to impaired cerebral perfusion. Here, MRI has been more useful than CT in diagnosing this type of ischemia. The advantage of MRI lies in the fact that multiplanar images, especially frontal views (FV) delineates more precisely the lesion most marked posteriorly (cortical and subcortical white matter necrosis).

In patients 4, 5 and 6, selective neuronal necrosis was considered. Comparing MRI to images obtained from CT and US scans, we noted that MRI was more useful in detecting the ischemic lesions. Indeed, on CT, a diffuse hypodensity was noted in patients 4 and 5 without any possibility to determine the noninjured area. Nevertheless, the CT scan pattern was abnormal: a diffuse hypodensity marked a neuronal injury probably associated with edema during the acute period. On US, altered parenchymal echogenicity was noted bilaterally.

This type of image is related to ischemia. However, US is not as useful as CT or MRI in the definition of cortical neuronal necrosis and lesions because this area is difficult to assess. On MRI, we have been able to more easily delimit the area of CNS involved by ischemia. A more severely injured brain was noted in patient 6: cortical, subcortical cerebral parenchyma and basal ganglia were necrosed. In patient 5, some of the cerebral parenchyma and the basal ganglia were spared. The latter area was not affected at all in patients 4 and 5. In all patients, brain stem centers were preserved.

When we analyzed MR images taken from these patients we noted that ischemic lesions affected the CNS differently. This led us to emphasize that perinatal asphyxia can occur with different levels of severity. Indeed, selective neuronal necrosis affects different sites of the neonatal CNS. However, there is a varying degree of vulnerability between areas within the CNS following asphyxia. It is well known that, after a hypoxemic event, an adaptive response occurs (increase in cardiac output and CBF) in order to maintain preferentially the intensity of vital brain stem centers. Thus, other areas of the CNS are less perfused. The area most severely affected by this adaptive response is the white matter. Moreover, the large amount of brain water and paucity of myelinated fibers makes the cerebrum parenchyma more vulnerable to dissolution. Regarding MR images taken from patients 4, 5 and 6, we concluded that perinatal asphyxia and the adaptive response occurred differently. They were more marked in patients 4 and 6 than in patient 5.

The outcome of all infants in group 1 was not favorable: two infants died and four are severely handicapped. Although MRI has provided additional information on ischemic lesions, neuropathologic features and pathophysiological events, the clinical status together with US scan, electroencephalogram, Doppler studies and electrophysiological measurements are sufficient to allow a prognosis. Nonetheless, MRI, if available, may be more useful than CT scans in such instances.

2.5.4 Group 2: Cerebral Leucomalacia

2.5.4.1 Patients and Results

Included in this group were 16 neonates whose gestational age (GA) ranged from 27 to 40 weeks and who were at risk of developing cerebral ischemic injury (Table 2.4). Cerebral leucomalacia was diagnosed by US in 14 neonates. In the remainder, an abnormal motor examination at 3 months of age led us to suspect a cerebral ischemic injury; this was confirmed by MRI. Also in this group, 12 infants were evaluated by MRI in early infancy, between 1 and 2 years of age (Table 2.4 and Figs. 2.55–2.107).

Of the 16 neonates studied, 13 were premature and 3 were term. In 2 full-term infants, occurrence of PVL was antenatal (patients 14, 16). Indeed, US, when applied early in the neonatal period, showed patterns of well progressed PVL.

Fig. 2.55. US scan at 36 weeks PCA, FV; patient 1. (1st twin). Bilateral periventricular parietal cysts (*arrows*)

Fig. 2.56. US scan at 36 weeks PCA, right parasaggital view; patient 1. (1st twin). Multiple periventricular parietal cysts (*arrows*)

Fig. 2.57. MRI at 36 weeks PCA, GE, 450/12 ms/90°, AV; patient 1 (1st twin). Bilateral periventricular parietal cysts

Fig. 2.58. Same as Fig. 2.57, right SV. Three periventricular parietal cysts

Fig. 2.59. Same as Fig. 2.57, FV. Bilateral parietal periventricular cyst

Fig. 2.60. US scan at 36 weeks PCA, left parasagittal view; patient 2 (2nd twin). Small periventricular parietal cysts (*arrows*)

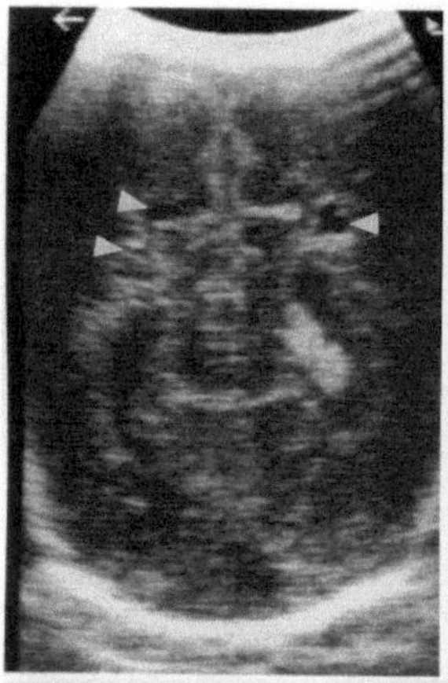

2.55

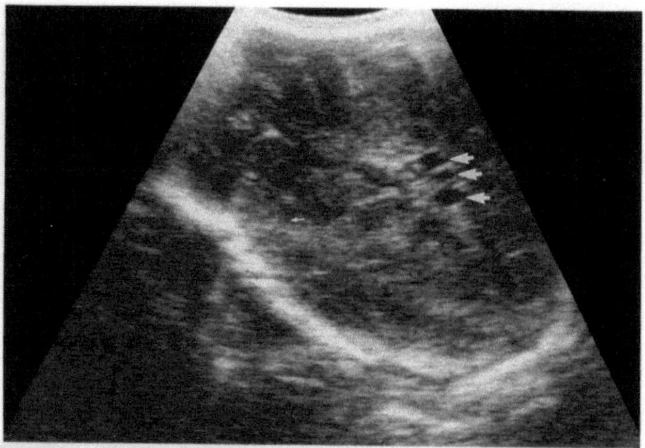

2.56

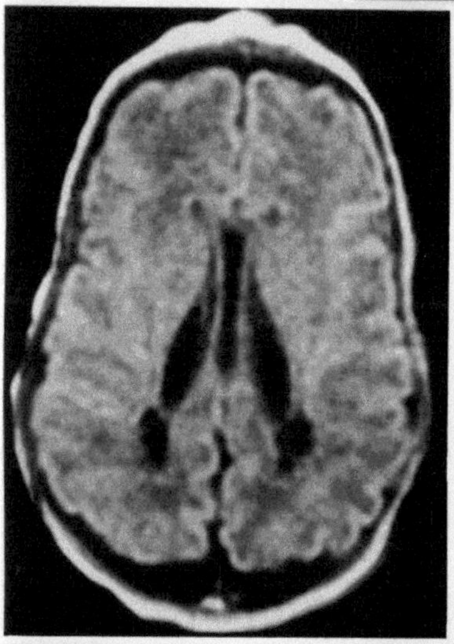

2.57

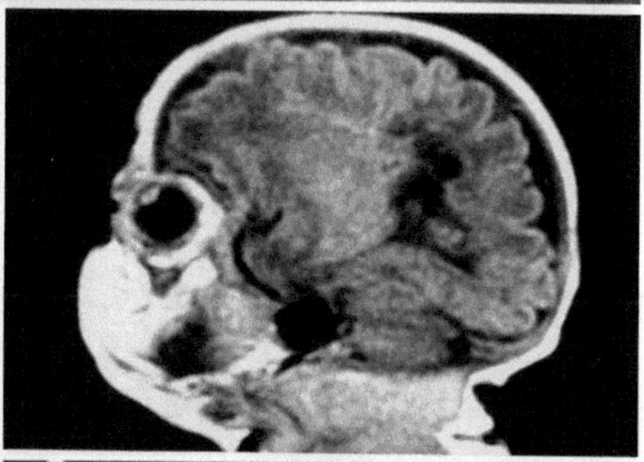

2.58

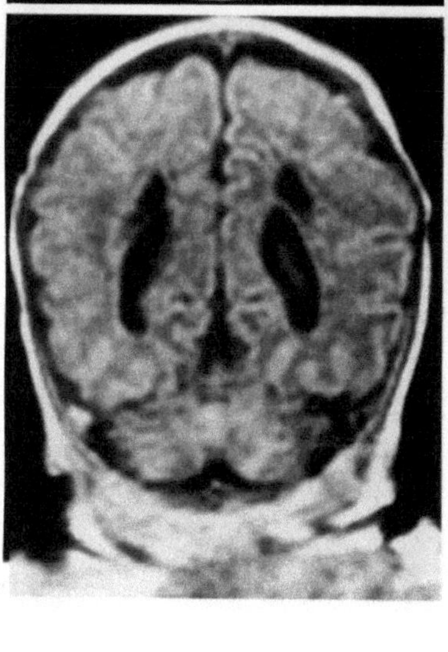

2.59

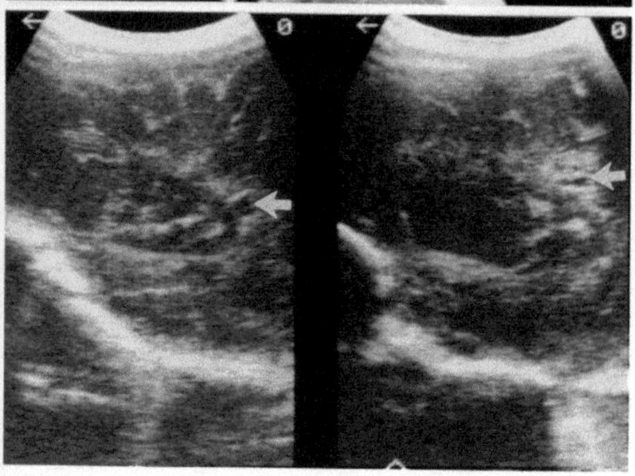

2.60

Table 2.4. Group 2: Perinatal data and patient outcome

Patient	GA (weeks)	Pregnancy	Events	Cerebral leucomalacia	Outcome
1	27	Twin	HMD, hypotension	Bilateral PVL	Spastic diplegia, squint
2	27	Twin	HMD, apnea	Bilateral PVL	Spastic diplegia
3	27	–	HMD, apnea	Bilateral hemorrhagic PVL + IVH	Spastic Quadriplegia, DQ < 50
4	27	–	HMD, hypotension	Bilateral PVL	Spastic diplegia
5	27	Twin, indocid	Mild HMD	Bilateral PVL	Spastic diplegia, squint
6	27	Twin, indocid	Mild HMD	Bilateral PVL	Spastic diplegia
7	28	–	Mild HMD, infection	Bilateral PVL	Spastic diplegia
8	29	–	Mild HMD, infection	Bilateral PVL	Spastic diplegia
9	29	–	Apnea, bradycardia	Bilateral PVL	Spastic diplegia
10	30	Twin	HMD	Unilateral PVL	Normal
11	31		Uneventful	Bilateral hemorrhagic PVL	Spastic quadriplegia, DQ < 50, visual loss
12	32		Apnea, bradycardia	Mixed hemorrhagic leucomalacia	Spastic quadriplegia, DQ < 50, visual loss
13	32	Twin, hypertension	Uneventful	Bilateral PVL	Spastic diplegia
14	38	IUGR	Uneventful	Unilateral PVL (antenatal)	Hemiparesis
15	40	Birth asphyxia	Seizures, hypotonia	Bilateral hemorrhagic PVL	Spastic quadriplegia, DQ < 50
16	40	IUGR	Infection	Bilateral PVL (antenatal)	Not known

HMD, hyaline membrane disease; IUGR, intrauterine growth retardation; IVH, intraventricular hemorrhage; indocid, indomethacin given during the 10 days before delivery; DQ, developmental quotient based on Brunet-Lezine test

Table 2.5. Neonatal classification of cerebral leucomalacia and its outcome

Classification	Outcome
Ultrasound	
Unilateral leucomalacia	Contralateral motor impairment
Bilateral leucomalacia	Bilateral motor impairment
Topography	
Periventricular PVL	Bilateral motor impairment
Subcortical SL	Bilateral motor impairment with visual loss
Mixed	Severe
Magnetic resonance imaging	
Localization	
Frontal	Uneventful short-term
Parietal	Motor impairment
Occipital	Visual impairment
Temporal	Auditory impairment
Number and diameter of cysts	Mild to severe
Pure leucomalacia	Moderate to severe
Hemorrhagic leucomalacia	Severe
Destruction of centrum semiovale	Moderate to severe

In one term baby, PVL occurred following birth asphyxia (patient 15). Classification of cerebral leucomalacia, as diagnosed by US in the 14 patients in the neonatal period was based on several criteria (Table 2.5):

- Uni- or bilateral leucomalacia
- Topography: periventricular, subcortical or mixed
- Location: frontal, parietal, occipital or temporal
- Number and diameter of cysts

Using MRI, we could add two criteria, which were rather difficult to assess by US (Table 2.5):

- Pure or hemorrhagic leucomalacia
- Evaluation of the destruction of the centrum semiovale

These criteria were applied in the neonatal period and correlated with neurodevelopmental outcome. Unilateral leucomalacia induced mild contralateral paresis without developmental delay; bilateral leucomalacia was always associated with spasticity, cognitive delay and motor and visual impairment. The severity of the neurodevelopmental outcome was related to:

1. Topography: Mixed leucomalacia had the worst outcome (quadriplegia, visual loss, DQ <50).
2. Location: Ischemia occurring in the parietal lobe was associated with spasticity and squinting. Ischemia in the frontal lobe occurred in our patients in association with other locations. In one patient it was not associated with contralateral abnormal development. A frontal location had no apparent deleterious short-term effects. Ischemia in the occipital lobe was associated with severe visual loss and cecity. We have found that an occipital location is rather difficult to diagnose by US, but using MRI it was easily identified. Temporal lobe ischemia did not occur in our patients. When ischemia occurred in multiple locations, the neurodevelopmental outcome was poor, with mental retardation, epilepsy and an abnormal motor exam. However,

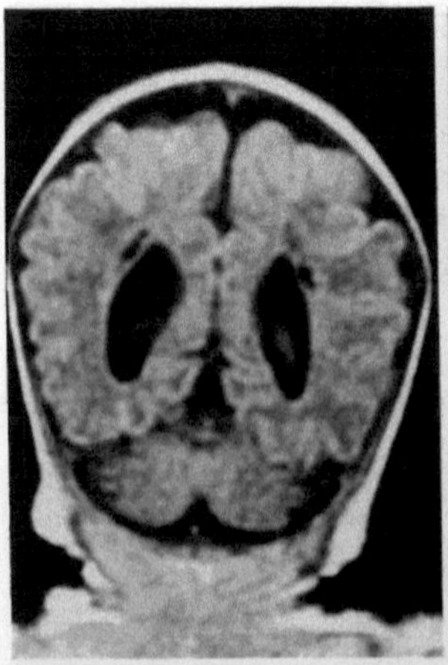

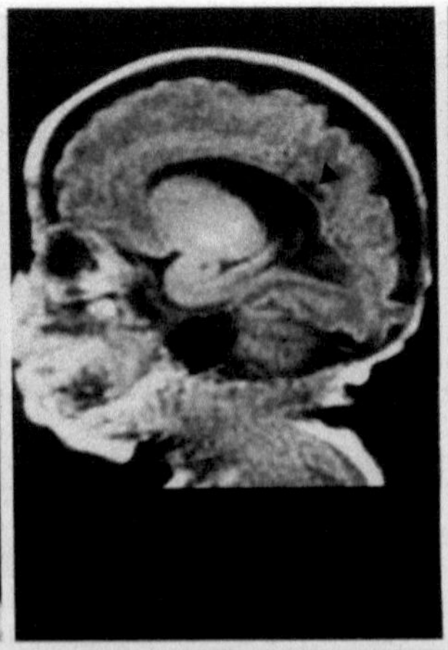

2.61, 62

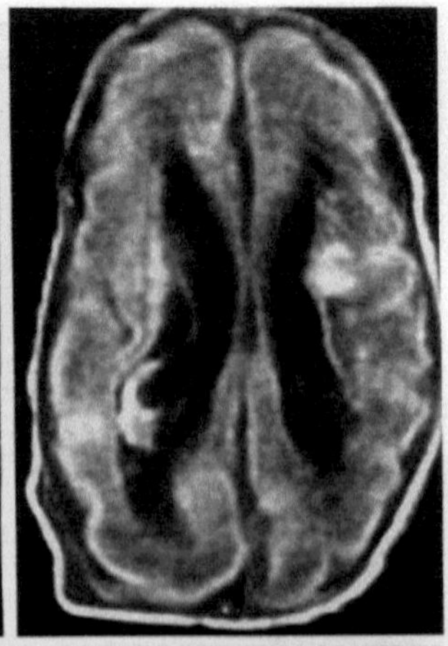

2.63

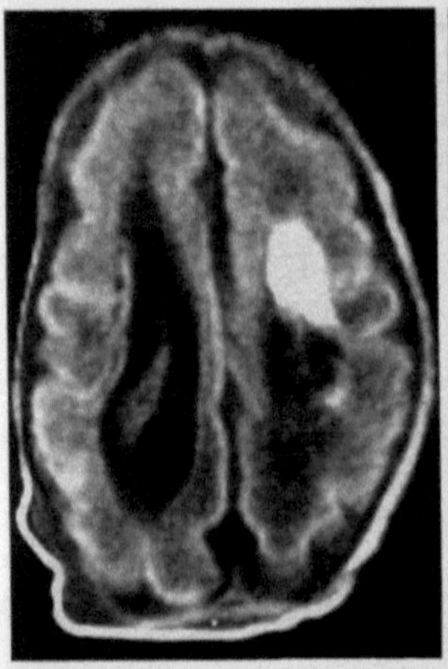

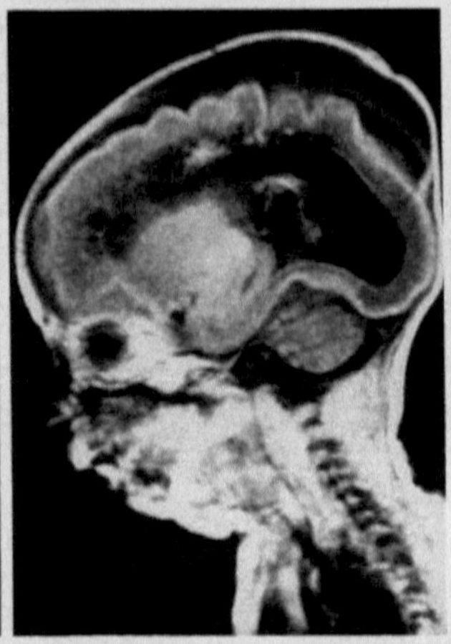

2.64, 65

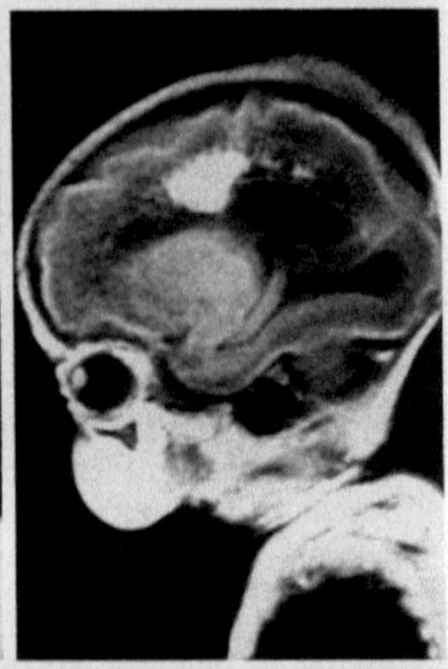

2.66

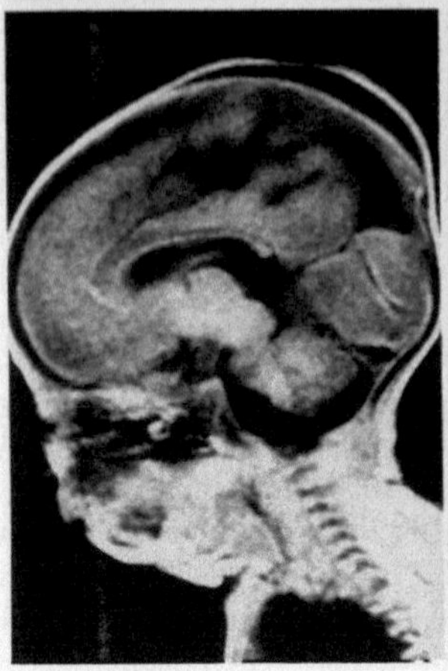

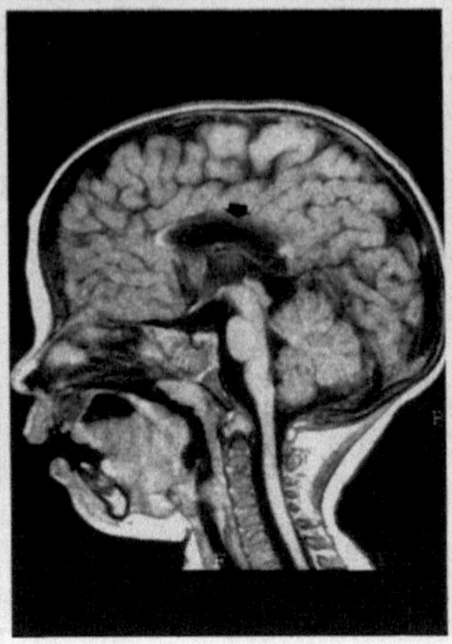

2.67, 68

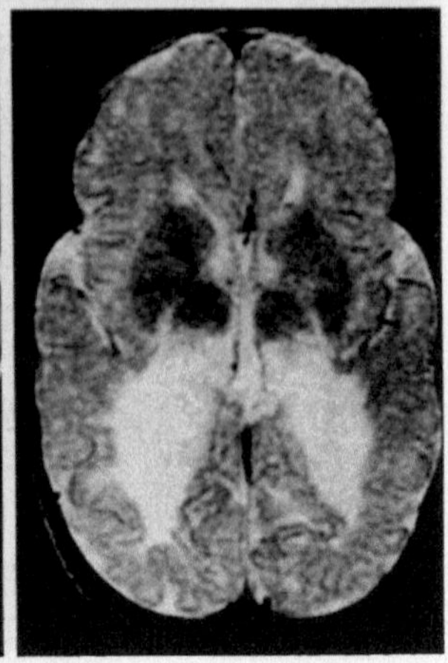

2.69

Fig. 2.61. MRI at 36 weeks WPCA, GE, 450/12 ms/90°, FV; patient 2 (2nd twin). Bilateral small periventricular cysts

Fig. 2.62. Same as Fig. 2.61, left SV. Small periventricular parietal cysts (*arrow*)

Fig. 2.63. GE, 450/12 ms/90°, AV; patient 3. Right intraventricular hemorrhage (hypersignal); left parenchymal parietal involvement with hemorrhagic component

Fig. 2.64. Same as Fig. 2.63, right periventricular ischemia (hyposignal); left parenchymal cerebral involvement; cerebral hemorrhagic leucomalacia (ischemia and hemorrhage)

Fig. 2.65. Same as Fig. 2.63, right SV. Periventricular leucomalacia involving frontal and parietal areas associated with a mild hemorrhagic signal

Fig. 2.66. Same as Fig. 2.65. Periventricular leucomalacia involving frontal and parietal areas associated with a very large hemorrhagic signal

Fig. 2.67. Same as Fig. 2.63, SV. Note the thickness of the corpus callosum (compare with Fig. 2.68)

Fig. 2.68. MRI at 1 year old, GE, 450/12 ms/90°, SV; patient 3. Severe atrophy of the corpus callosum (*arrow*)

Fig. 2.69. MRI at 1 year old, SET2, 2000/120 ms, AV; patient 3. Dilated ventricules with irregular walls; hypersignal of the posterior limb of the internal capsule

the neurological outcome was also related to the number and diameter of cysts (the more cysts and the larger their diameter, the more likely that the outcome will be poor).

3. Hemorrhagic leucomalacia, in our patients, was associated with a very poor neurological outcome compared to pure leucomalacia (Sect. 2.5.4.2; patients 3, 11, 12, 15).
4. Destruction of the centrum semiovale by ischemia was also one of the most important criterion determining neurological outcome.

Table 2.6. Effects of leucomalacia on brain development, based on MRI

White to gray matter differentiation not affected
Dilated lateral ventricles and reduction of white matter
Gliosis within the posterior limb of the internal capsule (severe leucomalacia)
Gliosis within the lenticular nuclei (severe leucomalacia)
Gliosis within the centrum semiovale
Iron accumulation within basal ganglia (severe leucomalacia)
Reduction of corpus callosum thickness (severe leucomalacia)

We can conclude that US provides important criteria by which the severity of the injury can be judged; furthermore, MRI has added useful information regarding neurological outcome. The two patients (14 and 19) who had abnormal motor exams in early infancy, had normal US exams in the neonatal period (Sect. 2.5.4.2).

MRI also provided the following information regarding brain anatomy and maturation during early infancy (Table 2.6):

1. The white to gray matter differentiation pattern was not affected in any of the patients.
2. Dilated lateral ventricles with irregular ventricular walls were due to resorption of cysts and associated with reduction of white matter (Figs. 2.70 and 2.80).
3. There was an abnormal signal from the posterior limb of the internal capsule (high intensity signal on SET2) (Figs. 2.69, 2.93, 2.106). However, this anomaly was obvious only in patients in whom spastic quadriplegia was noted (patients 3, 12, 15).
4. An abnormal signal within the centrum semiovale (high intensity signal on SET2) was observed (Figs. 2.73 and 2.107). The intensity of destruction of the centrum semiovale noted in the neonatal period correlated to the in-

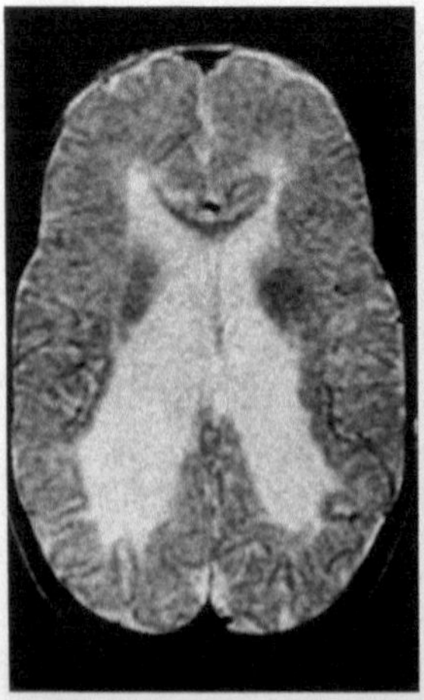
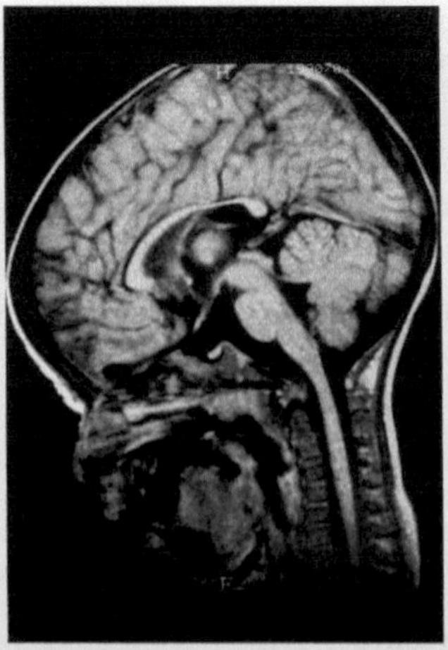

2.70, 71

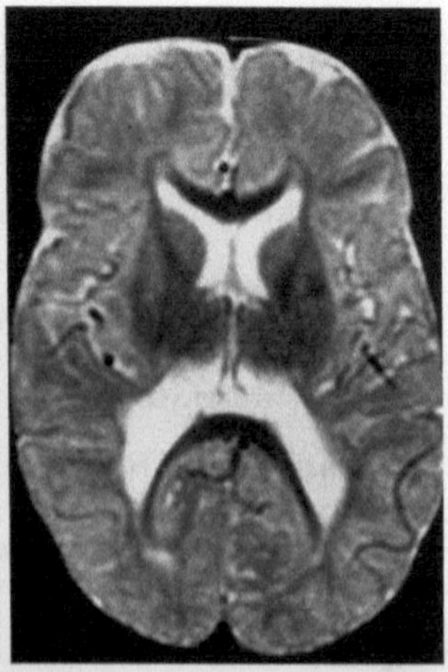

2.72 a

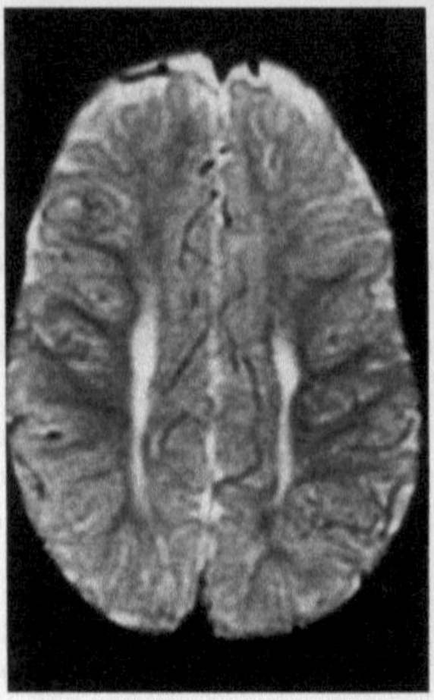
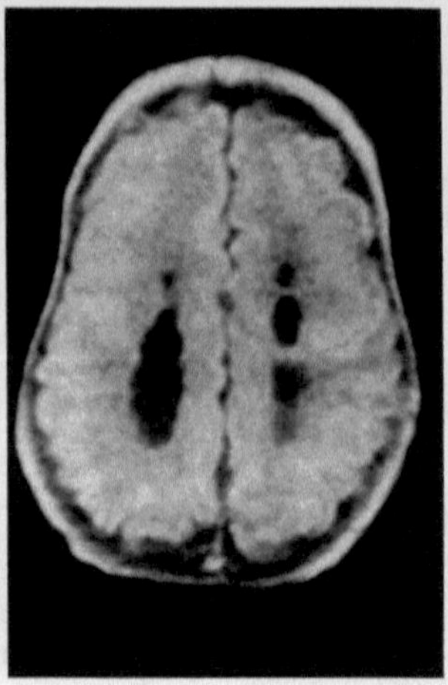

2.73, 74

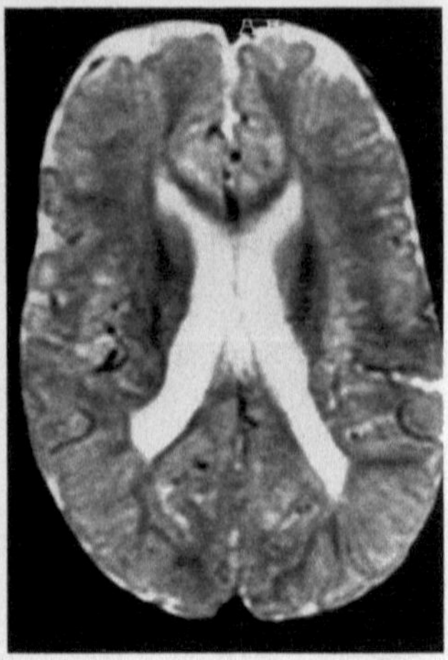

2.72 b

Fig. 2.70. Same as Fig. 2.69, AV. Corpus callosum is myelinated but atrophic; dilated ventricles with irregular walls

Fig. 2.71. GE, 450/12 ms/90°; patient 4. Corpus callosum seems normal

Fig. 2.72 a, b. MRI at 17 months old, SET2, 2000/120 ms, AV; patient 4. **a** Irregular ventricule walls; **b** normal myelination of internal capsule and corpus callosum

Fig. 2.73. Same as Fig. 2.72. Note hypersignal within the centrum semiovale most marked in the central and posterior regions

Fig. 2.74. GE, 450/12 ms/90°, AV; patient 5. Multiple bilateral cysts at the level of the centrum semiovale

tensity of the abnormal signal in early infancy and the severity of motor impairment (Fig. 2.95).

5. There was an abnormal signal within basal ganglia (low intensity signal on SET2). This was seen in only two patients (Fig. 2.92). A high intensity signal (on SET2) was also obvious in two patients in the lenticular nuclei (Fig. 2.106).
6. A reduced thickness of the corpus callosum was seen either on the anterior part (genu), the posterior part (splenium) or the medial part (Figs. 2.68, 2.81, 2.91). The severity of the corpus callosum injury was related to the severity of cerebral leucomalacia.

In the two patients who had normal neonatal US scans but who later exhibited abnormal motor exams, we were able to note only a high intensity signal on SET2 within the centrum semiovale, most marked posteriorly (Fig. 2.73). MRI features in early infancy were in general agreement with the neuromotor exams.

2.5.4.2 Discussion

Cerebral leucomalacia refers to necrosis of white matter. It can be located to the periventricular area (PVL) or to the subcortical white matter at the depth of the sulcus (subcortical leucomalacia).

Ischemia may involve either one hemisphere lobe or two and may be located either in the frontal, parietal, occipital or temporal lobes. The centrum semiovale is also involved. Corticospinal tracts, from their origin in the motor cortex, optic (occipital horn) and acoustic (temporal horn) radiations and the visual area, may also be affected by cerebral leucomalacia and are mainly responsible for the abnormal neuromotor outcome and neurosensorial loss. A serious complication that can occur and which seems to be deleterious is hemorrhage into the lesion (Figs. 2.66, 2.85).

An attempt to identify the injuries mentioned above and their characteristics and to link them to prognostic information is required in the neonatal period. Recently, using US, this goal has been achieved. There is a close relationship between cerebral leucomalacia as diagnosed by US and cerebral palsy later in infancy. Nonetheless, it is particularly difficult to predict minor impairments which may occur after the age of 5 years.

Questions about the accuracy of US in diagnosing cerebral leucomalacia have arisen. Indeed, some infants exhibited abnormal neuromotor exams but had supposedly normal US scans in the neonatal period. In some instances discrepancies were found between US results and anatomopathological studies. Although one might expect that US could misdiagnose cerebral leucomalacia, several arguments can be advanced to address this issue:

1. Interpreting US images depends on several factors; the examiner, if inexperienced, can misdiagnose PVL. Diverse pathologies, such as hemorrhage, gliosis, cerebral edema and infarction, produce a similar echo and thus increase the possibility of error.
2. The probe used is essential: with a 5 MHz transducer, small cysts (<3 mm) and proper evaluation of echo densities may be overlooked. These features can only be visualized with a 7.5 MHz or 10 MHz transducer.
3. Ischemic injury may also lie outside of the range of the detector (posteriorly or anteriorly).
4. Transient periventricular densities without subsequent evolution to cystic lesions could be ascribed to ischemic injury; however, they seem to correlate with less severe motor impairment than cerebral palsy. One must be cautious: periventricular densities lasting at least 10 days (prolonged periventricular flares) should be taken into consideration in evaluating neuromotor outcome. The timing of the US study is also of particular importance. Two US studies are necessary in the first week of life followed by once a week until discharge.

We can conclude that, with a good transducer and an experienced examiner, consistently normal US scans are reassuring and can accurately predict a normal neurologic outcome. In our patients, neonatal US scan was helpful in identifying cerebral leucomalacia even with small cysts (Figs. 2.55, 2.60, 2.96). It has allowed us to classify leucomalacia using the criteria mentioned above. It has also enabled us to accurately predict neurologic outcome in 12 patients.

MRI performed in the neonatal period has provided the same information ob-

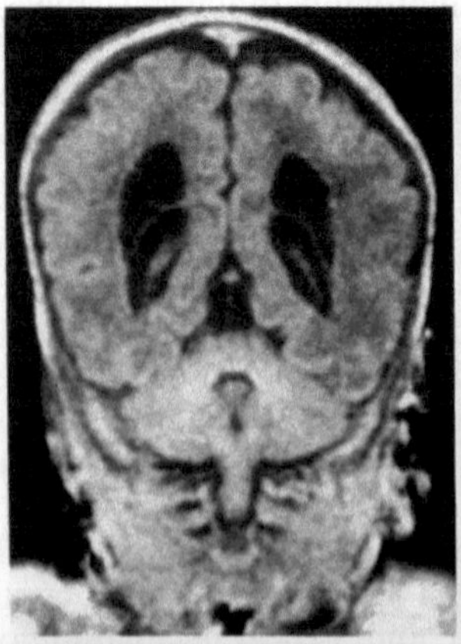
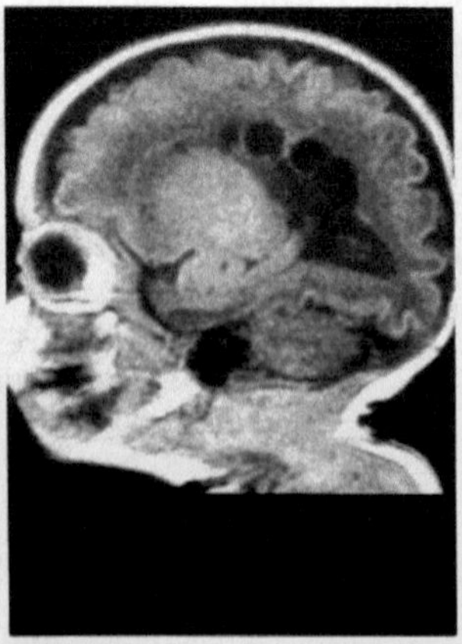

2.75, 76

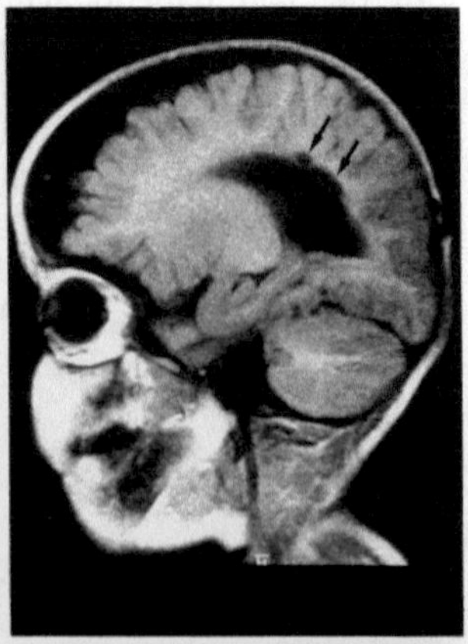

2.77

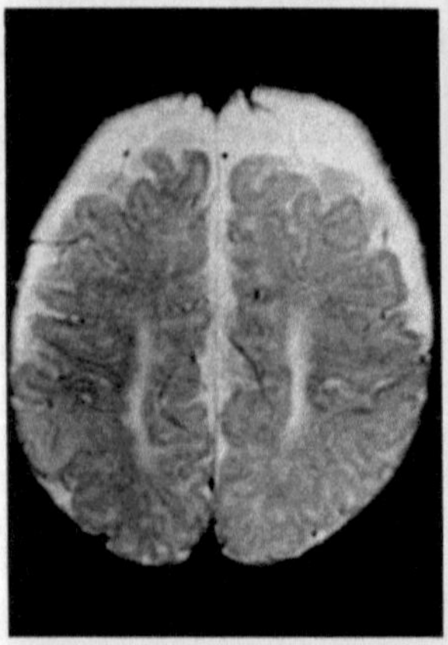
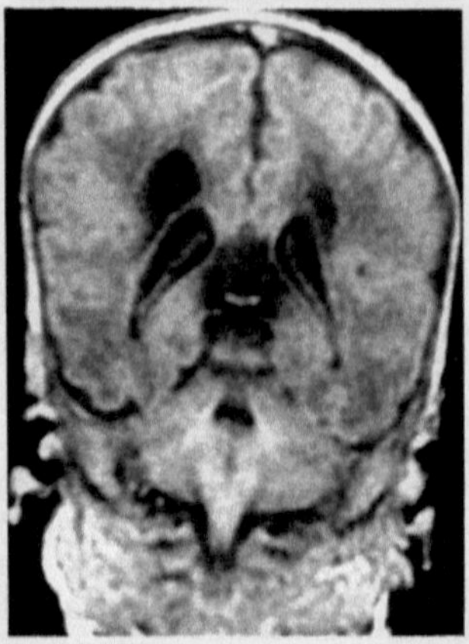

2.78, 79

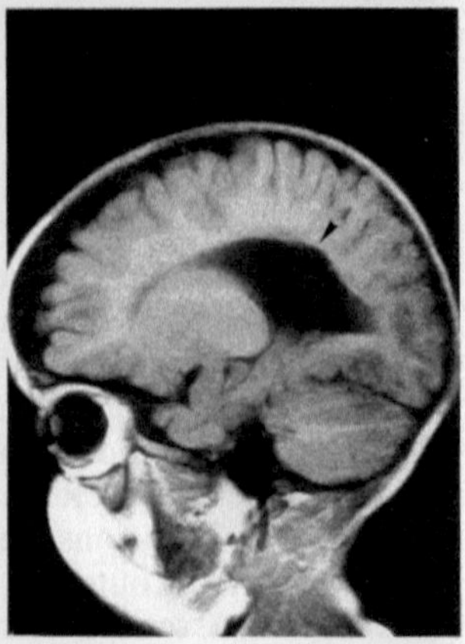

2.80

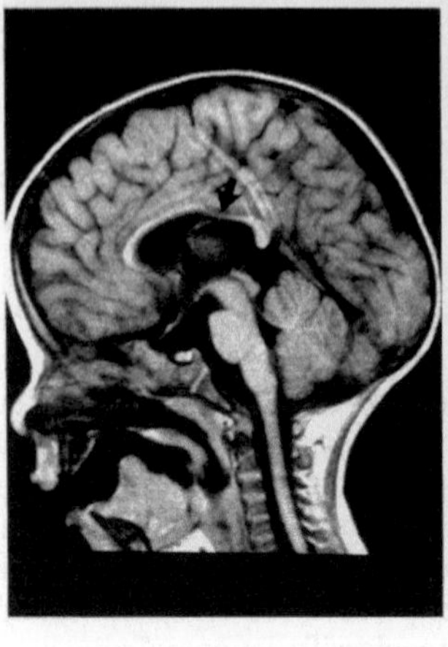
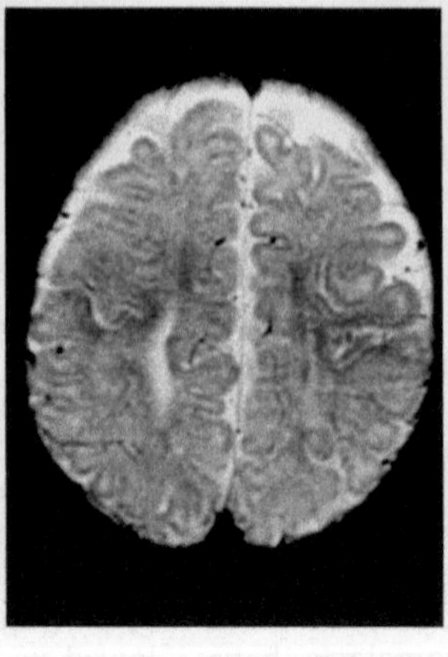

2.81, 82

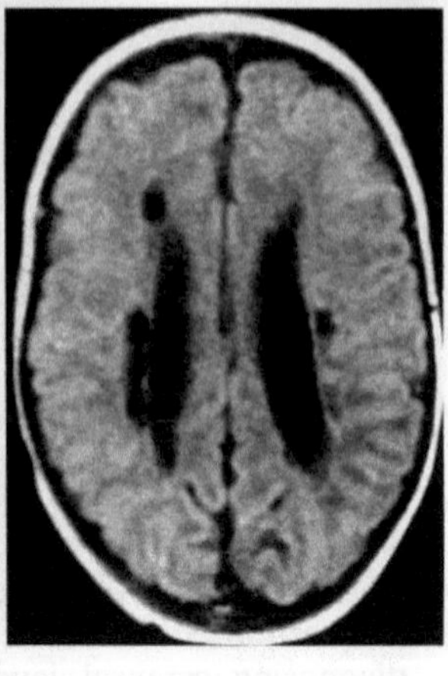

2.83

Fig. 2.75. Same as Fig. 2.74, FV. Bilateral cyst without communication with the lateral ventricles

Fig. 2.76. Same as Fig. 2.74, SV. Multiple cysts in the parietal periventricular area

Fig. 2.77. MRI at 15 months old, GE, 450/12 ms/90°, SV; patient 5. Cysts in the parietal periventricular area (*arrows*) are still visible without any resorption. Note also wide extracerebral space

Fig. 2.78. MRI at 15 months old, SET2, 2000/120 ms, AV; patient 5. Note the significant hypersignal in both centrum semiovale, most marked in the central and posterior portions

Fig. 2.79. MRI at 38 weeks PCA, GE, 450/12 ms/90°, FV; patient 6. Bilateral parietal cysts less significant in the left hemisphere and without communication with the lateral ventricles

Fig. 2.80. MRI at 15 months old, GE, 450/12 ms/90°, SV; patient 6. Cyst (*arrow*) still visible without communication with the lateral ventricle

Fig. 2.81. Same as Fig. 2.80. Mild atrophy of the corpus callosum (*arrow*)

Fig. 2.82. MRI at 15 months old, SET2, 2000/120 ms; patient 6. Right hypersignal most marked in the parietal portion of the right centrum semiovale

Fig. 2.83. MRI at 40 weeks PCA, GE, 450/12 ms/90°; patient 8. Bilateral periventricular leucomalacia with cysts at the right frontal and parietal area and on left parietal region

tained from US with two additional criteria that seem to contribute to predicting neurologic outcome (hemorrhagic leucomalacia and injury of the centrum semiovale). Hemorrhagic leucomalacia was associated with a very poor outcome. This is not surprising since hemorrhaging into the ischemic lesion occurs when the latter is the most critical. The process is referred to as hemorrhagic infarction (hemorrhage into reperfused ischemic areas). Some 25% of cerebral leucomalacias seem to be hemorrhagic. Hemorrhagic leucomalacia is suspected on US when a significant and very large echogenicity is exhibited (Figs. 2.86, 2.102). However, as emphasized above, a similar echogenicity could also be related to other brain pathologies. On MRI, hemorrhage shows a different signal than ischemia and can last for several weeks. Thus, hemorrhagic leucomalacia can be easily diagnosed. The other diagnostic criterion obtained from MRI is the destruction of the centrum semiovale. This area is of particular importance since all motor fibers descending from their origin cross it. MRI, by providing multiplanar images, contributes to the evaluation of the injury of the centrum semiovale. Its destruction is associated with severe motor impairment.

There are other benefits that can be obtained from MRI in the neonatal period:

1. Better location of leucomalacia, especially in the frontal and occipital lobes.
2. Determination of whether a periventricular area exhibiting increased echogenicity is due to ischemic injury or considered a normal variant (periventricular flares on US scan seem to exhibit an abnormal signal on MRI)
3. Better and easier identification of small ischemic lesions.

We can conclude that MRI is a useful tool for studying the pathology of the neonatal period since it provides information regarding diagnosis and prognosis. However, one must not neglect that it requires removal of prematures from their neonatal units and can thus be, in some instances, deleterious. MRI must be performed at a safe time in the neonatal period and in any instances in which cerebral leucomalacia is suspected (abnormal neuromotor exam and limited US data). Outside of the neonatal period, US is limited in the follow-up of such lesions with respect to the size of the anterior fontanelle. MRI is more helpful

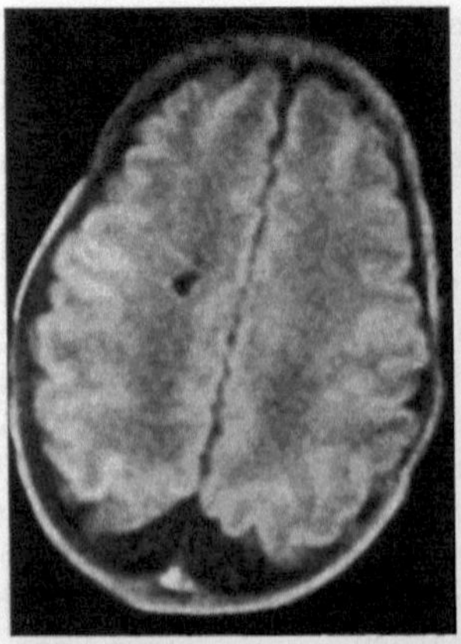
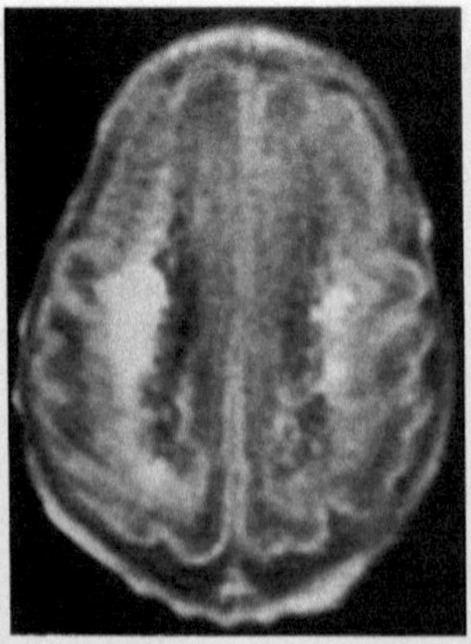

2.84, 85

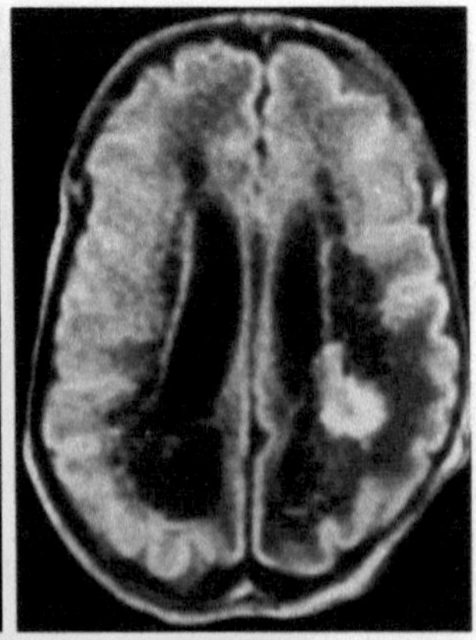

2.87

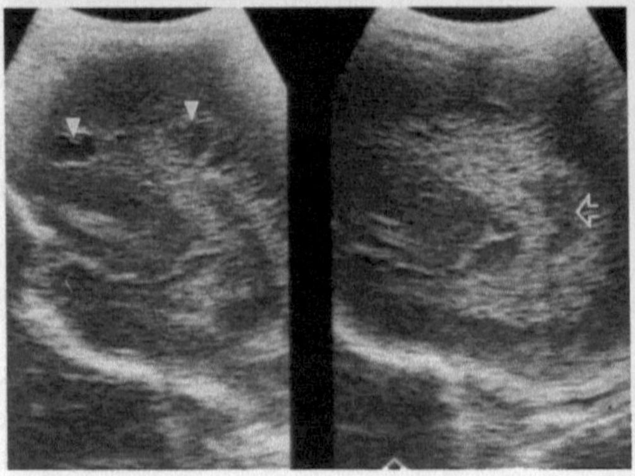

2.86

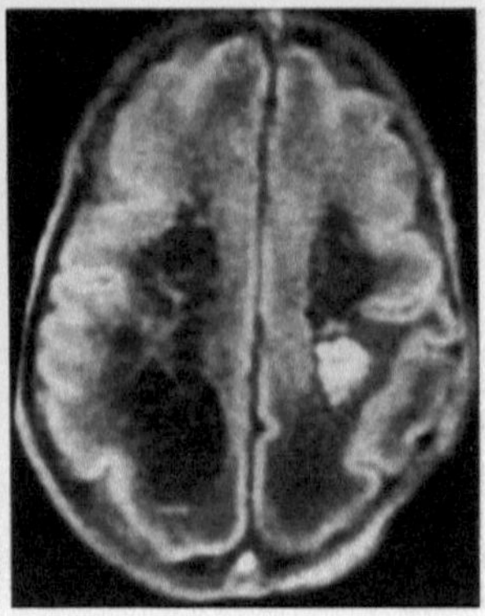

2.88

Fig. 2.84. MRI at 37 weeks PCA, GE, 450/12 ms/90°, AV; patient 10. Note cyst in the central portion of the centrum semiovale

Fig. 2.85. MRI at 32 weeks PCA, GE, 450/12 ms/90°, AV; patient 11. Note the significant ischemia at the level of the centrum semiovale associated with an hemorrhagic component

Fig. 2.86. US scan at 35 weeks PCA, right (*left*) and left (*right*) parasagittal view; patient 12. Note periventricular cysts on the right frontal and parietal periventricular area (*solid arrows*). Note the hyperechogenicity on the left periventricular area with an hypoechoic component (*open arrow*)

Fig. 2.87. MRI at 35 weeks PCA, GE, 450/12 ms/90° AV; patient 12. Note bilateral periventricular (hyposignal) ischemia most marked on the left and associated with a hypersignal corresponding to an hemorrhagic component

Fig. 2.88. Same as Fig. 2.87. Note the same bilateral ischemia at the level of the centrum semiovale associated with a left hemorrhagic component

Fig. 2.89. Same as Fig. 2.87, left SV. Note the significant periventricular and subcortical leucomalacia with an hemorrhagic signal

Fig. 2.90. Same as Fig. 2.87, right SV. Note the significant periventricular and subcortical leucomalacia

Fig. 2.91. GE, 450/12 ms/90°, SV; patient 12. Severe atrophy of corpus callosum

Fig. 2.92. MRI at 1 year old, SET2, 2000/120 ms; patient 12. Significant hyposignal in basal ganglia; dilated ventricles with irregular ventricle walls; reduction of white matter

Fig. 2.93. Same as Fig. 2.92. Hypersignal in the posterior limb of the internal capsule

Fig. 2.94. Same as Fig. 2.92. Dilated lateral ventricles; abnormal myelination

Fig. 2.95. Same as Fig. 2.92. Atrophy of the centrum semiovale with periventricular hypersignal

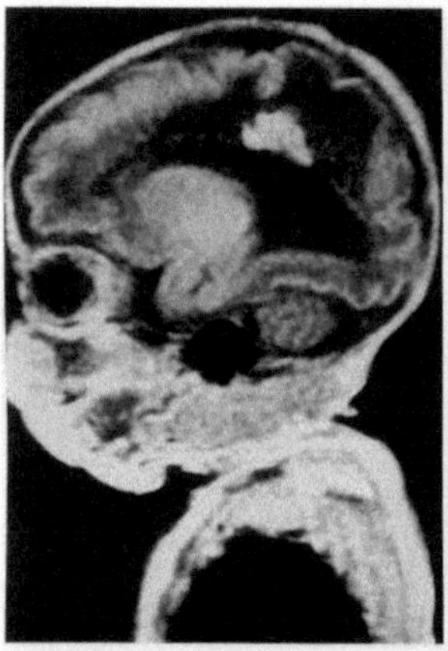

2.89

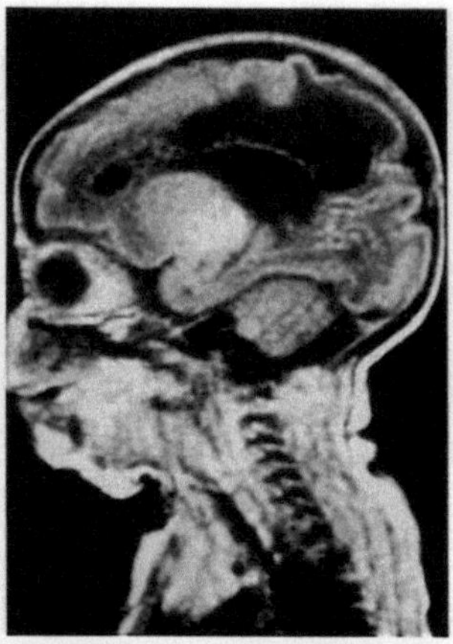

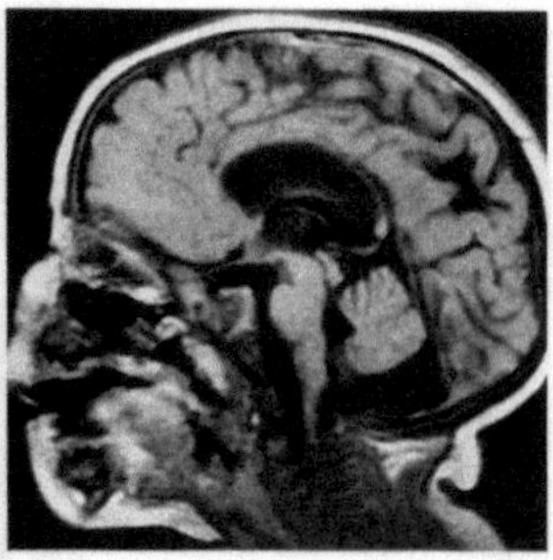

2.90, 91

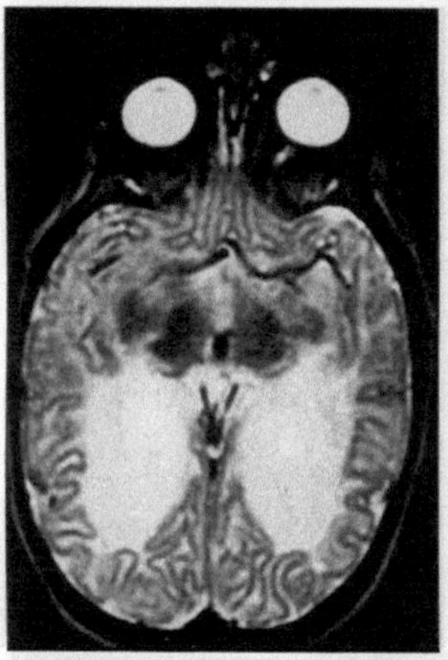

2.92

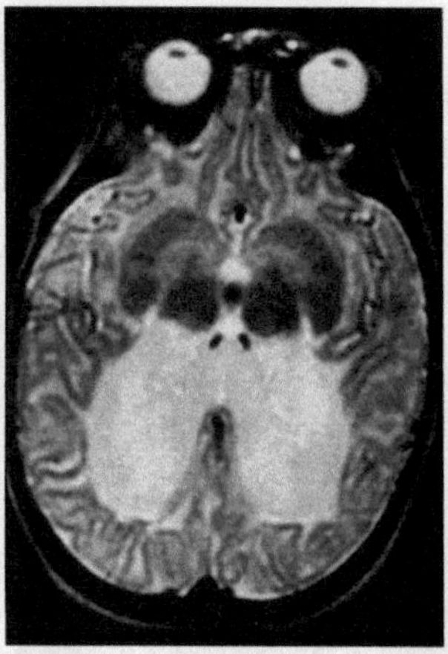

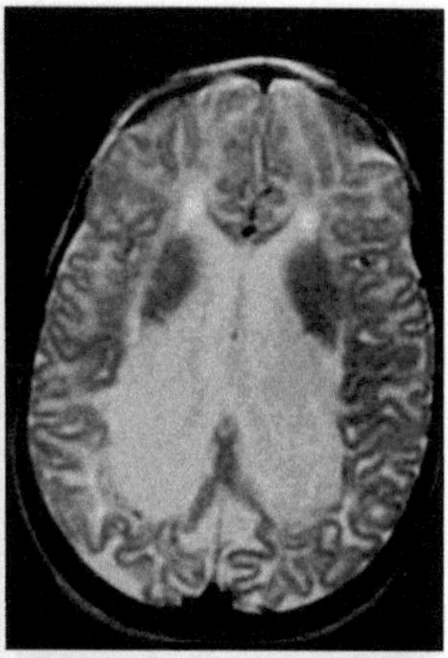

2.93, 94

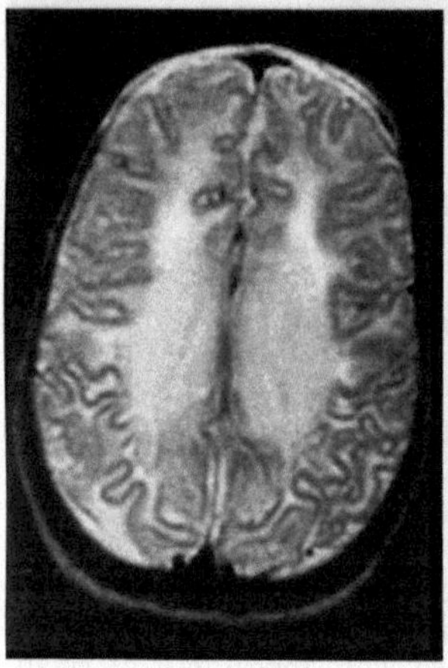

2.95

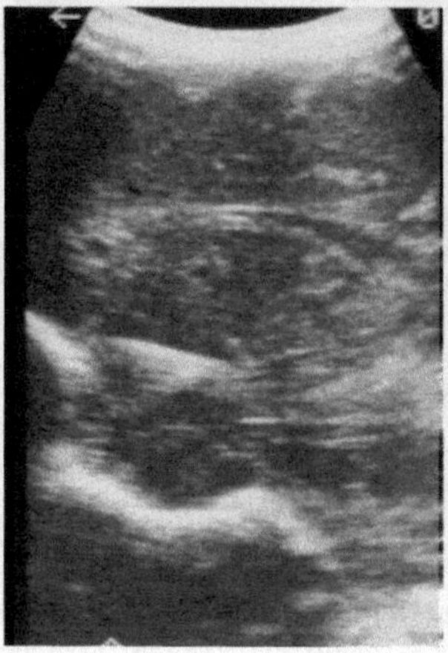

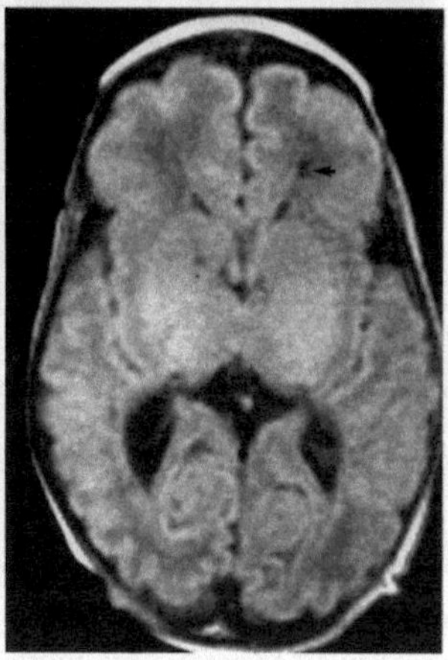

2.96, 97

Fig. 2.96. US scan, left parasagittal view at 35 weeks PCA; patient 13 (1st twin). Small left frontal cyst

Fig. 2.97. MRI at 38 weeks PCA, GE, 450/12 ms/90°, AV; patient 13 (1st twin). Small left periventricular frontal cyst (*arrow*)

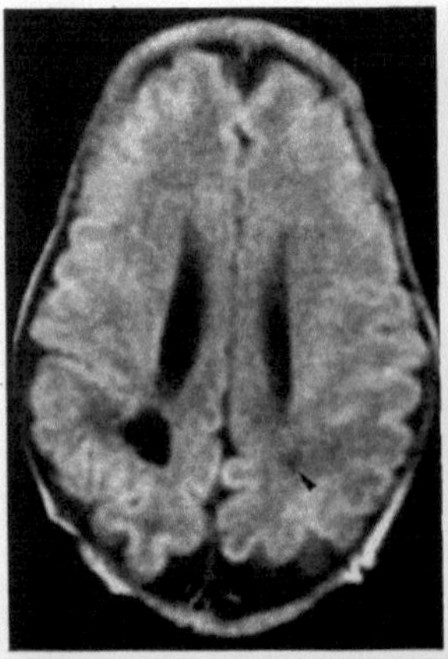
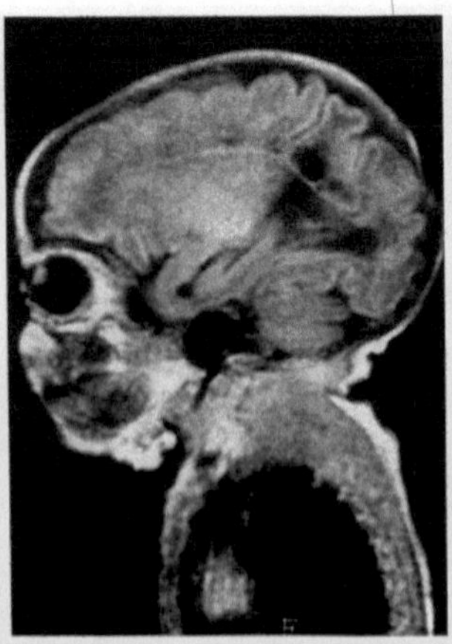

2.98, 99

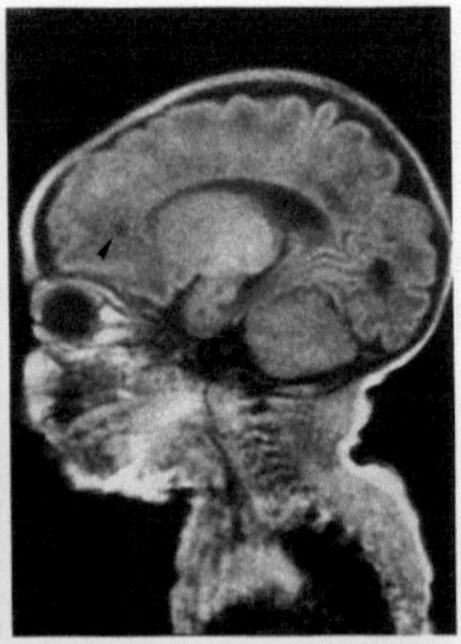

2.100

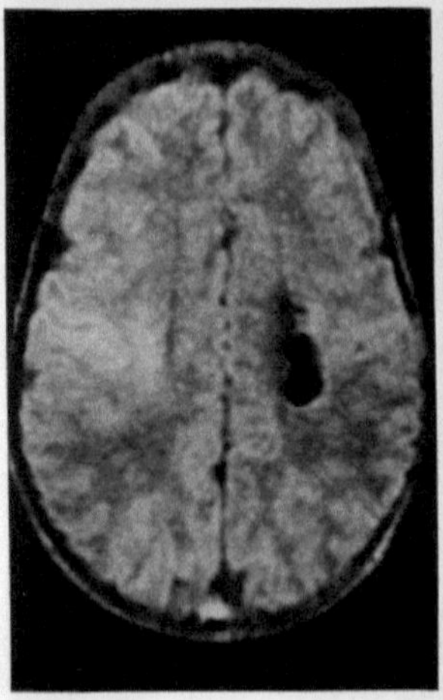
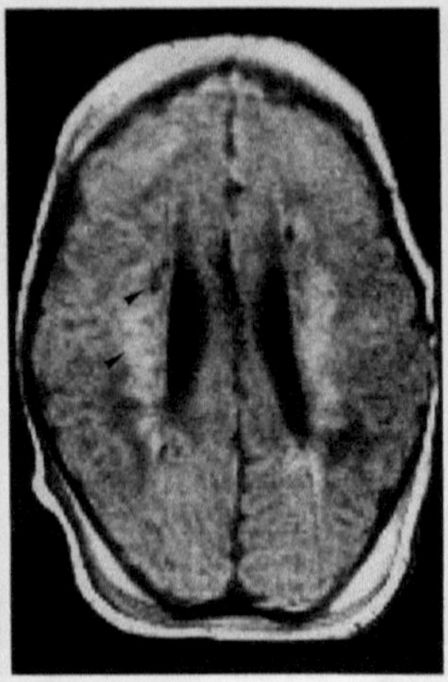

2.101, 103

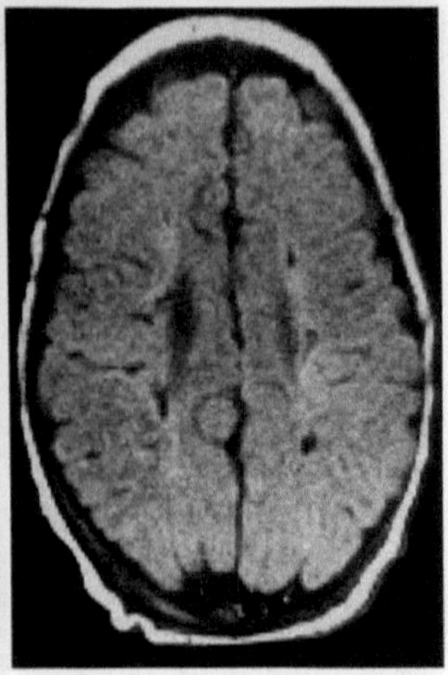

2.104

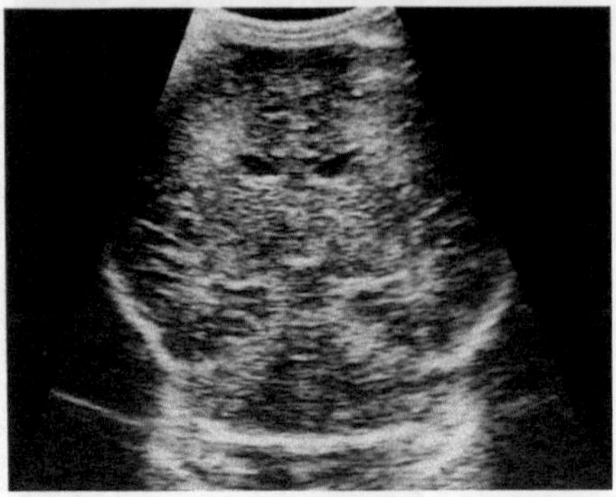

2.102

Fig. 2.98. Same as Fig. 2.97. Bilateral periventricular parietal cysts more significant at the right hemisphere (*arrow*)

Fig. 2.99. Same as Fig. 2.97, right SV. Multiple cysts of different diameters in the periventricular parietal area

Fig. 2.100. Same as Fig. 2.97, left SV. Small frontal cyst (*arrow*)

Fig. 2.101. MRI at day 7 GE, 450/12 ms/90°, AV; patient 14. Note cyst in the central portion of the left centrum semiovale probably due to antenatal leucomalacia

Fig. 2.102. US scan, day 12 after birth; patient 15. Note the bilateral periventricular hyperechogenicity

Fig. 2.103. SET1, 600/32 ms, AV, day 13 after birth; patient 15. Note the bilateral hypersignal found in the centrum semiovale (hemorrhage) associated with appearance of small cysts (*arrow*)

Fig. 2.104. SET1, 600/32 ms, AV, 2 months old; patient 15. Note small cyst within the centrum semiovale

2.105

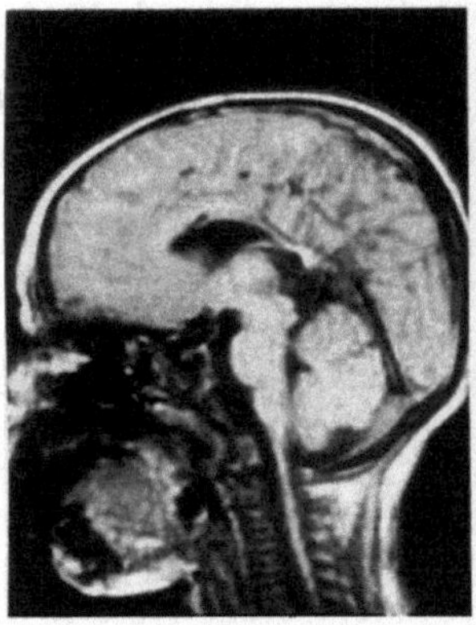

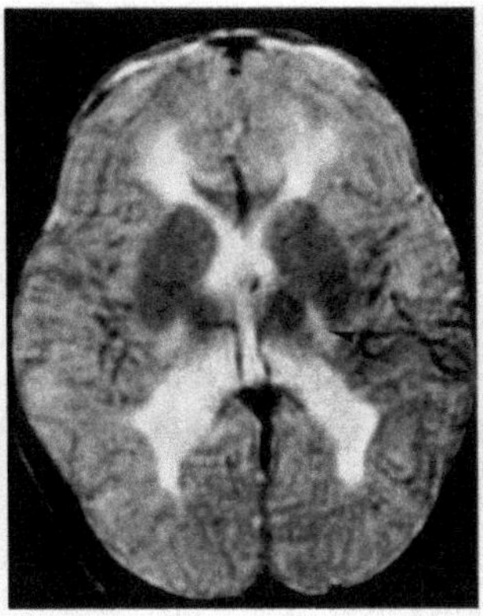

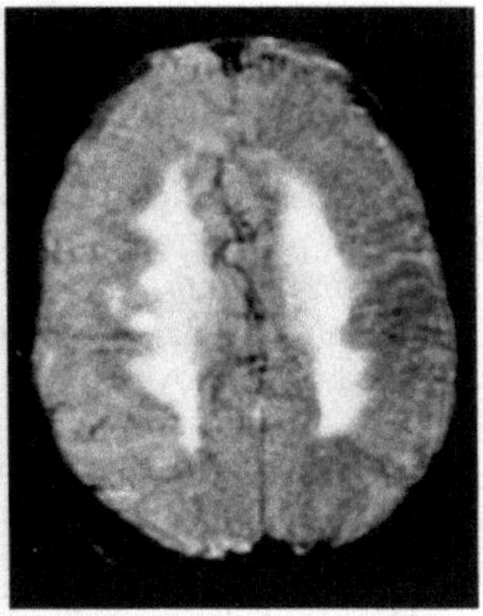

2.106, 107

Fig. 2.105. SET1, 600/32 ms, AV, 12 months old; patient 15. Note atrophy of corpus callosum

Fig. 2.106. SET2, 2000/120 ms, AV, 12 months old; patient 15. Note irregular ventricle walls; hypersignal in the posterior limb of the internal capsule and the lenticular nuclei (*arrow*)

Fig. 2.107. SET2, 2000/120 ms, AV; patient 15. Note the significant hypersignal in the centrum semiovale

in evaluating the effect of leucomalacia on anatomic changes and brain maturation. SET2 is the more reliable sequence to identify such changes. The findings from our patients are listed below:

1. The white to gray matter differentiation pattern was not affected by leucomalacia. This differentiation pattern is mainly due to the loss of brain water in early infancy and to the deposit of myelin in the white matter. The phenomenon seems to be independent of PVL and occurs within physiological ranges.
2. Dilated lateral ventricles with irregular ventricular walls and reduction of white matter were noted. This anatomic pattern is related to resorption of periventricular cysts within the ventricles (breakdown of ependymal separation) and loss of white matter by ischemic damage. However, in some patients, cysts do persist and are still obvious in early infancy without any reduction of white matter. Although these aspects were found with cystic leucomalacia, it seems that they are absent in noncavitated leucomalacia.
3. A high intensity SET2 signal, coming from the posterior limb of the internal capsule and within the lenticular nuclei, was noted in patients with severe cerebral leucomalacia. This is mainly related to loss of tissue and gliosis rather than to a delay in myelination. The location of these abnormalities correlates well with the distribution of cysts and clinical motor impairment. In fact, descending corticospinal fibers of the lower and upper limbs cross over the posterior limb of the internal capsule.
4. Damage to the centrum semiovale was also noted in early infancy and correlated with MRI data obtained in the neonatal period. Significant loss of white matter was seen in severe cerebral leucomalacia. The tissue was replaced by gliosis, which exhibits a high intensity signal on SET2. With mild or moderate cerebral leucomalacia, this SET2 hypersignal was most marked posteriorly in the centrum semiovale, which is crossed mainly by descending motor fibers of the lower limbs. This could explain why moderate leucomalacia is associated with diplegia, whereas severe leucomalacia induces quadriplegia.

5. An abnormal signal (low intensity SET2 signal) within the basal ganglia was caused by iron accumulation induced by abnormal transfer of iron from basal ganglia towards subcortical white matter (associative fibers). The abnormal transfer is due to the breakdown of axonal transport since axons are damaged by ischemia. This pattern was only seen in two patients with severe cerebral leucomalacia.
6. Damage to the corpus callosum is also a consequence of ischemia. Indeed, cerebral leucomalacia occurs near the corpus callosum and can disturb its development. A reduction in the thickness of the corpus callosum, either on its anterior, medial or posterior part, was noted. Damage to the corpus callosum also correlated with the severity of cerebral leucomalacia.

MRI data were also in general agreement with the neurodevelopmental outcome. The MRI features described above are characteristic of cerebral leucomalacia in early infancy. This allows "a posteriori" diagnosis of cerebral leucomalacia in an infant presenting with abnormal motor development despite a normal US scan in the neonatal period. Furthermore, MRI enables us to distinguish between disorders of myelination: primary disturbances (dysmyelinating diseases) or perinatal insults (demyelinating diseases). In the latter, abnormal white matter is located periventricularly, whereas in the former anomalies are widespread.

In conclusion, the effects of cerebral leucomalacia on brain maturation can be readily evaluated by MRI. Severe leucomalacia is associated with all of the features described above, whereas mild or moderate leucomalacia shows some abnormal cerebral maturation. MRI data correlates well with neuromotor examination results.

2.5.5 Group 3: Cerebral Focal Ischemia

Cerebral focal ischemia or focal infarction (CI) refers to necrosis within an area supplied by one of the major cerebral arteries: posterior (PCA), anterior (ACA), or middle cerebral artery (MCA). In the neonatal period, few if any symptoms occur. Generally, the diagnosis is suspected in early infancy based on unilateral motor impairment and confirmed by brain imaging. Such incidences of CI are often attributed to perinatal asphyxia without any proof. However, several types of CI occur antenatally. Brain imaging plays an important role in the diagnosis of CI in the neonatal period. Here, we will try to determine to what extent MRI may be helpful in diagnosing this pathology.

2.5.5.1 Patients and Results

Five infants were included (Figs. 2.108–2.122). Their perinatal data are summarized in Table 2.7. As shown, no evidence of perinatal asphyxia was noted. In two patients, focal seizures were the main symptoms that led us to perform brain imaging. In the remainder, CI was diagnosed by routine US scan. Brain imaging was performed during the periods listed in Table 2.7.

We could divide our patients into three subgroups:

- Group 1: CI of the MCA (patients 1 and 2)
- Group 2: CI of distal branches of the MCA (patients 3 and 5)
- Group 3: CI of the MCA, PCA and ACA (patient 4)

Images from patients 1, 2 and 4 are shown in order to illustrate the pathology of CI and to define the role of MRI in the neonatal period.

In patients 1 and 2, brain imaging was performed in the early neonatal period, shortly after the day of birth. Comparing images from these two patients is very beneficial since we were not able to dif-

Table 2.7. Group 3: Perinatal data, brain imaging and patient outcome

Pregnancy	GA	Apgar at 5 min	Events	US[a]	CT scan[a]	MRI[a]	Outcome
Hypertension	38	10	Seizures (focal)	D3	D4	D3	Hemiparesis, squint
IUGR	40	10	Normal	D3	D5	D3	Hemiparesis, squint
Normal	40	7	Normal	D27	D26	D24	Normal
IUGR	40	10	Hypotonia	D18		D18	Hemiparesis, squint
Normal	40	10	Seizures (focal)	D7	D7	D30	Normal

GA, gestational age; IUGR, Intrauterine growth retardation
[a] Day (D) after birth of US, CT scan and MRI exams

ferentiate between them based only on US and CT data (compare Figs. 2.110–2.117 and Figs. 2.111–2.116).

Both exhibited the same radiologic anomaly on US and CT, along with hemorrhagic omponent in the lesion of patient 2. On MRI, different signals were noted. In patient 1, the signal exhibited was related to the early phase of infarction (Fig. 2.108), whereas in patient 2 a cystic appearance was evident (Fig. 2.114). Moreover, the hemorrhagic component in the latter patient, as displayed by MRI, was comprised of a fresh and an old hemorrhage (Fig. 2.115). This led us to emphasize that in patient 1 CI occurred perinatally, whereas in patient 2 hemorrhagic CI occurred antenatally associated with a hemorrhage perinatally.

In patient 4, ischemia of the distal branches of the MCA was considered. A cystic appearance was obvious on MRI scan, whereas on US an altered echogenicity was noted (Figs. 2.118, 2.121).

Infant victims of CI of the distal branches of the MCA (patients 3, 5) had normal neurologic exams at 2 years of age. On MRI scans, CI was replaced by a porencephalic cavity without any effect on brain maturation (Fig. 2.122). In subgroups 2 and 3, contralateral motor impairment was noted. On MRI, porencephaly and atrophy were noted with a delay in myelination in the internal capsule and optic radiation (Figs. 2.112 and 2.113). These findings correlated well with neuromotor and visual impairments.

2.5.5.2 Discussion

The evolution of CI can be divided into two overlapping stages, the edematous stage, which lasts for 10 days, followed by the atrophic stage. Based on reports in the literature and on our own patients we have summarized CI brain imaging data (Tables 2.8 and 2.9). A CI signal is the most reliable sign allowing recognition of ischemia. Although US allowed diagnosis of CI, only MRI enabled us to differentiate the two stages. On GE or SET1, in the edematous stage, a homogeneous signal, less intense than that of white matter, is found. This is followed by a cystic appearance in the atrophic stage. Data from US and CT regarding CI signals were the same in the first and second stages. A cystic appearance on US scan is not obvious until 3–4 weeks after the insult. However, the distinction between the two stages can be based on US and CT findings when other radiological signs are analyzed. They are considered indirect signs and thus require particular attention.

We can conclude that MRI seems to be a sensitive method for detecting of CI either in the edematous or atrophic stage. Moreover, the evolving stage, from necrosis to liquefaction (cystic appearance),

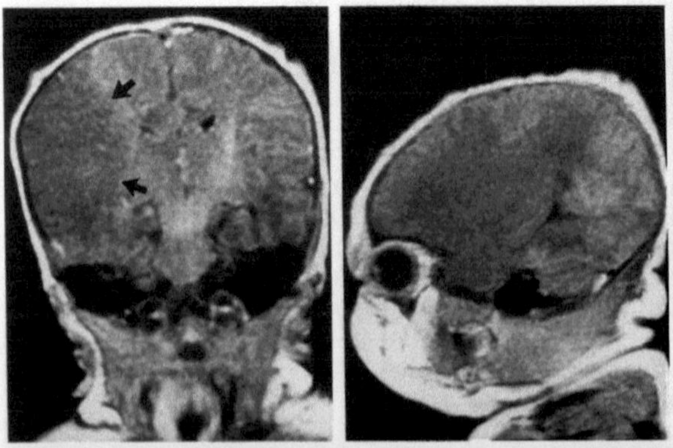

2.108, 109

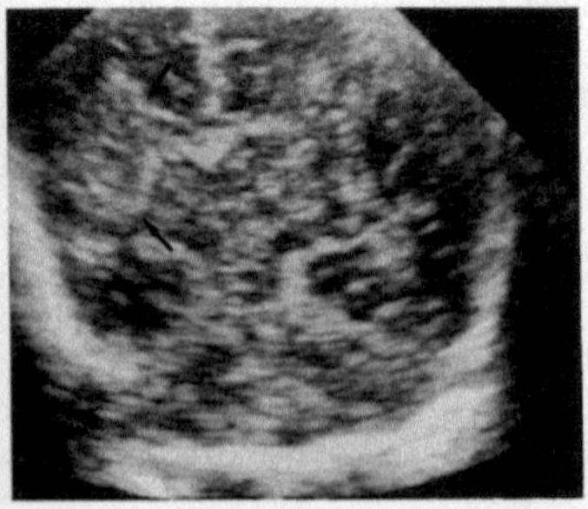

2.110

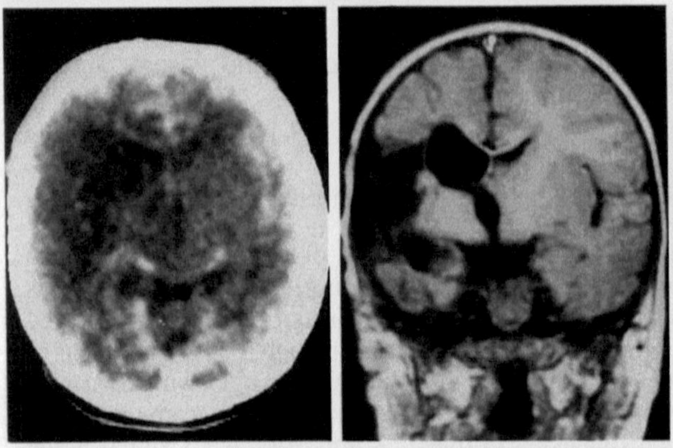

2.111, 112

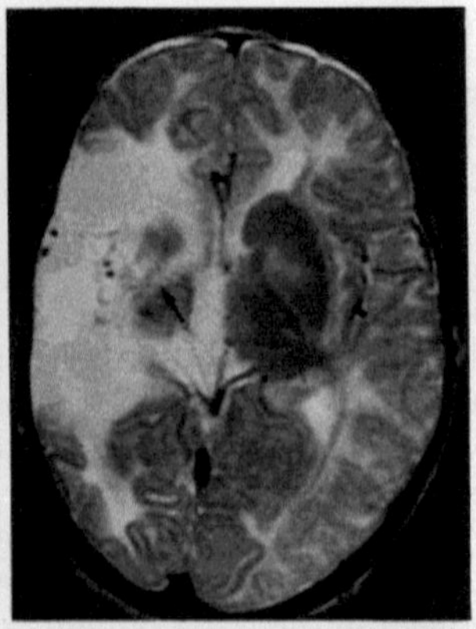

2.113

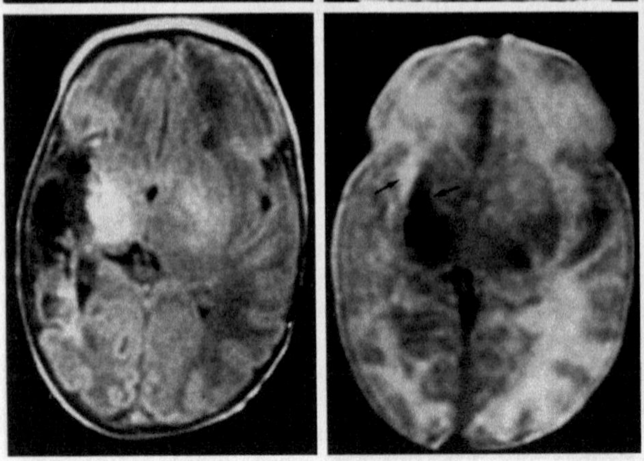

2.114, 115

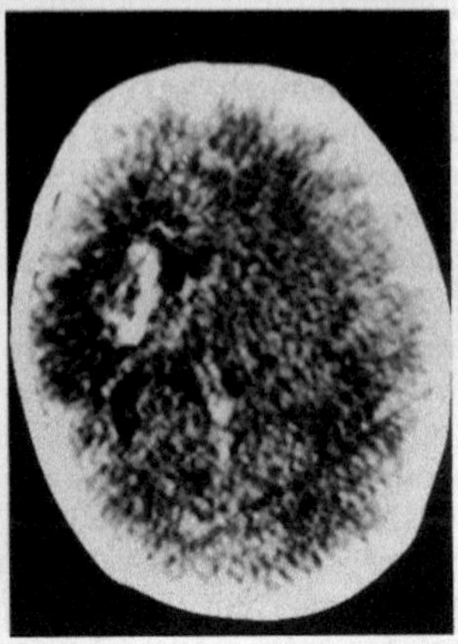

2.116

Fig. 2.108. Right MCA infarction, GE, 450/12/90°, day 3, FV; patient 1. Note the right triangular signal (*arrows*) different from the white matter and myelin signals and corresponding to the early phase of ischemia in the area of the MCA. Basal ganglia are spared

Fig. 2.109. Same as Fig. 2.108, right SV. Note the disparity in the gyral definition and the alteration of the white matter signal

Fig. 2.110. Right MCA infarction, US scan, 5 MHz, day 3; patient 1. Note right triangular wedge (*arrows*) representing an altered echogenicity of the cerebral parenchyma

Fig. 2.111. Right MCA infarction, CT scan, day 4; patient 1. Note right triangular hyposignal

Fig. 2.112. GE, 450/12/90 ms, FV, patient 1. Note right ventricular dilatation with atrophy, right MCA infarction (hyposignal). Basal ganglia are spared

Fig. 2.113. MRI at 7 months old right MCA infarction, SET2, 2000/120 ms, AV; patient 1. Note right triangular hypersignal with delayed myelination of the right internal capsule (*arrows*) and optic radiations (hypersignal)

Fig. 2.114. Right MCA infarction, GE, 500/12/90°, day 3 after birth, AV; patient 2. Note right cerebral infarction (hyposignal) of the area supplied by the MCA; basal ganglia are spared. Note the hypersignal corresponding to a hemorrhage adjacent to the CI

Fig. 2.115. Right MCA infarction, SET2, 2000/120 ms, day 3, AV at the same level as Fig. 2.108; patient 2. Adjacent to the right cerebral infarction note a hypersignal (old hemorrhage) beside a hyposignal (fresh hemorrhage) (*arrows*)

Fig. 2.116. Right MCA infarction, CT scan, day 5; patient 2. Note the hypodensity of CI associated with a hemorrhagic signal (hyperdensity) corresponding to a fresh hemorrhage

Table 2.8. Brain imaging in the oedematous phase of cerebral infarction

	US	CT	MRI
Infarction signal	Altered echogenicity	Hypodensity	Abnormal signal
Arterial pulsations	absent	–	–
Gyral disparity	±	–	+
Midline shift	+	+	+
Hemorrhage	–	+	+

+, good definition; –, bad definition

Table 2.9. Brain imaging in the atrophic stage

	US	CT	MRI
Infarction signal	Altered echogenicity, late cystic appearance	Hypodensity	Cystic appearance
Arterial pulsations	present	–	–
Ventricular dilatation	+	+	+
Hemorrhage	–	–	+

+, good definition; –, bad definition

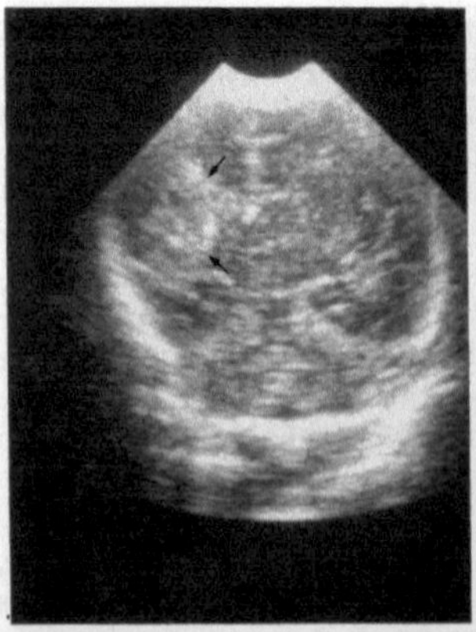

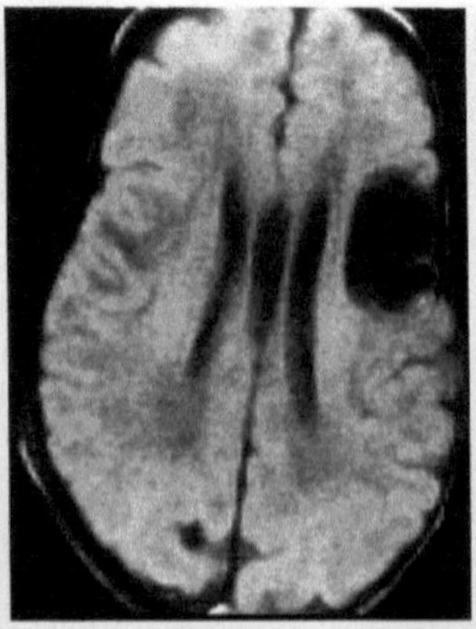

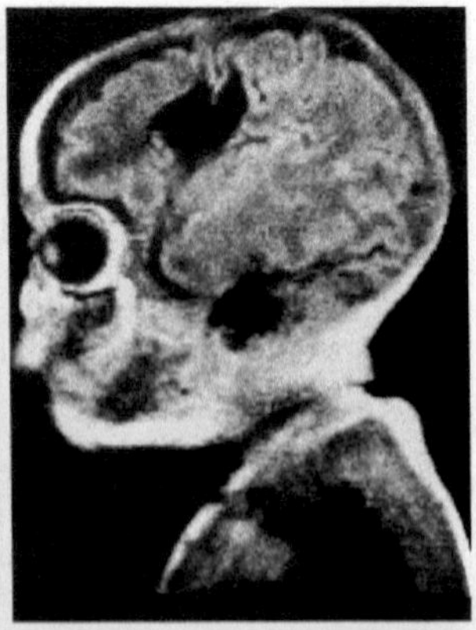

2.117, 118

2.119

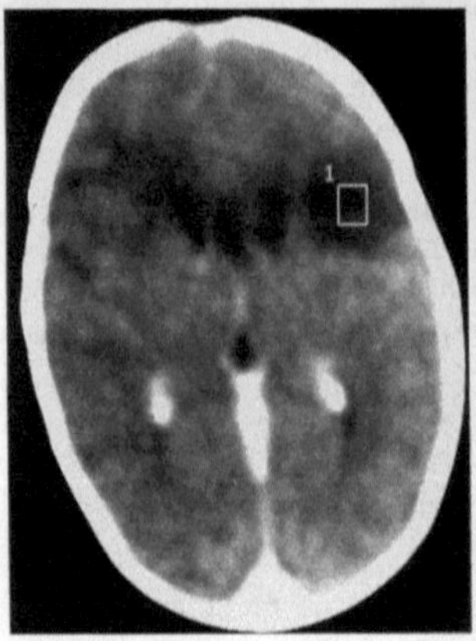

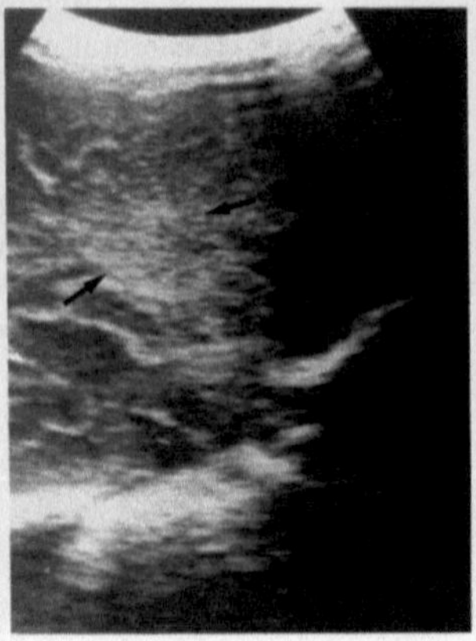

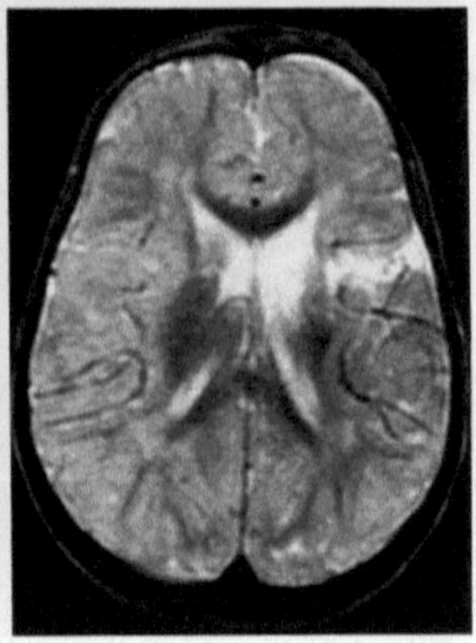

2.120, 121

2.122

Fig. 2.117. Right MCA infarction, US scan, day 3 after birth; patient 2. Note the right triangular altered echogenicity of the cerebral parenchyma

Fig. 2.118. Left MCA infarction (ischemia of distal branches) SET2, 200 ms/40 ms, day 25, AV; patient 4. Left cerebral ischemia (hyposignal) in the area supplied by the distal branches of the MCA

Fig. 2.119. Left MCA infarction (ischemia of distal branches), SET1, 450 ms/14 ms, left sagittal view; patient 4. Note the infarction (hyposignal) with cortical necrosis

Fig. 2.120. Left MCA infarction (ischemia of distal branches) CT scan, day 26, AV at the same level as Fig. 2.119; patient 4. Note hypodensity (*open square*) in the same location as Fig. 2.119

Fig. 2.121. Left MCA infarction (ischemia of distal branches), US scan, 5 MHz, day 27, left parasagittal view; patient 4. Note the hyperechogenicity of the infarction

Fig. 2.122. MRI at 20 months old, left MCA infarction, SET2, 2200/120 ms, AV at the level of the centrum semiovale and major and minor fornix; patient 4. Note the left hypersignal (necrosis with gliosis) at the same location as the focal ischemia in the neonatal period is better evaluated by MRI than by US and CT. Furthermore, as noted in patients 1 and 2, MRI allowed us to date the occurrence of CI by distinguishing the edematous from the atrophic stage. It can thus be expected that by performing brain imaging, especially MRI, early in the neonatal period, the occurrence of CI can be more precisely dated. The results will most likely show that, in most cases, CI occurs antenatally.

2.6 Intracranial Hemorrhage

Intracranial hemorrhage (ICH) is an important clinical problem in the neonatal period. Major factors implied in the pathogenesis of ICH are perinatal asphyxia, coagulation defect, trauma, vascular defect (aneurysm), arteriovenous malformation, etc. Several types of neonatal ICH are encountered (Table 2.10) and US and CT have proven to be useful in their diagnosis. In this section, we will try to determine to what extent MRI can be useful in identifying ICH in the neonatal period.

2.6.1 Patients and Results

From the neonates admitted to our unit, we have selected ten patients, evaluated by MRI, in order to illustrate this pathology (Tables 2.11, 2.12 and Figs. 2.123–2.153). Perinatal data are summarized in Table 2.9. The hemorrhagic signal was studied at different stages using SET1 and SET2:

1. *Acute Phase of Hemorrhage:* On SET1, hemorrhage exhibits an isosignal in the first 24–48 h, followed by the appearance of a high intensity signal. On SET2, acute hemorrhage is marked by the appearance of both an isosignal and a low intensity signal in the first 24–48 h (Fig. 2.115).

2. *Subacute Phase of Hemorrhage:* In this phase, the hemorrhage begins to exhibit a high intensity signal on both SET1 and SET2 (Fig. 2.142).

3. *Chronic Phase of Hemorrhage:* After 2 weeks, the hemorrhage exhibits a high intensity signal on both SET1 and SET2 which can last for several weeks even in the ventricular system (Figs. 2.125–2.127).

Development of Hematoma

The characteristic MRI patterns during the development of a hematoma are as follows: There is a central hypointensity on SET2 during the acute stage and an isosignal on SET1. The change to hyperintensity, initially on SET1 and then on

Table 2.10. Types of ICH in the neonatal period

	Frequency	Full-term	Prematures
Pericerebral hemorrhage			
Subarachnoidal	Common	±	+
Subdural	Uncommon	+	−
Intracerebral hemorrhage	Uncommon	+	−
Parenchymal involvement	Common	−	+
Thalamic hemorrhage	Uncommon	+	−
Periventricular-intra-ventricular hemorrhage	Common	−	+
Intracerebellar hemorrhage	Uncommon	±	+

+, specific; ±, less specific; −, not specific

Table 2.11. Perinatal data and developmental outcome of newborns suffering from intracranial hemorrhage

Patient	GA (weeks)	Type of hemorrhage	MRI	Neurodevelop-mental outcome
1	30	Right SEH + PE	37 WPCA	Hemiparesis
2	28	Right IVH + PE	40 WPCA	Normal
3	35	Right IVH + PE	37 WPCA	Hemiparesis
4	37	Left T, IVH + PE	40 WPCA	Spastic diplegia
5	40	Right T	41 WPCA	Normal
6	40	Left parietal hematoma + SD	41 WPCA	Normal
7	40	SD	43 WPCA	Unknown
8	29	Right IVH + PE	30 WPCA	
9	40	Right IVH + ventricular dilatation	D4	Hemiparesis
10	40	Right IVH + PE	41 WPCA	Mild hemiparesis

GA, gestational age; SEH, subependymal hemorrhage; T, thalamic hemorrhage; IVH, intraventricular hemorrhage; SD, subdural hemorrhage; PE, parenchymal involvement; WPCA, weeks postconceptional age; D, day

Table 2.12. Sensitivity of CT, US and MRI different stages of hemorrhage

	Acute	Subacute	Chronic
Pericerebral hemorrhage			
Subarachnoidal	CT > MRI > US	MRI ≥ CT > US	MRI > CT > US
Subdural	CT > MRI > US	MRI ≥ CT > US	MRI > CT > US
Parenchymal hemorrhage	CT ≥ MRI ≥ US	MRI ≥ CT > US	MRI > CT > US
Thalamic hemorrhage	CT = MRI ≥ US	MRI ≥ CT > US	MRI > US > CT
PV-IVH	US > CT > MRI	US > MRI > CT	MRI ≥ US > CT
Intracerebellar	CT > MRI > US	MRI ≥ CT > US	MRI > CT > US

SET2, extends from the hematoma periphery inward in the subacute phase (Figs. 2.144, 2.145). The rim of parenchymal hypointensity on SET2 abutting the hematoma is found during both the subacute and chronic stages.

Pericerebral hemorrhage is well displayed on MRI; however, differentiation between subdural and subarachnoidal hemorrhage remains a challenge since they are often interrelated in the newborn. Generally, subdural hemorrhages lead to compression of the cerebral parenchyma (Fig. 2.146). Subarachnoidal hemorrhages fill the convolutions and gyri and are often present in the sylvian fissure and the subarachnoidal space of the posterior fossa. It seems that SET1 is more sensitive than SET2 in detecting pericerebral hemorrhages, especially in differentiating subdural from subarachnoidal hemorrhages (compare Figs. 2.144 and 2.145).

2.6.2 Discussion

The appearance of hemorrhage on MRI is complex and mainly related to the breakdown of oxyhemoglobin to deoxyhemoglobin to methemoglobin. Fresh hemorrhage (acute phase), made up of essentially deoxyhemoglobin, is not detected by SET1; however, on SET2, it

2.123
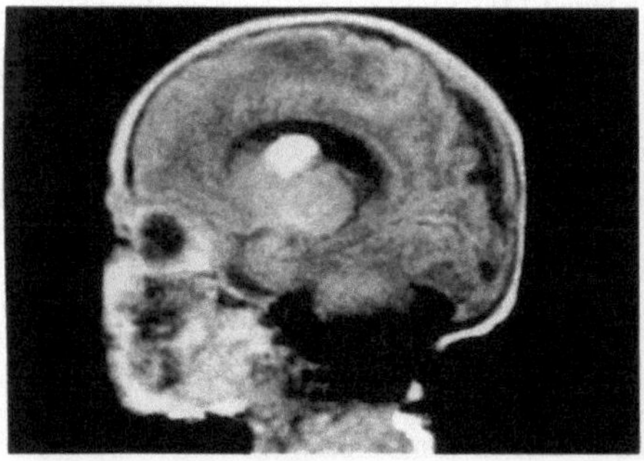
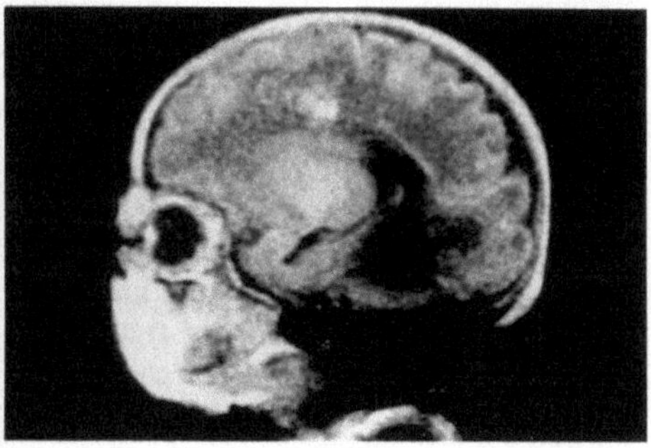
2.124

2.125
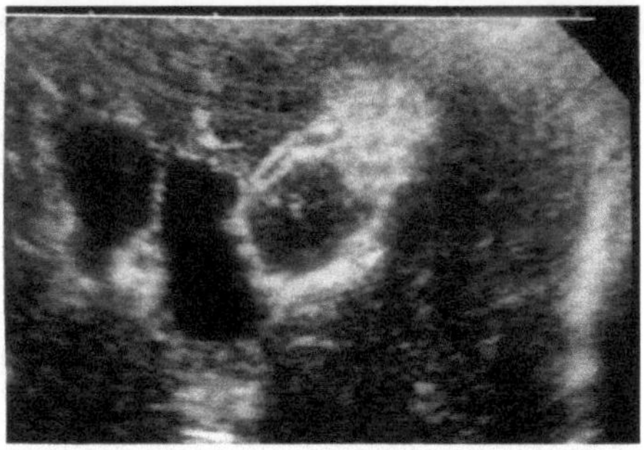

Fig. 2.123. GE, 450/12 ms/90°, medial SV; patient 1. Subependymal germinal matrix hemorrhage (hypersignal)

Fig. 2.124. Same as Fig. 2.123, right SV. Parenchymal involvement seems to be a venous infarction with hemorrhagic signal (hypersignal)

Fig. 2.125. US scan, day 10; patient 1. Subependymal hemorrhage with parenchymal involvement

exhibits a low intensity signal easy to detect since the high intensity signals of the unmyelinated cerebral parenchyma and the CSF provide an ideal background to the low intensity of fresh hemorrhage.

After the first few days (subacute phase), the hemorrhage is more easily identified by MRI. Visibility of the hemorrhage depends on the formation of methemoglobin, which begins 24–48 h after the hemorrhage occurs and increases during the first week. An intermediate to high intensity signal is seen on both SET1 and SET2. At this stage SET1 provides better recognition of the hemorrhage, since it exhibits a hyperintensity signal different from that of cerebral parenchyma. On SET2, confusion can result due to the signal exhibited by unmyelinated cerebral parenchyma or CSF.

The increased intensity of hemorrhage during the chronic phase, on SET1 and SET2, is most likely due to the continued presence of methemoglobin. At this stage, SET1 and SET2 are equally sensitive in detecting hemorrhage. With respect to the appearance of hematoma, the signal due to hemorrhage is also related to oxyhemoglobin, deoxyhemoglobin and methemoglobin as described above. The hypointense rim found in the subacute and chronic stages is due to hemosiderin.

Regarding pericerebral hemorrhage, it seems that the signals exhibited do not last as long as those of intracerebral or periventricular-intraventricular hemorrhages (PV-IVH) (Fig. 2.146).

PV-IVH are of particular importance in the premature baby. They occur early in the neonatal period and can lead to cerebral impairment. The current classification of PV-IVH is as follows: Grade 1: subependymal hemorrhage (germinal matrix hemorrhage) from which the blood enters the ventricles (Fig. 2.123); grade 2: IVH with blod covering 10%–50% of the ventricular area; grade 3: IVH with blood covering more than 50% of the ventricular area with ventricular dilatation.

US is highly effective in diagnosing grades 1, 2 or 3. Grades 1 and 2 are generally associated with a good outcome, whereas grade 3 is often associated with a poor outcome. However, the outcome with PV-IVH depends essentially on the absence or presence of complications which can alter the course of the lesion, e.g. hydrocephalus and parenchymal involvement (Figs. 2.129, 2.130). Regarding hydrocephalus, there is no doubt that early diagnosis leads to early treatment and to a better outcome. The most reliable technique to diagnose hydrocephalus is US, which identifies ventricular dilatation that occurs before the appearance of clinical signs. Parenchymal involvement refers to hemorrhagic infarction or hemorrhagic leucomalacia. Here again, US is highly effective in diagnosing such lesions. MRI adds useful information by more acurately depicting ischemia (Figs. 2.129, 2.130). However, MRI requires removal of sick premature babies from their neonatal care units. Thus, US seems the most reliable technique in diagnosing PV-IVH in prematures due to its safety and the possibility of performing serial exams. Moreover, decisions concerning continuous intensive care (prognosis) in patients with PV-IVH are mainly based on US; here, CT and MRI are neither beneficial nor desirable. In Table 2.12, we have compared the sensitivity of US, CT and MRI in the detection of hemorrhage. We can conclude that MRI is a useful tool in detecting hemorrhage in the subacute and chronic stages. It allows one to date the occurrence of the hemorrhage, as for patients 8, 9 and 10, in whom it occurred antenatally. Indeed, MRI applied early in the neonatal period enabled us to detect a hemorrhagic signal within the ventricles compatible with an old hemorrhage (Figs. 2.151, 2.152). Findings of parenchymal involvement in those patients also led us to conclude that IVH occurred antenatally.

Fig. 2.126. SET1, 600/32 ms, right SV; patient 2. Parietal porencephalic cyst communicating with extracerebral space associated with blood clot signal (hypersignal)

Fig. 2.127. Same as Fig. 2.126, AV. Note right intraventricular blood clot (hypersignal) with porencephalic parietal cyst

Fig. 2.128. Same as Fig. 2.126, FV. Parietal porencephalic cyst with blood clot (hypersignal)

Fig. 2.129. GE, 450/12 ms/90°, AV; patient 3. Right intraventricular blood (hypersignal) associated with right parenchymal frontoparietal involvement (ischemic and hemorrhagic). Hemorrhagic signal within the parenchymal involvement is comprised of two signals: a peripheral hypersignal surrounding a central hyposignal. Note the dilated ventricles

Fig. 2.130. SET2, 2000/120 ms; patient 3. Hemorrhage exhibits the same signal as on GE (Fig. 2.129). Parenchymal ischemia exhibits a hypersignal on the frontal and parietal lobes

Fig. 2.131. SET1, 500/28 ms, AV; patient 4. Note left intraventricular blood clot. Left parenchymal cerebral involvement seems to be ischemic only on the parietal lobe (hyposignal)

Fig. 2.132, Same as Fig. 2.131. Note left hemorrhagic thalamic signal with dilated left lateral ventricle; intraventricular blood clot exhibits a hypersignal

Fig. 2.133. SET2, 2200/120 ms, AV at the same level as Fig. 2.131; patient 4. Not left hemorrhagic thalamic signal (hypersignal) and intraventricular blood clot

Fig. 2.134. US scan, left parasagittal view; patient 4. Intraventricular blood clot with a hypoechoic center and hypoechoic thalami (*arrow*)

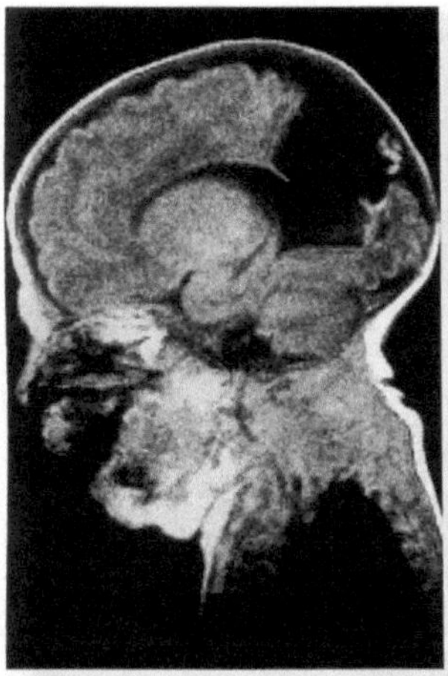

2.126

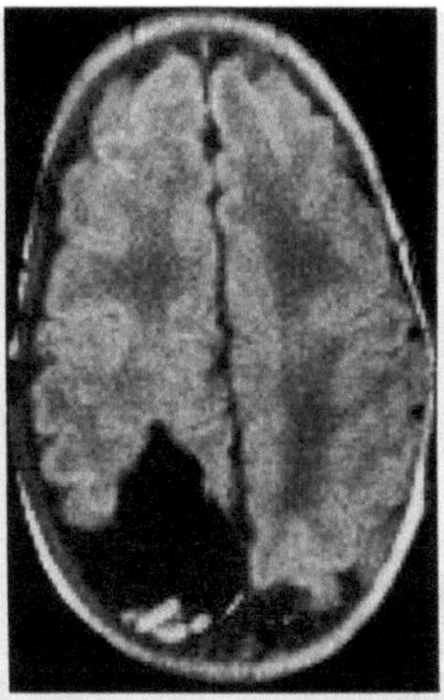

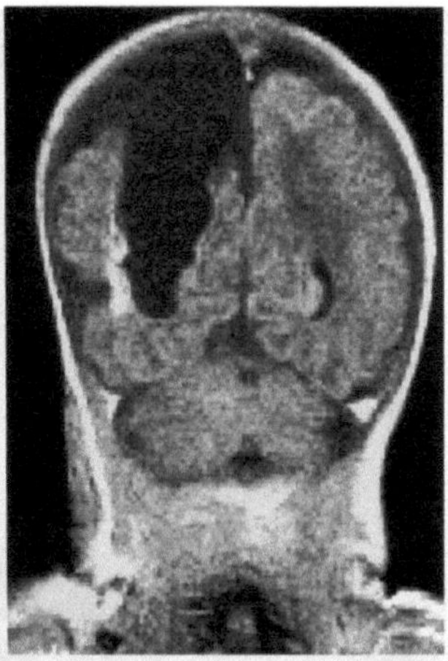

2.127, 128

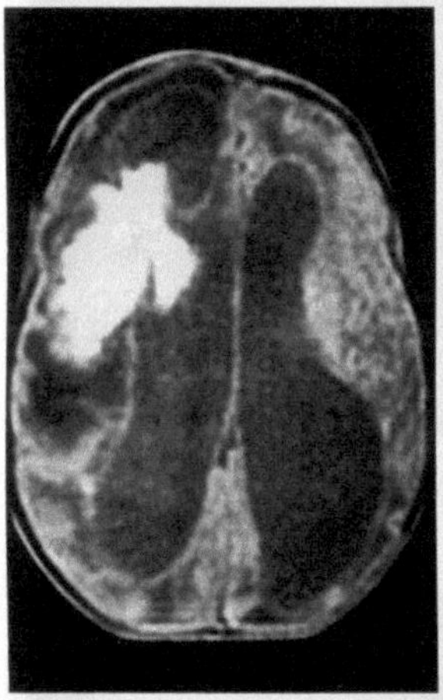

2.129

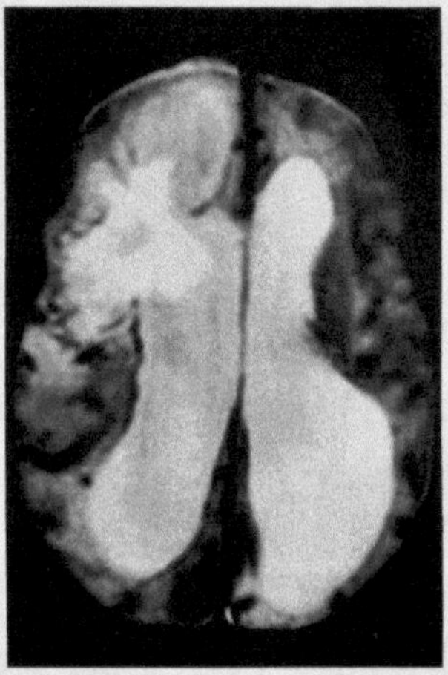

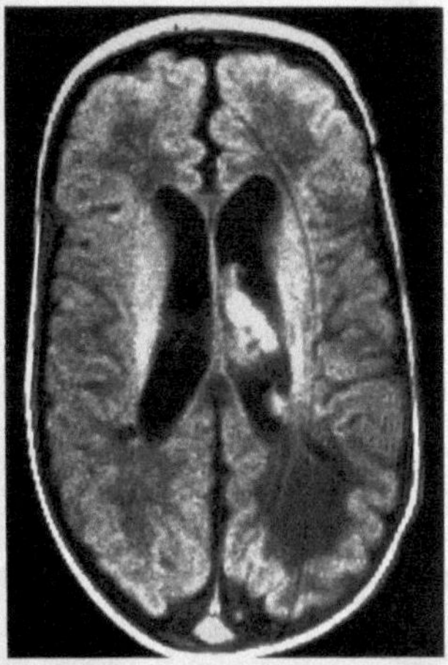

2.130, 131

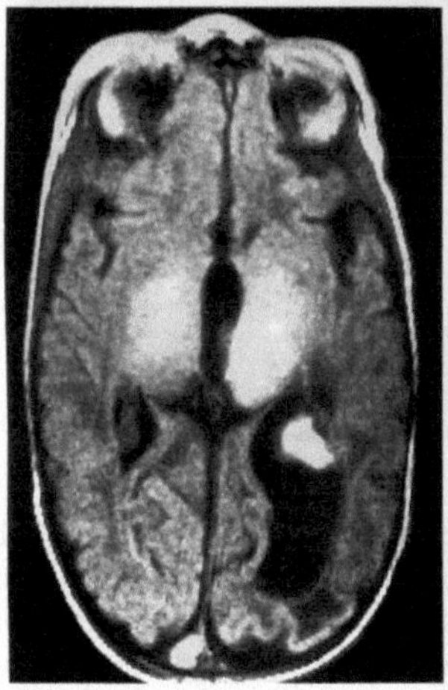

2.132

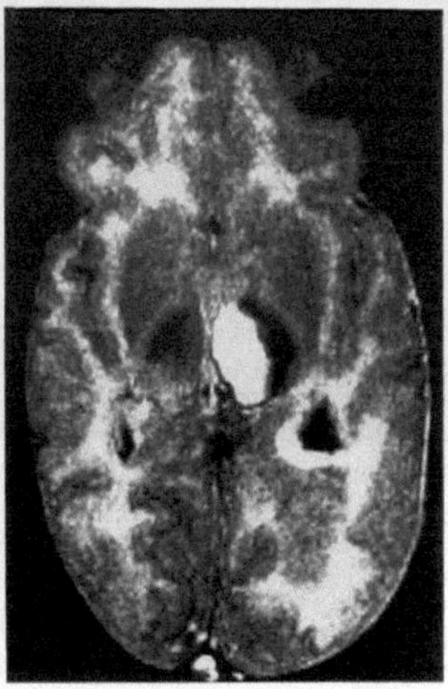

2.133

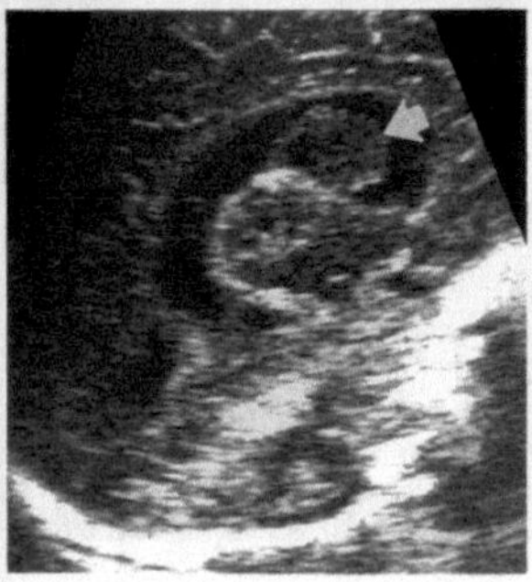

2.134

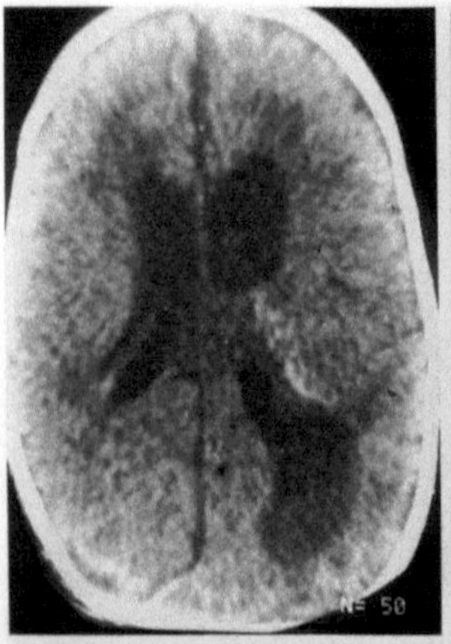
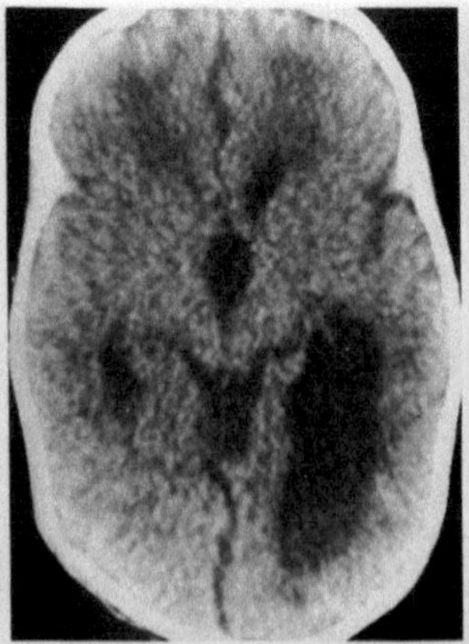

2.135, 136

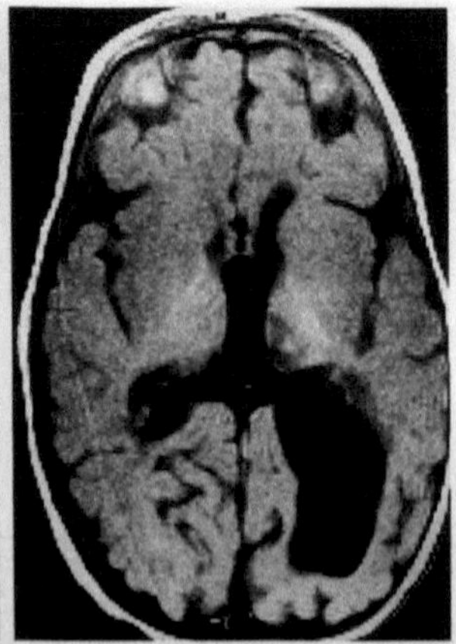

2.137

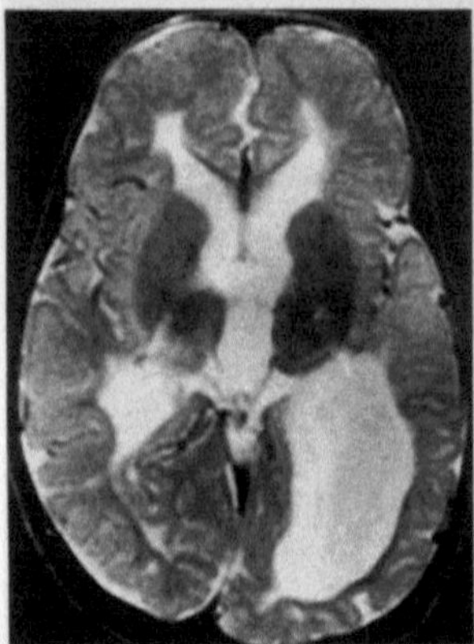
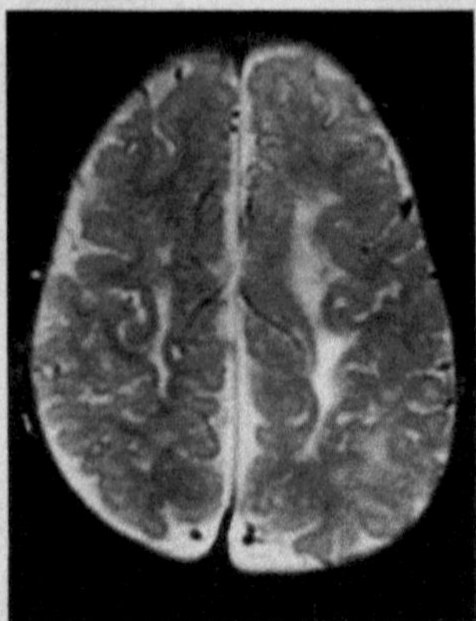

2.138, 139

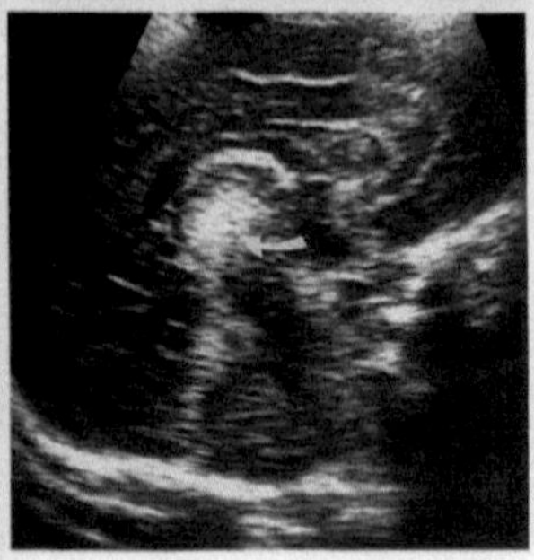

2.140

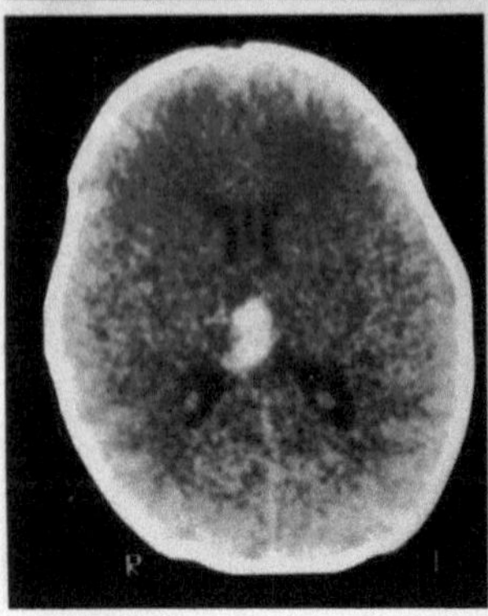
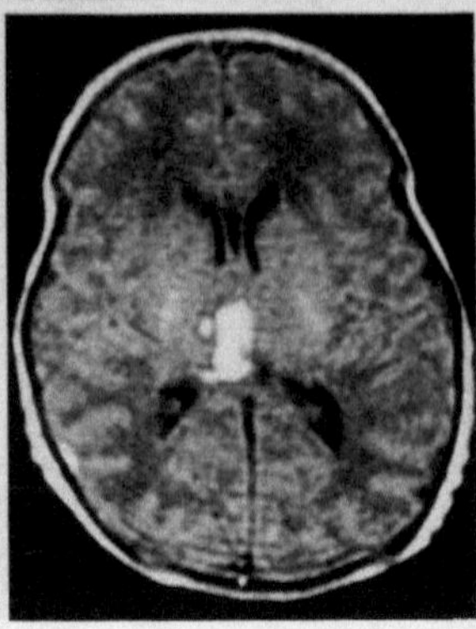

2.141, 142

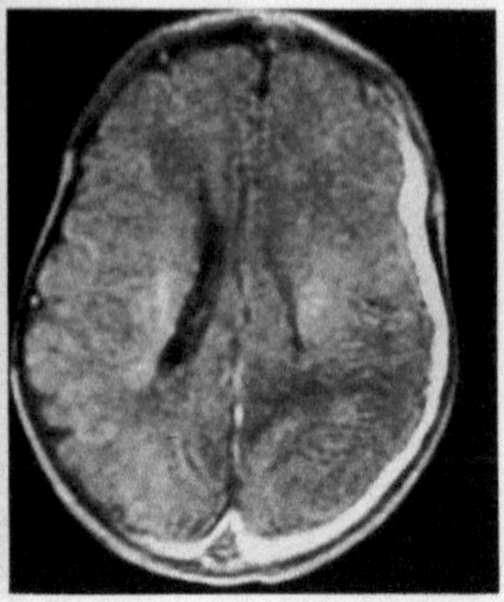

2.143

2.7 CNS Infections

2.7.1 Introduction

Neonatal CNS infections are induced by several agents: bacteria, viruses, protozoa and fungi. Of these bacterial organisms are the most common; however, all infectious agents are of major clinical importance since they are responsible for severe illness and mortality in the neonatal period. The clinical course of neonatal CNS infections, especially bacterial meningitis, is often complicated by the fol-

Fig. 2.135. CT scan, day 30, AV; patient 4. Note dilated left ventricle associated with a mild hyperdensity (old hemorrhage)

Fig. 2.136. CT scan, AV; patient 4. no abnormal signal on the left thalamus or in the left dilated ventricle

Fig. 2.137. MRI at 4 months old, SET1, 600/32 ms; patient 4. Note dilated left ventricle and hyposignal of the left thalami at the same location as the neonatal hemorrhage

Fig. 2.138. MRI at 18 months old, SET2, 2000/120 ms, AV; patient 4. Note dilated left ventricle with asymmetric cerebral hemisphere volume; delay in myelination in both internal capsules with abnormal signal in the posterior limb

Fig. 2.139. MRI at 18 months old, AV; patient 4. Note delay in myelination in both centrum semiovale associated with abnormal signal in the posterior portion on the left (demyelination?)

Fig. 2.140. US scan, day 3, SV; patient 5. Hyperechoic signal in the region of the thalamus (*arrow*)

Fig. 2.141. Cerebral CT scan, day 5, AV; patient 5. Hemorrhagic signal (hyperdensity) in the region of right basal thalamus

Fig. 2.142. MRI, day 12, GE, 450/12 ms/90°, AV; patient 5. Hemorrhagic signal (hypersignal) at the same location as in Fig. 2.140

Fig. 2.143. MRI, day 8, GE, 450/12 ms/90°, AV; patient 6. Subdural hemorrhage (hypersignal)

lowing events: (a) parenchymal involvement; (b) abscess; (c) ventriculitis with intraventricular purulent material and ventricular compartmentalization and (d) hydrocephalus.

Early diagnosis of CNS infections and complications is essential in order to allow rational patient management. Identification of the CNS complications mentioned above is mainly done by brain imaging. Several US and CT radiologic findings have been reported in the literature. In this section, we will discuss MRI data on CNS infections.

2.7.2 Patients and Results

Ten newborn term infants, who exhibited clinical signs of CNS infections, were studied. Agents recovered from their CSF fluid were: Streptococcus B ($n=4$); *Escherichia coli* ($n = 3$); Coxsackie B viruses ($n=3$). With respect to bacterial meningitis, hydrocephalus was noted in four patients (two with *Streptococcus* B, two with *E. coli*), ventriculitis was noted in two patients (one with *Streptococcus* B, one with *E. coli*); parenchymal involvement was observed in one patient with an *E. coli* infection.

Concerning viral infections, two patients exhibited viral meningitis and one meningoencephalitis; in the latter, white matter necrosis was noted. The results of brain imaging are shown in Figs. 2.154–2.158.

2.7.3 Discussion

As mentioned above, neonatal CNS infections are often associated with complications that lead to neuromotor impairment. Of the ten patients reported on here, seven exhibited CNS complications, six of them due to bacterial meningitis. The most frequent event encountered with bacterial meningitis was acute hydrocephalus. Ventriculitis, parenchymal involvement and abscess were less frequent; however, these events can be interrelated. In one patient with coxsackie B encephalitis, periventricular white matter damage was seen.

Acute hydrocephalus is related to an obstruction of CSF flow, either inside the ventricular system secondary to ventriculitis or outside the ventricular system

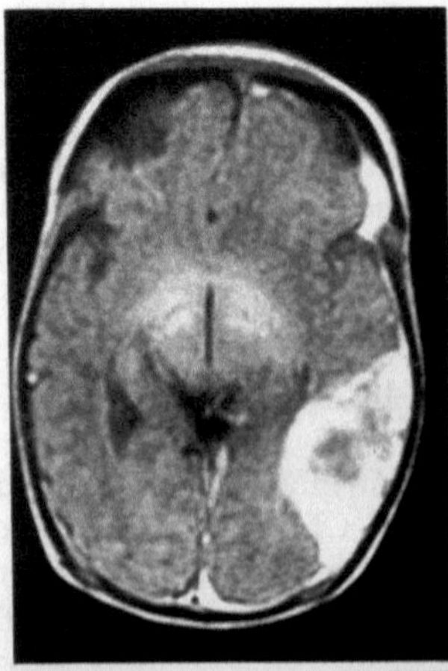

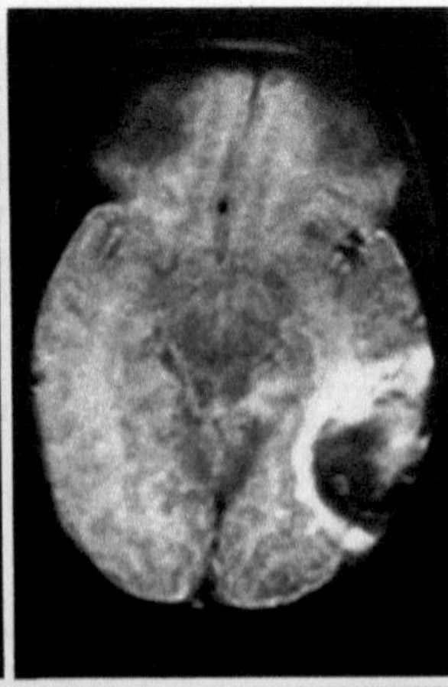

2.144, 145

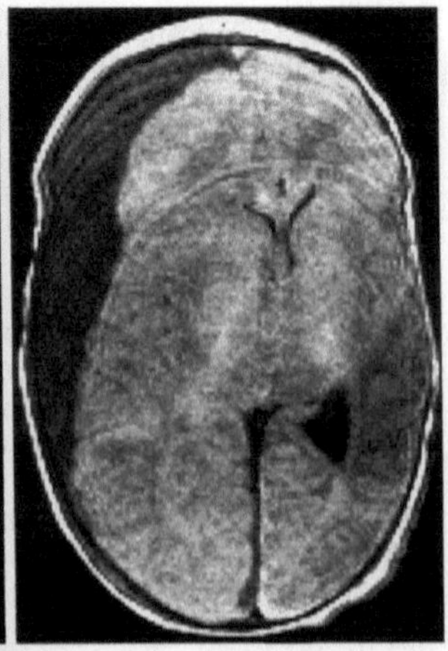

2.146

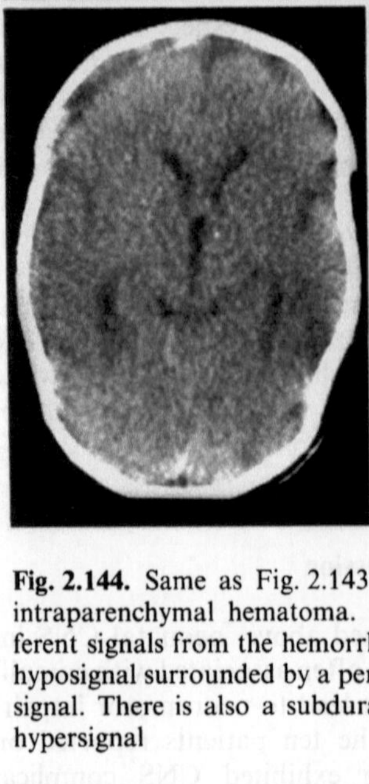

2.147

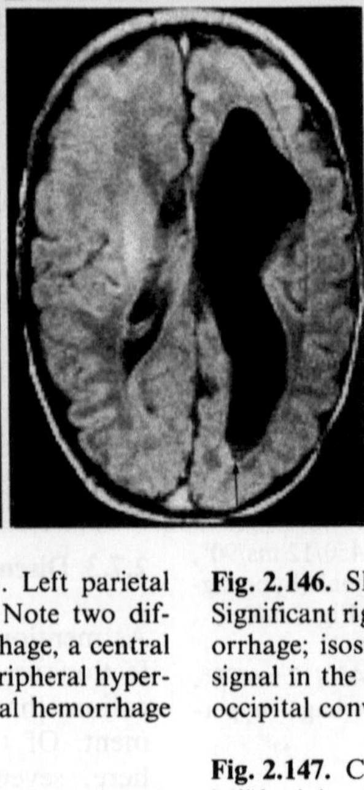

2.150

Fig. 2.144. Same as Fig. 2.143. Left parietal intraparenchymal hematoma. Note two different signals from the hemorrhage, a central hyposignal surrounded by a peripheral hypersignal. There is also a subdural hemorrhage hypersignal

Fig. 2.145. SET2, 2000/120 ms, AV; patient 6. Left parietal intraparenchymal hematoma. Two different signals are noted: a very large central hyposignal surrounded by a thin peripheral hypersignal. The extracerebral hemorrhage is difficult to identify

Fig. 2.146. SET1, 600/32 ms, AV; patient 7. Significant right subdural collection (old hemorrhage; isosignal) with a fresh hemorrhagic signal in the subarachnoidal space at the left occipital convexity

Fig. 2.147. CT scan, day 15, AV; patient 7. Mild right frontal extracerebral collection (isodense)

Fig. 2.150. SET1, 600/32 ms, left SV; patient 9. Note the dilated ventricle associated with a mild hemorrhagic signal (intraventricular blood clot). Note also the reduction of white matter on the frontoparietal region

2.148 2.149

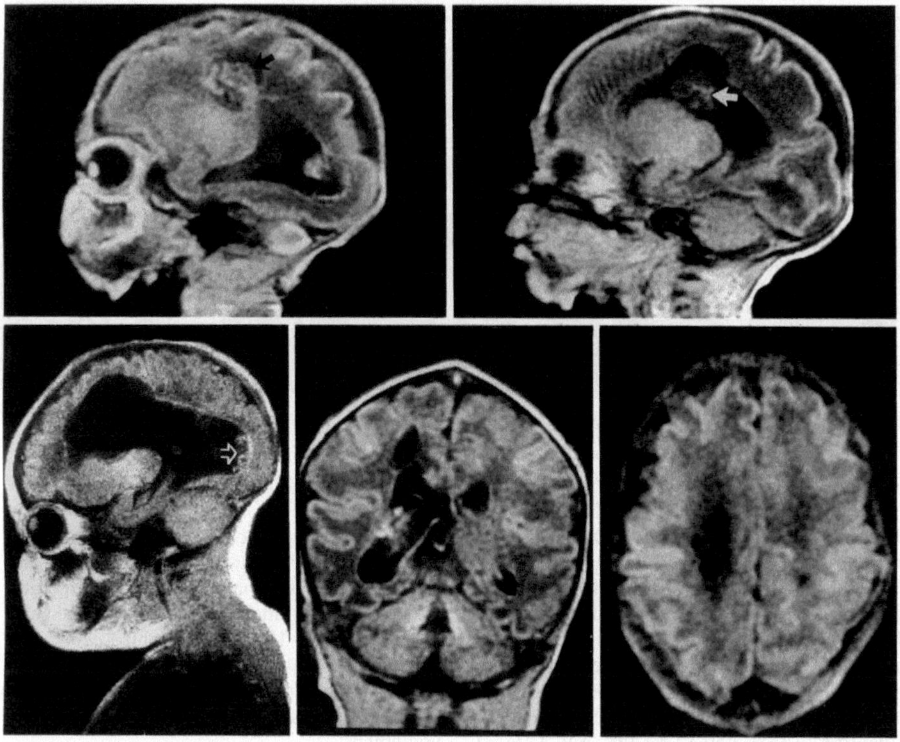

2.151 2.152, 153

Fig. 2.148. GE, 450/12 ms/90°, right SV; patient 8. Right parenchymal cerebral involvement with a hemorrhagic signal surrounded by a peripheral hyposignal (*arrow*), associated with intraventricular blood clot obvious in Fig. 2.149

Fig. 2.149. Same as Fig. 2.148. Intraventricular blood clot associated with a porencephalic parietal cavity (*arrow*)

Fig. 2.151. SET1, 600/32 ms, AV; patient 9. Note dilated left ventricle in the frontoparietal region and intraventricular blood clot

Fig. 2.152. GE, 450/12 ms/90°, FV; patient 10. Right intraventricular blood clot (hypersignal) associated with parietal periventricular cavity

Fig. 2.153. GE, 450/12 ms/90°, AV; patient 10. Multiple cysts in the right centrum semiovale in the central portion

2.154
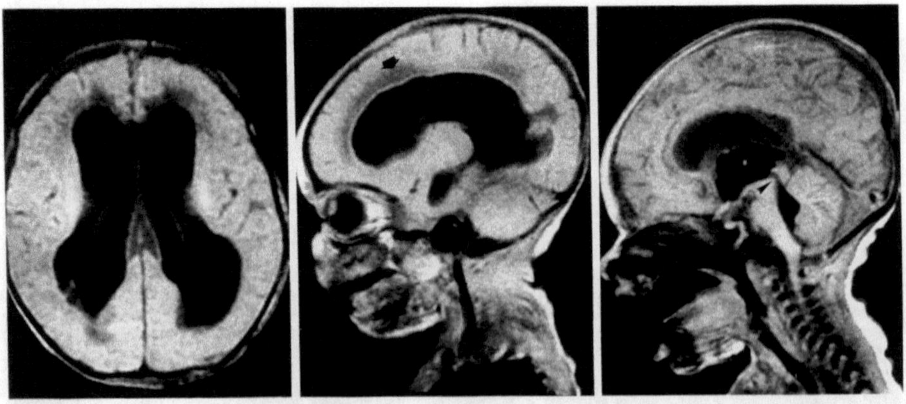

a b c

Fig. 2.154 a–c. Patient 1; *E. coli* meningitis, full-term baby, imaged at day 20; outcome: died. **a** GE, 450/12 ms/90°, AV. Dilated lateral ventricles; periventricular hyposignal (edema). Note purulent material and ventricle compartmentalization; **b** GE, 450/12 ms/90°, SV. Thickened ventricular wall with increased signal (ventriculitis); dilated ventricles; periventricular hyposignal (edema) (*arrows*). Note purulent material and ventricle compartmentalization. **c** GE, 450/12 ms/90°, SV. Dilated third ventricle; aqueduct of Sylvius filled with purulent material (*arrows*); fourth ventricle moderately dilated

Fig. 2.155. Patient 2; *Streptococcus* B meningitis, MRI at day 14; outcome: at 1 year normal
GE, 510/12 ms/90°, AV. Note dilated ventricles (*white arrow*) and purulent material (*black arrow*)

Fig. 2.156 a–d. Patient 3; *E. coli* infection full-term baby, MRI at day 30; outcome: severe developmental delay. **a** SET1, 400/26 ms, SV. Multiple left frontal abscesses (*arrow*). **b** SET1, 400 ms/26 ms, SV. Note left multiple frontal abscesses with pericerebral subdural collection (hemorrhage). **c** SET2, 1800/40 ms, first echo, AV. Note left pericerebral subdural collection (hemorrhage); right posterior parenchymal necrosis (hyposignal); left frontal parenchymal involvement (abscess). **d** SET2, 1800/120 ms, third echo, AV. Left pericerebral collection with right occipital (*arrow*) and left frontal (*arrow*) involvement (abscess) and right occipital (*small arrows*) involvement

Fig. 2.157. Patient 4; Premature baby of 28 weeks gestational age MRI at 41 weeks, outcome: normal
450/12 ms/90°, SV. Dilated lateral ventricles with thickened walls; periventricular edema (hyposignal)

Fig. 2.158 a, b. Patient 6. Coxsackie B virus intracranial infection, outcome: mild left hemiparesis. **a** SET1, 500/28, AV, 1 month old. Right periventricular white matter necrosis (hyposignal). **b** SET2, 2000/120 ms. AV, 7 months old. Dilated right lateral ventricle; delayed myelination of right internal capsule (*upper and lower arrows*)

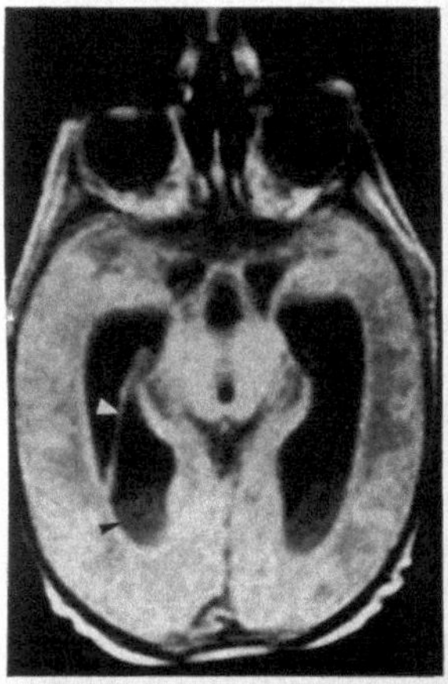

155

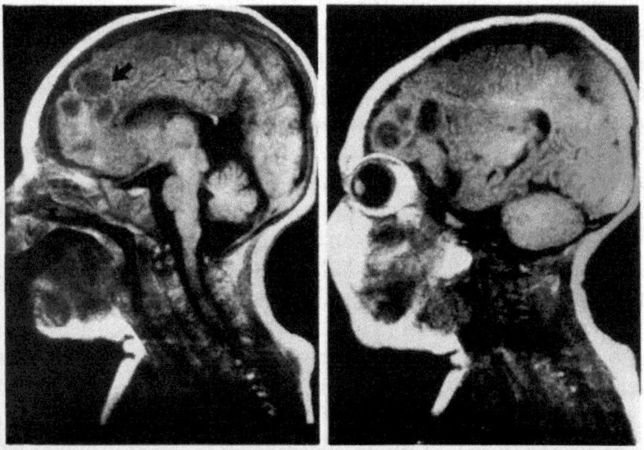

2.156 a, b

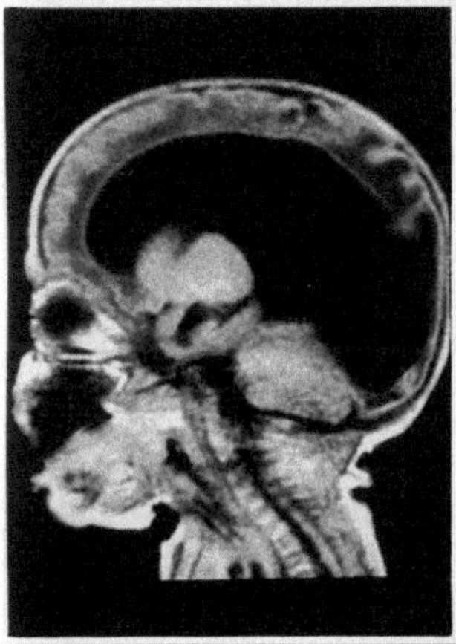

157

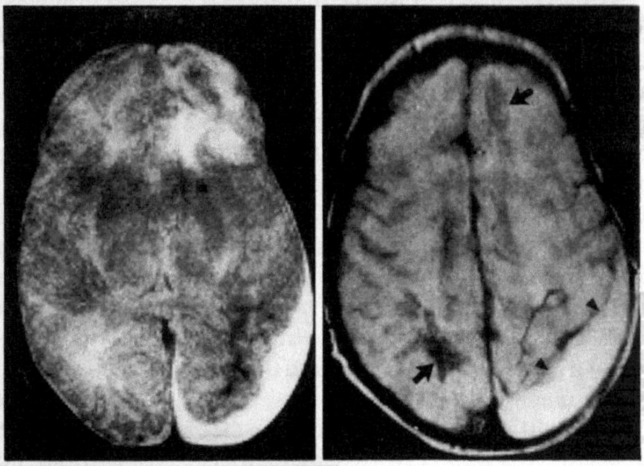

2.156 c, d

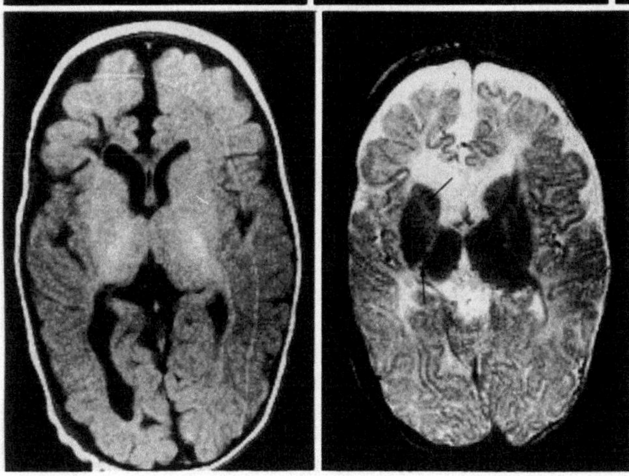

58 a

b

secondary to arachnoiditis. It is well known that hydrocephalus occurs before the advent of clinical signs. Thus, the most reliable diagnostic technique is US, assessing ventricular size in serial studies. MRI provides information on the location of the obstruction, since, in SV, the foramen of Monro, the aqueduct of Sylvius and the third and fourth ventricles are displayed. Periventricular edema is a consequence of hydrocephalus and is easily visualized by MRI (Fig. 2.154a). It exhibits a low intensity signal around the lateral ventricles on GE (patients 1 and 4). Periventricular edema is difficult to assess by US or CT in the neonatal period. Thus, its recognition constitutes useful information in order to achieve rational patient management.

In patient 1, in whom hydrocephalus was associated with ventriculitis and intraventricular septa, we were able to locate the obstruction of CSF flow at two levels. The aqueduct of Sylvius was filled with purulent material inducing dilatation of the lateral and third ventricles (Fig. 2.154c). However, arachnoiditis was also considered since the fourth ventricle was moderately dilated.

Ventriculitis most often follows bacterial meningitis and is caused by exuberant inflammation of the ependymal line. It is also associated with hydrocephalus caused mainly by obstruction of the aqueduct of Sylvius. MRI findings included ventricular dilatation with irregular and thickened margins (Fig. 2.154b; high intensity signal on GE). Periventricular edema was obvious and exhibited a low intensity signal on GE. The significance of periventricular edema with ventriculitis is difficult to interpret. Whether this signal is related to acute hydrocephalus or periventricular involvement by the bacterial agent remains to be determined. Perhaps by using MRI enhancement, this issue will be clarified. Intraventricular septa formation, which resulted in intraventricular compartmentalization, were also seen on MRI. The purulent material in the ventricles exhibited a different signal intensity than that of CSF on GE (Fig. 2.155). This different signal allowed us to locate the purulent material in the aqueduct of Sylvius in patient 1 (Fig. 2.154c).

Parenchymal involvement with bacterial meningitis includes formation of an intra- or extracerebral collection, necrosis or infarction, with or without a hemorrhagic component, and subdural effusion.

In patient 3, we noted multiple parenchymal abscesses which exhibited a different signal on GE or SET2 than either white matter or CSF. A pericerebral collection was well visualized and was located at the subdural space. The signal exhibited by this collection led us to conclude that it was due to hemorrhage. In fact, on SET1, it exhibited a high intensity signal compatible with that of a hemorrhage.

Viral CNS infection can lead to serious neurologic consequences. Several viruses may be recovered: Cytomegalovirus, Herpesviridae, Rubella viruses and Enteroviruses (Coxsackie A, B and Echovirus).

In the patients studied here, three intracranial infections were related to coxsackie B viruses. Two exhibited meningitis without any CNS damage. The remainder showed signs of meningoencephalitis associated with periventricular white matter necrosis obvious on MRI (Fig. 2.157a). MRI performed at 7 months of age (Fig. 2.157b) showed dilated ventricles and a delay in myelination of the internal capsule and correlated with the neuromotor exam. MRI allowed recognition of the CNS necrosis and the effect on brain maturation.

Based on data from the literature and our own experience, we can conclude that, due its safety and capacity for serial studies, US is still the most reliable technique to define the complications of CNS infections in the neonatal period. However, MRI can add useful information on hydrocephalus, ventriculitis and parenchymal involvement thereby leading to adequate therapeutics.

2.8 Conclusions and Perspectives

MRI has proven to be useful in the evaluation of brain disorders in neonates. However, recommendation of a MRI exam in the neonatal period should be carefully considered. The limits of the method are numerous:

- MRI is not a bedside exam; thus, it requires removing neonates from their neonatal care units. In critically ill infants, it may be deleterious.
- MRI requires perfect immobility of the infant to gain better images. Thus, sedation is often needed. Surveillance of vital parameters is essential when a sedative protocol is used. The proper equipment may be difficult to assemble and must be well isolated from the ferromagnetic component of the MR imager.
- The duration of the exam, the noise induced by the intermediate or high field magnet and the relatively high cost of the exam must be taken into consideration.
- There is still a lack of MRI facilities in many hospitals.
- Cerebral calcifications are misdiagnosed by MRI.
- Interpreting images requires thorough knowledge of cerebral disorders in the neonate, including neuropathology, pathogenesis and clinical and laboratory features.

Nonetheless, the advantages of this technique are significant. First, MRI constitutes a noninvasive technique and provides images in several planes: axial, coronal and sagittal. Second, MRI explores all regions of the CNS without difficulty. Third, MRI signals are specific and contribute to a better definition of cerebral disorders. Finally, MRI seems to be helpful when other brain imaging data are of limited value.

The future is promising: rapid acquisition of images, tridimensional reconstruction, MRI angiography, diffusion-perfusion techniques, CSF dynamics, use of enhanced contrast, etc. Although these new methods are now being applied in the adult, their application in neonates is under investigation.

We hope that we have given an overview of MRI in the exploration of the neonatal CNS, that the horizons of the reader have been widened and that the technique has been made easier to perform in the neonate. While US is still the first brain imaging exam to perform in a neonate in order to diagnose cerebral injury, MRI constitutes a very useful and complementary technique.

Acknowledgements. The authors thank Henri Gallin for providing the photo proofs and Patricia Stephan and Simone Mathern for the secretariat help. The authors also thank Nestle-France and especially Mr. Pierre Jozeau and Mr. Georges Corron for financial support.

List of Abbreviations

W.G.A.	Weeks Gestational Age
W.P.C.A.	Weeks Post Conceptional Age
MRI	Magnetic Resonance Imaging
SET1	Spin Echo T1 weighted Images
SET2	Spin Echo T2 weighted Images
GE	Gradient Echo
CT	Computed Tomography
US	Ultrasound examination
AV	Axial view
SV	Sagittal view
FV	Frontal view
CSF	Cerebrospinal fluid
CNS	Central nervous system
PET	Positron Emission Tomography
CBF	Cerebral blood flow
N.O.	Neurodevelopmental outcome
D.Q.	Developmental quotient drawn from Brunet-Lezine Test
M.C.A.	Middle cerebral artery
PCA	Posterior cerebral artery
ACA	Anterior cerebral artery
CI	Cerebral infarction
ICH	Intracranial hemorrhage
PV – IVH	Periventricular – intraventricular hemorrhage
D	Day after birth of Brain Imaging Exam.

References

Baker L, Stevenson DK, Enzmann D (1988) End stage periventricular leucomalacia: MR evaluation. Radiology 168:809–815

Barkovich JA, Norman D (1988) Anomalies of the corpus callosum: correlation with further anomalies in the brain. AJR 151:171–179

Barkovich JA, Chuang SH, Norman D (1988) MR of neuronal migration anomalies. AJR 150:179–187

Barkovich JA, Kjos BO, Norman D, Edwards M (1989) Revised classification of posterior fossa cysts and cysts like. Malformations based on the results of multiplanar MR imaging. AJR 153:1289–1300

Carson SC, Hertzberg BS, Bowie JD, Burger P (1990) Value of sonography in the diagnosis of intracranial hemorrhage and periventricular leucomalacia. AJR 155:595–601

Dietrich R, Bradley WG (1988) Iron accumulation in the basal ganglia following severe ischemic anoxic insults in children. Radiology 168:203–206

Elster A (1990) Cranial imaging with Gd-DTPA in neonates and young infants: preliminary experience. Radiology 176:225–230

Flodmark O, Lupton B, Li D, Stimag G, Roland E, Hill A, Whitfield M, Norman M (1989) MR imaging of periventricular leucomalacia in childhood. AJR 152:583–590

Haddad J, Christmann D, Roy E, Messer J, Willard D (1990a) Cerebral magnetic resonance imaging in the neonate. Pediatrie 45:665–675

Haddad J, Messer J, Gut JP, Chaigne D, Christmann D, Willard D (1990b) Neonatal echovirus encephalitis with white matter necrosis. Neuropediatrics 21:215–217

Hernantz-Schulmann M, Cohen W, Geneiser NB (1988) Sonography of cerebral infarction in infancy. AJNR 9:131–136

Levene MI (1990) Cerebral ultrasound and neurological impairment: telling the future. Arch Dis Child 65:469–471

McArdle C, Richardson JC, Hagden KC, Nicholas D, Crofford M, Amparo EG (1987a) Abnormalities of the neonatal brain, part I: intracranial hemorrhage. Radiology 163:387–394

McArdle C, Richardson JC, Nicholas D, Mirfakhree M, Hayden KC, Amparo EG (1987b) Developmental features of the neonatal brain: MR imaging, part II: ventricular size and extracerebral space. Radiology 162:230–234

Seidenwurm D, Meng TK, Kowalski A, Weinreb JC, Kricheff I (1989) Intracranial hemorrhage lesions: evaluation with spin echo and gradient refocused. MR imaging at 0.5 and 1.5 T. Radiology 172:189–194

Sipponen JT, Seponnen RE, Sivula A (1983) Nuclear magnetic resonance imaging of intracerebral hemorrhage in the acute and resolving phases. J Comput Assist Tomogr 7:954–959

Volpe J (1987) Neurology of the newborn. Saunders, Philadelphia

Wilson DA, Steiner RE (1986) Periventricular leucomalacia: evaluation with MRI. Radiology 160:507–511

Yakovlev PI, Lecours AR (1967) The myelogenetic cycles of regional maturation of the brain. In: Minkowski A (ed) Regional development of the brain in early life. F.A. Dans, Paris, pp 3–70

Zimmermann RD, Heier LA, Snow BR, Liu DPL, Kelly AB, Deck MD (1988) Acute intracranial hemorrhage. Intensity changes on sequential MR scans at 0.5 T. AJR 150:651–661

3 Ultrasound

C. L. Fawer and A. Calame

CONTENTS

3.1 Introduction

Before the advent of brain imaging, the approach to detecting lesions in the CNS in the neonatal period was restricted either to indirect methods or to the post-mortem examination because of the lack of appropriate techniques. Over the last decade, technological developments and modifications both in resuscitation criteria for managing patients and in defining the viability and limits of survival of clinically ill infants implied a need for brain imaging. Computerized tomography (CT), in 1977, and cerebral ultrasonography, in 1979, made it possible for the first time to accurately detect cerebral lesions. Since then, real time ultrasonography has been used in many neonatal units as a research tool and it has now become an invaluable routine investigative procedure. The widespread use of ultrasound (US) is due to its portability, safety, ease of use and good correlation with neuropathology. For most neonatologists, concerned about patient assessment and the outcome of neonatal intensive care, direct access to the neonatal brain represented a major advance not only in investigating brain structures, but also in offering a rapid improvement in the understanding of cerebral injury.

The validity of US for the diagnosis of germinal layer and intraventricular haemorrhages was rapidly recognized by most medical centres. However, its use for the identification of ischaemic lesions and more particularly, white matter injury has been much more controversial. Haemorrhage, necrosis, venous infarction, congestion, gliosis and microcalcifications may all appear as increased echogenicities in the periventricular white matter, even though they may all coexist in the same brain and differ in their topography. Their recognition and interpretation rely on the quality of the equipment, the timing of scannings and the investigator's experience.

Nevertheless, conflicting conclusions have been drawn regarding the predictive value of cerebral US. Such disparate and controversial results can be explained by differences in the populations studied and variations in classifications of US abnormalities. Also, US definitions have been regularly modified by technological progress, the availability of high frequency transducers and clinicopathologic correlations.

Despite newly available imaging techniques, ultrasonography remains the method of first choice in neonatal units because of the ease of making a quick bedside diagnosis of major haemorrhagic and ischaemic lesions and other cerebral pathologies, such as malformations and congenital and acquired infections. It should be part of the management of all sick preterm and term infants and it should not only help provide the best medical care, but also the best quality of survival for the baby.

Fig. 3.1. Relationship between sound-velocity, wavelength and frequency. Velocity (v) does not change in most biological tissues; thus, if the wavelength (λ) increases, the frequency (f; *amplitude*) must decrease

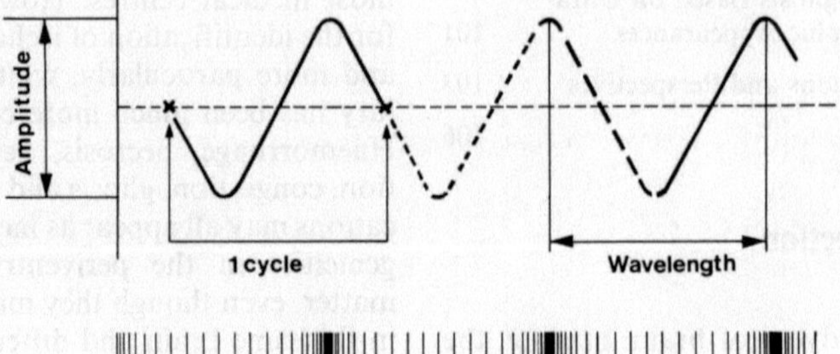

3.2 The Physics of US

Ultrasonic waves are mechanical vibrations similar to audible sound waves. The only difference between US and audible sound is the frequency of vibrations. Sound travels through a medium in the form of a wave by inducing compression and rarefaction of the space between molecules of the medium. The distance between two compression regions is the wavelength. The sound velocity (v) depends on the wavelength (λ) and frequency (f). This is illustrated by the relationship (Fig. 3.1):

$$v = \lambda \times f \quad (3.1)$$

Furthermore, sound propagation will also depend on the *characteristic impedance* of the tissue, on *attenuation* and on *absorption*. Sound velocity does not change significantly for most biological soft tissues (1540 m/s).

An echo is produced when the wave passes two media at differing *acoustic impedances*. When the wave meets the acoustical interface in a perpendicular plane, complete reflection occurs. However, most often in biological structures, the beam strikes the interface obliquely, resulting in reflection, refraction and scattering. These phenomenon explain some artefacts which are likely to be created in producing an US image.

Similar processes of reflection, refraction and scattering affect the echoes re-

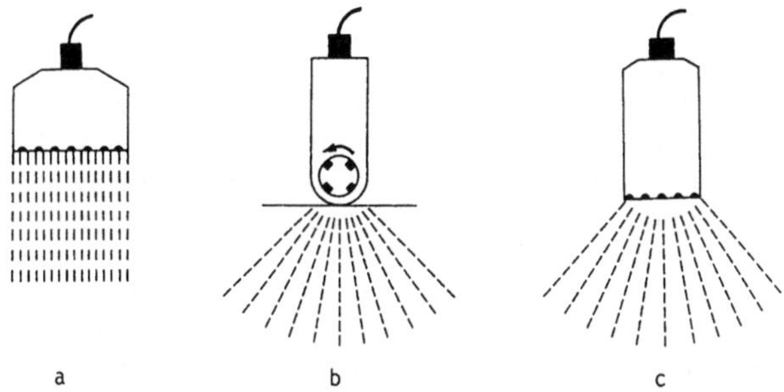

Fig. 3.2. Linear array transducer (**a**), mechanical sector scan (**b**) and multielement phased array (**c**)

turning to the transducer. It follows that the echoes from deeper structures will be smaller than those reflected by surfaces nearer the transducer. Therefore, adjustment of the time-gain compensation (TGC) curve allows a gradually increasing amplification of deeper echoes while suppressing the relatively strong near echoes.

US waves are generated by a piezoelectric crystal. The transducer converts short electrical impulses into high frequency sound and vice versa, so that echoes are converted into electrical signals. In medicine, crystals of lead zirconate and lead titanate are used. Crystals are selected so that they resonate electrically and acoustically at their nominal frequencies. The range of frequencies used for diagnostic US is limited by two principal constraints: At high frequency, there is better resolution but poorer depth penetration (because of shorter wavelength) and, at low frequency, there is poorer resolution, but better depth penetration (because of longer wavelength).

A compromise between these two conditions will guide the investigator in the choice of the transducer to be used.

The most commonly used frequencies for medical diagnosis range from 2.5 million cycles per second (2.5 MHz) up to 10 million cycles per second (10 MHz).

The width of the US beam and its focussing to correct the distal divergence are also important in the quality of image production. *Axial resolution* and *perpendicular resolution* refer to the ability to distinguish two reflecting structures located along or perpendicularly to the beam's axis. These two properties are essential for displaying anatomic features as clearly as possible.

To produce a two-dimensional US image, the reflected signal is detected by the transducer. Then, the distance from the acoustic interface to the transducer is calculated by the velocity of sound in the tissue and the time required by the echo to strike the transducer. Successive images can be then rapidly displayed and erased on the screen, permitting the visualization of structures in real time.

3.3 Methods

3.3.1 Equipment

The movements of the sound beam are obtained by *mechanical* or *electronical means*. The form of the image is either a rectangle of lines or a fan-shaped sector scan (Fig. 3.2).

Real time US images may be produced by several devices. In the late 1970s, a multiple series of crystals placed side by side in a housing was used. Such *linear array* transducers visualize a large volume of tissue, resulting in a rectangular scan (Fig. 3.2 a). However, a long contact area (long window) is necessary, thus limiting its use over the anterior fontanelle.

Another type of instrumentation consists either of a conventional single oscillating crystal or of two or more conventional elements rotating in a spindle thereby generating a *sector scan* (Fig. 3.2b). This system is more suitable for the neonatal brain. The small size of the transducer enables it to be angled into the convexity of the skull. More recently, a *multielement phased array* utilizes a block of identical elements which are electronically excited at different instants, resulting in angled or sectored views needing only a small acoustic window. It can also be used to focus the sound beam to a selected depth in the area of interest (Fig. 3.2c).

3.3.2 Safety

As with any widely used diagnostic technique, the topic of safety is of fundamental importance in ultrasonography. To provide a perspective of safety, the American Institute of Ultrasound in Medicine Bioeffects Committee has formulated, over the last 15 years, a number of statements regarding heat generation, cavitation, epidemiology and in vitro biological effects.

As US propagates through tissue, a thermal mechanism occurs, part of the US energy being progressively absorbed and converted into heat. However, diagnostic US of low intensity produces little increase in temperature and can be used without reservation in clinical examination. Acoustic cavitation describes the interactions of sound waves with microscopic gas bodies in a biological medium. There is, as yet, no direct evidence that cavitation causes any adverse biological effects in human subjects under diagnostic conditions.

Mechanical vibration effects on macromolecules such as DNA are possible. Yet, epidemiological studies have shown no causal association of diagnostic US with any of the adverse fetal outcomes studied.

A review of in vivo mammalian bioeffects data concluded that there have been no independently confirmed, significant adverse effects on mammalian tissues exposed to unfocussed US with intensities below 100 mW/cm^2 or to focussed US below 1 W/cm^2.

Quality control in commercial production allows maximal energy output to be in the range of $1-50\ mW/cm^2$. The American Institute of Ultrasound in Medicine released, in 1988, the following statement on clinical safety: "No confirmed biological effects on patients or instrument operators caused by exposure at intensities typical of present diagnostic ultrasound instruments have ever been reported. Although the possibility exists that such biological effects may be identified in the future, current data indicates that the benefits to patients of the prudent use of diagnostic ultrasound outweigh the risks, if any, that may be present".

3.3.3 Imaging

Cranial US sans are commonly performed in two standard planes, coronal and sagittal, obtained through the anterior fontanelle. An additional scan series can be obtained in the axial plane through the temporoparietal bone or through the posterior fontanelle.

In the coronal plane, the transducer is angled progressively from anterior to posterior to obtain several sequential sections:

1. Anterior coronal section through the frontal lobes
2. Anterior coronal section through the frontal horns
3. Coronal section at the level of the foramen of Monro and third ventricle
4. Coronal section through the trigone of the ventricles at the level of the choroid plexus
5. Posterior coronal section through the occipital lobes;
6. Sagittal section through the midline to the right or to the left hemisphere towards the Sylvian fissures

7. Midline section including the corpus callosum, third ventricle, fourth ventricle and posterior fossa
8. Parasagittal sections through the lateral ventricles
9. Extreme parasagittal sections through the insula

As a result of the indisputable advantages of ultrasonography, i.e. portable instrumentation, lack of ionizing radiation, unknown side effects and relatively low cost, US scanning has become a routine imaging procedure in most medical centres and is systematically and sequentially performed among preterm infants in intensive care units. Over our 10 year experience, this procedure has allowed us to detect cerebral lesions, to establish their incidence, evolution and resolution and to evaluate a "lesion profile" over time. It has also enabled us to identify etiopathogenic factors, to monitor treatment, to assign a prognosis and to provide additional guidelines in making decisions in intensive care.

In order to achieve the most accurate US diagnosis, one must consider the indications, the timing of scanning and the pathology looked for (Table 3.1).

Table 3.1. Current indications for US examination, timing of scannings and pathology looked for

Indication	Timing of scannings	Pathology looked for
Preterm infants (≤34 weeks gestation)	1st week	Germinal layer haemorrhage, intraventricular haemorrhage, PVL (acute stage)
	2nd–3 rd week	Cystic PVL or persistent echogenicities
	2nd–8 th, 12 th weeks	Assessment of ventricular size after intraventricular haemorrhage
Mature infants (>34 weeks gestation)		
With perinatal asphyxia	1st–3rd and 4th weeks	Hypoxic-ischaemic lesions
	1–3 months	Leucoencephalomalacia, cerebral atrophy
With abnormal neurological signs	1–3 weeks	Hypoxic-ischaemic and haemorrhagic lesions, malformations
Dysmorphic signs, chromosomic abnormalities	Birth	Cerebral malformations
Congenital infections	Birth	Calcifications, cysts, ventricular dilatation
Intrauterine growth retardation	Birth	Calcifications, prenatal vascular anomalies
Meningitis	Acute phase	Ventriculitis, echogenic sulci, parenchymal lesions, enlargement of CSF spaces
	2nd–3rd week to several months	Assessment of ventricular size
Rapid growth of head circumference		Subdural, subarachnoid haemorrhage, hygroma, external or internal hydrocephalus, arachnoid cysts
Suspicion of battered child		Subdural haematoma

3.4 Normal Anatomy from Premature to 40 Weeks Gestational Age

3.4.1 Preterm US Images

By 10 weeks gestation, cerebral hemispheres, thalamic structures, midbrain and cerebellum can be differentiated. The ventricular cavity is filled by a proliferating choroid plexus. The increasing volume of the cerebral hemispheres is associated with progressive development of the sulci. During the first 18–20 weeks, the ventricular system is relatively large and then reduces progressively in size. However, prominent lateral ventricles are normally found up to 32 weeks gestation.

At 26 weeks gestation, on coronal section through the middle fossa, there is a normal widening of the Sylvian fissures due to incomplete operculisation of the insula (Fig. 3.3). Subarachnoid spaces are physiologically enlarged and the external surfaces of the hemispheres are very smooth. Basal ganglia appear as slightly hyperechogenic structures. The cavity of the septum pellucidum is open. More posteriorly, at the level of the posterior fossa, a large cisterna magna is normally visualized (Fig. 3.4). The cerebellar hemispheres, with their hyperechogenic surfaces, and the vermis are clearly distinguished. The cavum vergae, under the splenium of the corpus callosum, is still open. Hyperechogenic zones are often noted on the occipital lobes, which are separated by the straight, vertical interhemispheric fissure (Fig. 3.5).

On parasagittal section, the glomus of the choroid plexus, which is prominent, should not be mistaken for an intraventricular haemorrhage or a haemorrhage of the choroid plexus. The parenchyma appears as a uniformly echogenic structure without any sulci or gyri (Fig. 3.6). The midline sagittal plane clearly displays the corpus callosum, the open cavum of the septum pellucidum and the cavum vergae (Fig. 3.7).

Fig. 3.3. Coronal scan (26 weeks gestation) through the middle fossa at the level of the sphenoid bone showing a normal widening of the Sylvian fissures (*large arrows*). The cavity of the septum pellucidum (*cs*) below the corpus callosum is open. The external surface of the hemispheres is very smooth (*small arrows*)

Fig. 3.4. Coronal scan (26 weeks gestation) through the posterior fossa. A large cisterna magna is normally visualized below the hyperechogenic cerebellum. The cavum vergae is still open (*cv*)

Fig. 3.5. Coronal scan (26 weeks gestation) through the occipital lobes. Hyperechogenic zones are normally observed

Fig. 3.6. Parasagittal scan (26 weeks gestation) through the ventricular system. The parenchyma is a uniformly echogenic structure without sulci or gyris. The glomus of the choroid plexus is prominent

Fig. 3.7. Midline sagittal scan (26 weeks gestation) with the main landmarks: corpus callosum, open cavum of septum pellucidum (*cs*) and cavum vergae (*cv*) and the enlarged cisterna magna (*arrow*)

Fig. 3.8. Parasagittal scan (32 weeks gestation) showing the presence of the straight callosomarginal sulcus. The ventricles have decreased in size. The glomus of the choroid plexus is less prominent

Progression of brain development is evidenced by an increase in the number and depth of sulci appearing in the parenchyma. By 32 weeks gestation, on parasagittal plane, the callosomarginal sulcus is clearly visible (Fig. 3.8) and the glomus of the choroid plexus has reduced in size. Ventricles may be variable in size.

3.4.2 Term US Images

At term, the margins of the sylvian fissures have approached because of the development of the parietal and temporal lobes and have acquired the characteristic y-shaped form. A number of sec-

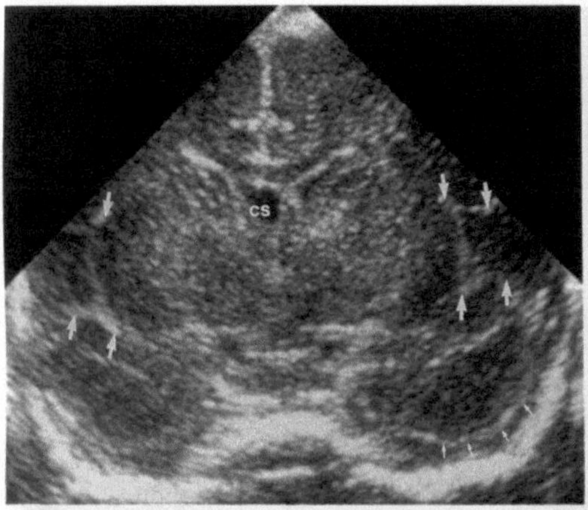

3.3

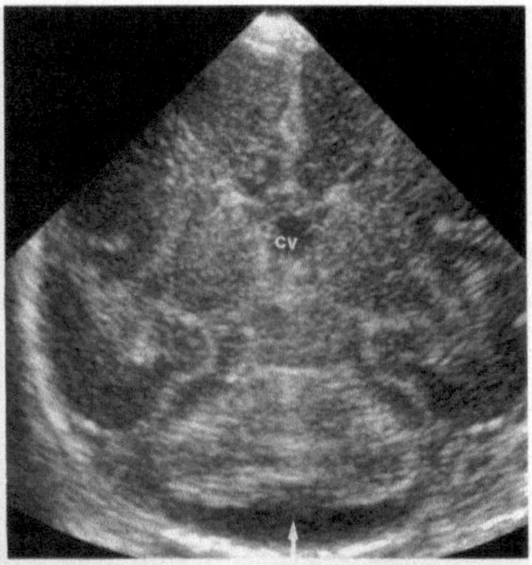

3.4

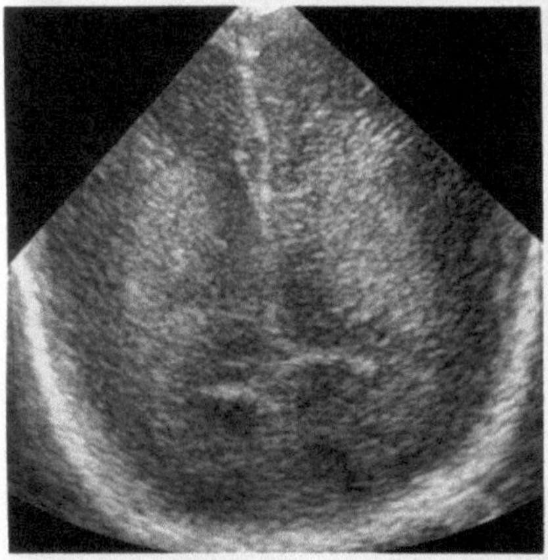

3.5

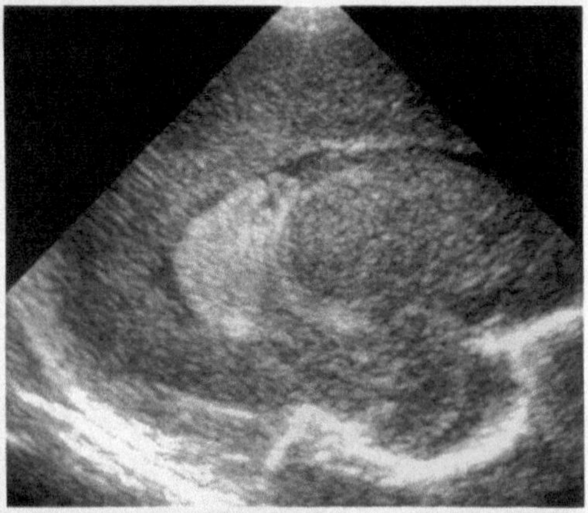

3.6

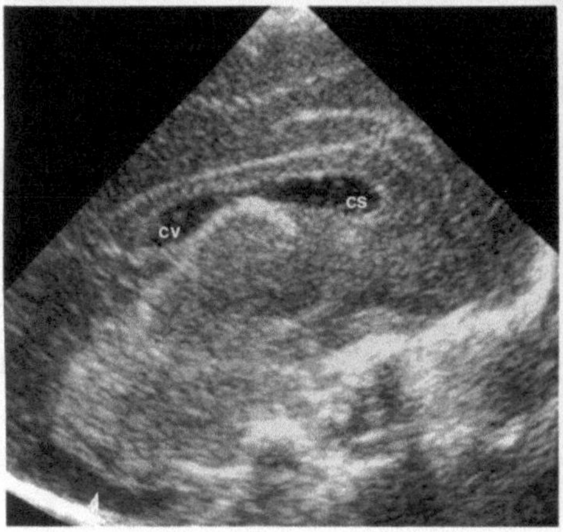

3.7

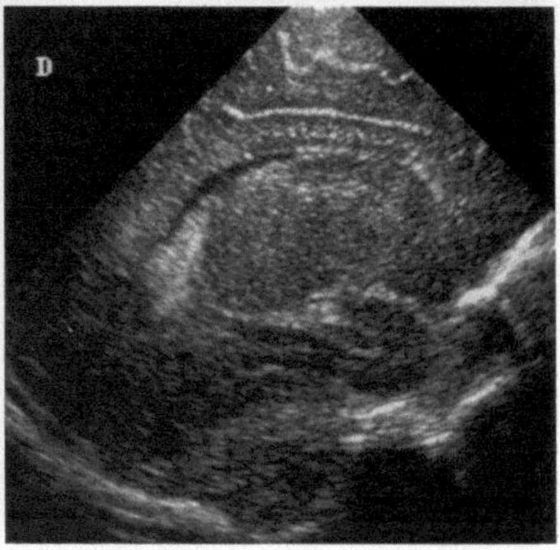

3.8

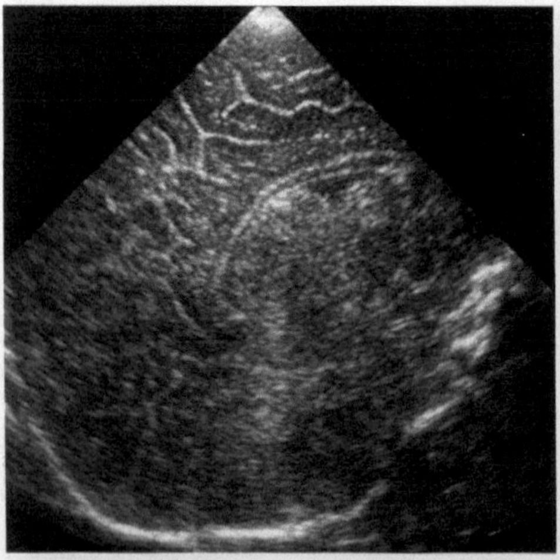

3.9

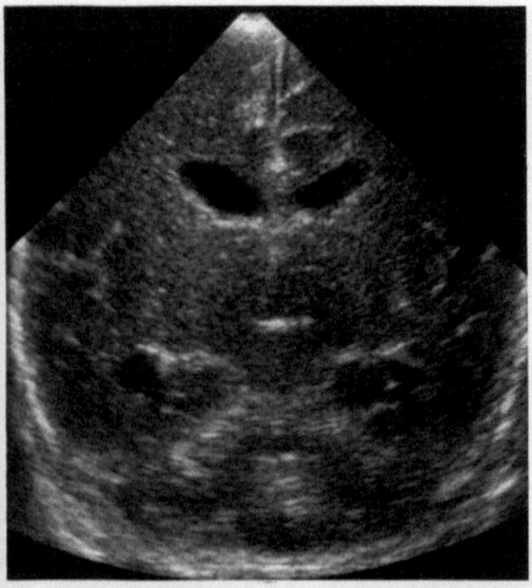

3.10

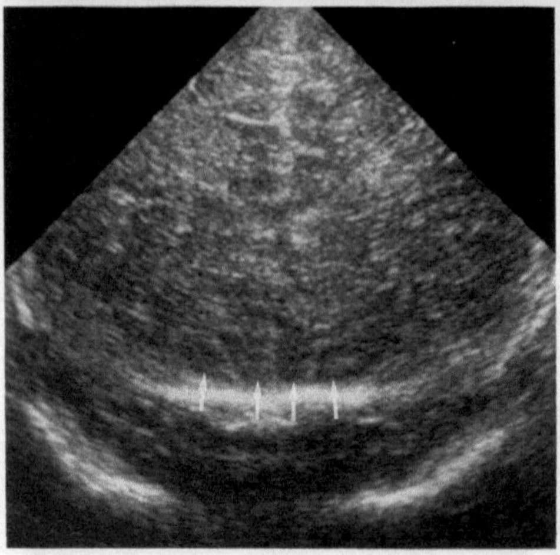

3.11

Fig. 3.9. Middle sagittal section (40 weeks gestation) showing the corpus callosum and a great number of secondary and tertiary sulci

Fig. 3.10. Coronal section at the level of the posterior fossa. The interhemispheric fissure appears anechoic (because it is slightly enlarged) and the cerebrum falxis displayed. An asymmetrical, moderate ventricular dilatation is also noted in this infant

Fig. 3.11. Frontocoronal scan (40 weeks gestation). Anterior to the corpus callosum and to the frontal horns, the frontal corpus callosum and to the frontal horns, the frontal lobes are slightly hyperechogenic. The normal interhemispheric fissure is hyperechoic and demonstrates many gyri. Over the sphenoid bone, the orbital and olfactory sulci are distinguished (*arrows*)

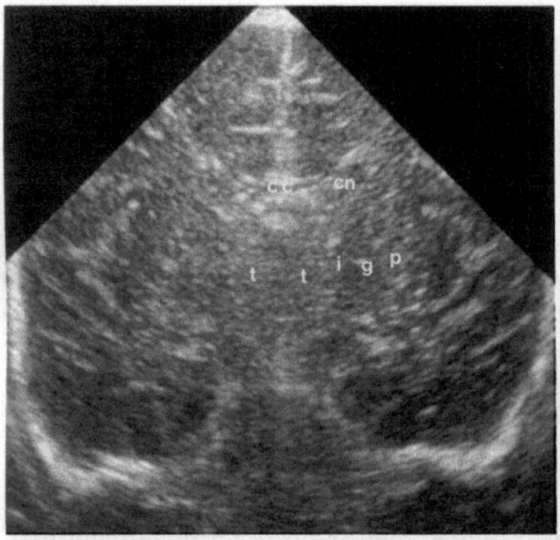

3.12

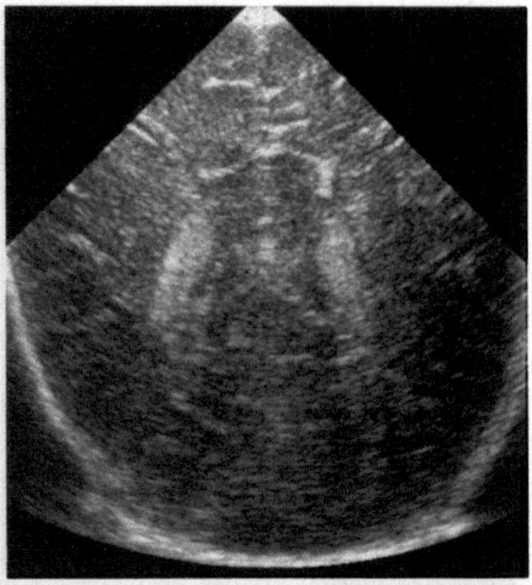

3.13

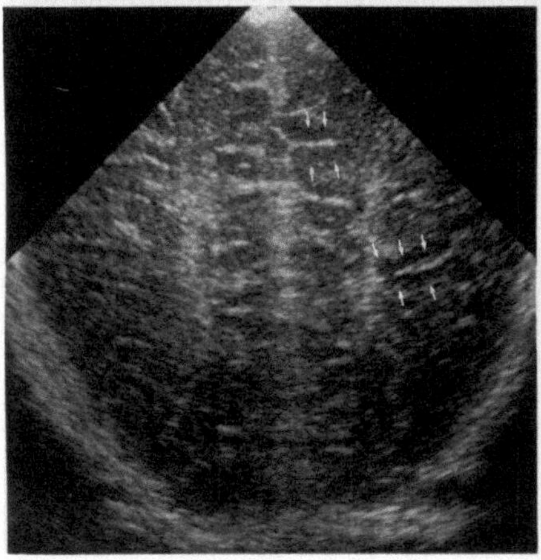

3.14

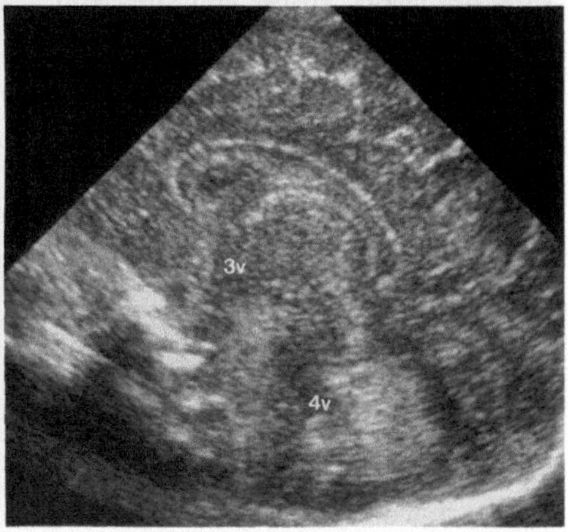

3.15

Fig. 3.12. Parietocoronal scan (40 weeks gestation). The ventricles are virtual spaces; the Sylvian fissures have their characteristic y-shaped form. Corpus callosum (*cc*), caudate nucleus (*cn*), thalami (*t*), internal capsule (*i*), globus pallidum (*g*) and putamen (*p*) are visualized

Fig. 3.13. Coronal parieto-occipital scan displaying the bright choroid plexus

Fig. 3.14. Coronal occipital scan showing numerous sulci and gyri and the normal, slightly hyperechoic central zones of both occipital lobes. The hypoechogenic ribbon of grey matter (*small arrows*) is clearly seen

Fig. 3.15. Middle sagittal scan (40 weeks gestation) with the main landmarks: corpus callosum, a small open cavity of septum pellucidum, a narrow third ventricle (*3v*), the parieto-occipital sulcus and the posterior fossa with the cerebellum and the small, triangular fourth ventricle (*4v*)

ondary and tertiary sulci have developed with bifurcations and a great variability in sinuosity (Fig. 3.9). Recent improvements in US equipment allows the display of many anatomic structures of the term neonatal brain, not identifiable previously.

Grey matter and white matter in very immature infants is poorly differentiated. As gestational age increases, the thin cortical layer of grey matter will appear as a relatively hypoechogenic ribbon on the brain surface and in each gyrus. In mature infants, the grey-white matter junction is normally recognizable on US (Fig. 3.14). Normally, the sulci and fissures are virtual spaces and appear hyperechogenic. If they are wider, they appear hypoechogenic because of the presence of anechoic CSF. The cerebrum falx can also be demonstrated as a straight echogenic vertical line within the interhemispheric fissure (Fig. 3.10).

On frontocoronal sections, slightly hyperechogenic zones in the frontal lobes, due to the presence of vessels, are noted (Fig. 3.11). Olfactory and orbital sulci can also be identified. More posteriorly, on parietocoronal section, the interhemispheric fissure with numerous gyri over the hypoechogenic corpus callosum is demonstrated. By 40 weeks gestation, the lateral ventricles are generally visualized as very narrow spaces. The following anatomical structures of basal ganglia may be clearly displayed: caudate nucleus, thalami, internal capsule, putamen and globus pallidus. The third ventricle is barely visible. The temporal lobes with both hippocampuses are easily defined as relatively low echogenic structures (Fig. 3.12).

At the level of the posterior fossa, the choroid plexus appears as two hyperechogenic masses; the ventricular walls are generally not visualized (Fig. 3.13). Far posteriorly, the occipital lobes are seen with their numerous gyri and sulci (Fig. 3.14).

Figure 3.15 is a midline sagittal section showing the major landmarks of this plane: the corpus callosum and the small cavitas septi pellucidi. The third ventricle is a thin cleft, frequently visible on US only as a hypoechogenic triangle limited by a bright echogenic roof, the choroid plexus, and anteriorly by the supraoptic and infundibular recesses. The posterior fossa is occupied by the cerebellar vermis and the cisterna magna. The fourth ventricle is a small cavity appearing as a small anechoic triangle, with its apex directed into the vermis.

Although gyri and sulci are variable in their topography, the observation of unusual architecture, with regard to the main landmarks of the midline sagittal plane, may indicate an underlying malformation. Furthermore, the cortical surface should also be carefully explored and the absence or presence of gyri and sulci has to be interpreted with reference to the stage of the developing brain. Also, the extracerebral spaces and the cisterna equally vary in size throughout gestation. Pachygyri, lissencephaly and abnormal gyration may be suspected based on a relative paucity in the number of sulci and gyri.

Demonstration of the neuroanatomic structures and the normal ultrasonographic appearance of the brain depends on the type and length of utilization of the equipment, the size of the fontanelle and the investigator's skill. Knowledge of normal US images requires time, experience and a good understanding of neonatal neurology and pathology. This is an essential point, for the dividing line between normal and abnormal images may be difficult to make, especially in the term infant.

3.5 Applications in Pathologic Situations

The onset and nature of brain lesions depends on several factors: type of insult, timing of event and, more particularly, the gestational age. Blood supply follows the structural development and, at 28 weeks gestation, there is a predominance of vessels in the central structures of the brain. At 32–34 weeks, there is peripheral development of blood vessels along with rapid growth of the cortex and white matter. Basic forms of brain damage may be understood in terms of anatomic maturation of the CNS together with changes in vascular distribution. In addition, cerebral lesions detected in the fetus and in the neonate actually represent an endstage of a series of pathologic processes such as anoxia, hypoxia and ischaemia, representing a "continuum of casualties". Also, vigorous resuscitation at birth and modern management of sick newborns have tremendously modified both the chance of immediate and long-term survival and the spectrum of brain lesions reported following neuropathologic examinations of infants who have died.

In the following sections US abnormalities are presented with regard to brain maturation, because the timing of scanning, brain lesions looked for, criteria for engagement of intensive care and medical attitude differ between preterm and term infants. Finally, the correlation between US changes and pathologic processes will be discussed as far as possible.

3.6 Haemorrhagic and Hypoxic-Ischaemic Lesions in Preterm Infants

Early application of US was mainly concerned with the diagnosis of germinal layer haemorrhage and intraventricular haemorrhage. Later, involvement of brain parenchyma was also recognized due to its major prognostic value. However, the exact nature of the parenchymal injury, demonstrated in its early phase as increased echogenicities, is still very much debated. Several neuropathologic and ultrasonographic correlation studies are currently being performed to further explore the wide spectrum of these histological changes.

Since the advent of US, the terminology used to refer to haemorrhage has varied from one study to another. Intraventricular haemorrhage (IVH), germinal layer haemorrhage (GLH), and peri-intraventricular haemorrhage (P-IVH) have been used to describe the same condition. Furthermore, classification systems for grading the haemorrhage have also been controversial. We have decided to describe haemorrhagic and ischaemic lesions with respect to the normal anatomic landmarks, the areas involved and the extent of the lesions.

3.6.1 Germinal Layer Haemorrhage

This condition refers to a bleeding confined to the germinal layer. Most haemorrhages occur into the germinal layer at the head of the caudate nucleus adjacent to the foramen of Monro. The haemorrhage appears on US as an echogenic area identified in both coronal and sagittal planes over the head of the caudate nucleus (Figs. 3.16 and 3.17). GLHs are frequently bilateral. Bleeding may extend far anteriorly into the caudate nucleus or may remain localized in the caudothalamic notch. Small haemorrhages of 1–2 mm in size will be detected by US. A haemorrhage may also occur in the anterior part of the choroid plexus, particularly among very immature infants, which may be difficult to differentiate from a GLH. A rupture of a GLH with small bleeding into the ventricles may be missed on US as fresh blood is anechoic and ventricles of preterm infants are normally prominent. Serial sonography demonstrates that GLH resolves over a period of a few weeks. The most frequent sequel to GLH is the development of a subependymal cyst (Fig. 3.18).

3.16 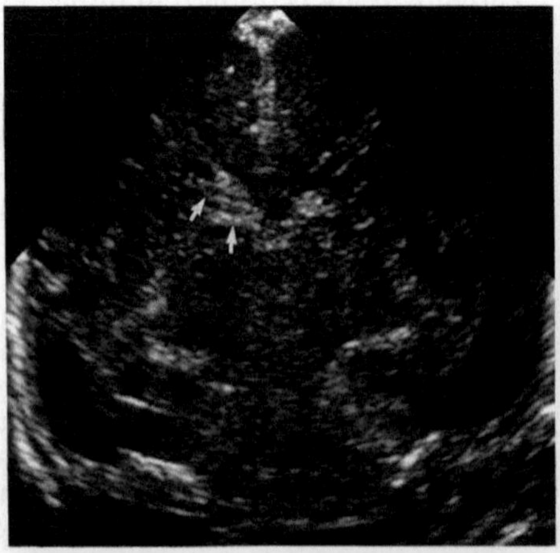

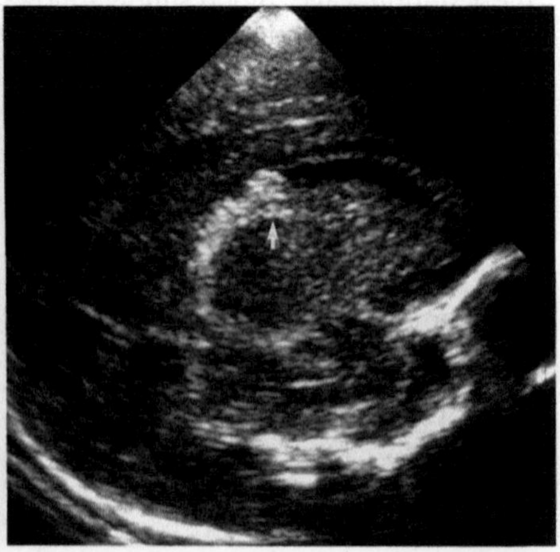 3.17

3.18 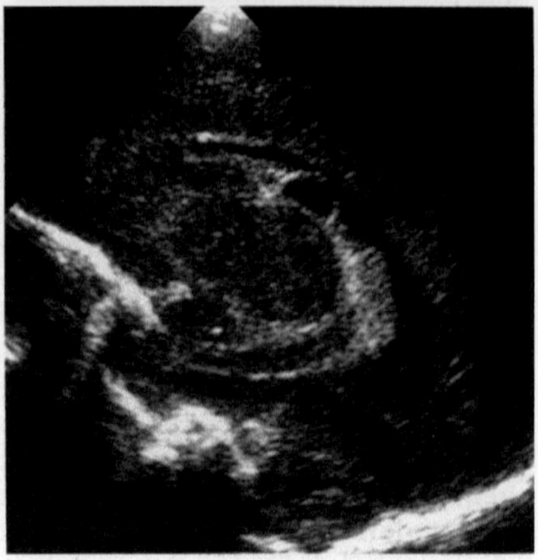

Fig. 3.16. Coronal scan showing a germinal layer haemorrhage (grade I). A focal echogenic area is noted in the floor of the left ventricle (*arrows*)

Fig. 3.17. Left parasagittal scan demonstrating a germinal layer haemorrhage (*arrow*)

Fig. 3.18. Parasagittal scan showing a subependymal cyst, signature of a previous germinal layer haemorrhage

3.6.2 Intraventricular Haemorrhage

A GLH may rupture the overlying ependyma, filling and distending the ventricular system. IVH may also arise from a primary choroid plexus haemorrhage. Blood may also spill into the subarachnoid spaces and the cisterna. A recent IVH is anechoic but becomes rapidly echogenic over a few hours. Clots develop, adhere to the choroid plexus and are indistinguishable from it on US (Fig. 3.19). The IVH will then form a cast of the ventricular system. In some patients, IVH is suspected when an echogenic clot collects in the occipital horns or when the surface of the choroid plexus is irregular and in close contact with the roof of the ventricles. Scannings must then be performed regularly in each newborn infant who has a diagnosis of IVH, as posthaemorrhagic ventricular dilatation is a frequent complication which occurs a few days to several weeks after the initial bleeding. The severity and course of dilatation is variable and not easily predictable.

3.6.3 Intraparenchymal Haemorrhage

In our experience, intraparenchymal haemorrhage (IPH) occurs most often in very immature infants and coexists with a moderate or a large IVH. It appears on US as a very marked increased echogenicity in the periventricular white matter in continuity with the IVH (Fig. 3.20). There is a progression from a GLH to an intraventricular bleeding extending to the parenchyma which will be detected by repeated scannings.

There are several mechanisms which are nowadays postulated to explain parenchymal haemorrhagic involvement. In the early 1980s, a direct extension from IVH was incriminated. Parenchymal haemorrhage has also been related to a previous underlying white matter ischaemia, favouring extension from the distended ventricles. Finally, the venous cerebral circulation might also play a role in the pathogenesis of parenchymal haemorrhagic involvement. A large IVH with distended ventricles is frequently associated with venous stasis and obstruction, which may result in venous infarction. At the present time, there is good evidence that these mechanisms may coexist in the same brain and result in various types of haemorrhagic parenchymal involvement (Fig. 3.21).

Whatever the pathologic processes, the evolution of the parenchymal haemorrhagic involvement will be similar. The large, uniformly echogenic intraparenchymal haematoma will resolve over a period of 2–3 weeks with a progressive reduction in the density of echoes. There is a retraction of clots, and thrombi within the ventricles become detached, gradually disappearing. Large porencephalic cysts opening into the ventricular system replace the parenchymal haematoma (Fig. 3.22). It is noteworthy that haemorrhagic parenchymal lesions are most often associated with a massive IVH and will be accompanied in surviving patients by a progressive hydrocephalus.

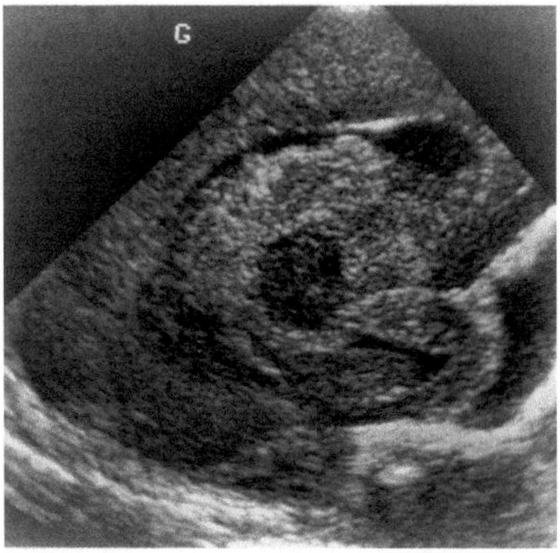

Fig. 3.19. Parasagittal scan demonstrating a huge intraventricular haemorrhage forming an echogenic clot adherent to the choroid plexus

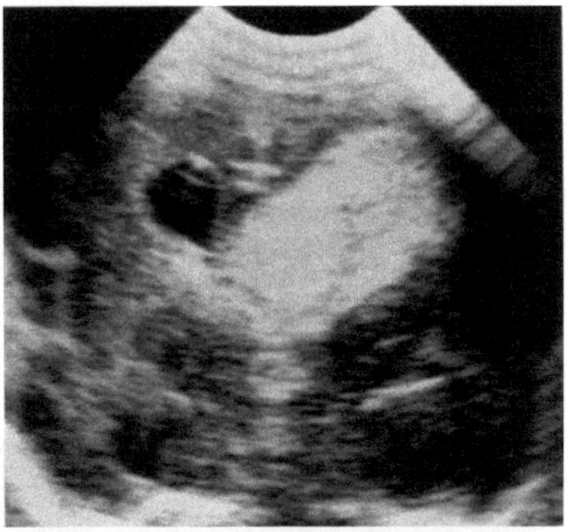

Fig. 3.20. Coronal scan of an intraparenchymal haemorrhage associated with an intraventricular haemorrhage

3.6.4 Periventricular Leucomalacia

For many years, neonatologists' interests focussed mainly on the diagnosis of germinal layer and intraventricular haemorrhages. Periventricular leucomalacia (PVL) had already been a well recognized entity in neuropathology books. However, it was only with the advent of sector scan and high frequency transducers, allowing one to explore and visualize more peripheral areas of the brain, that investigators started to discover sonographically periventricular white matter lesions.

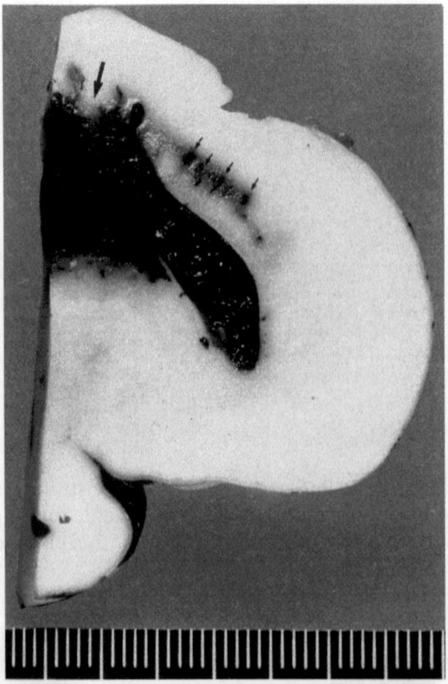

Fig. 3.21. Post-mortem, frontal parietal parasagittal section showing the frontal horn filled with blood, a venous congestion (*small arrows*) and, more posteriorly, a rupture of the ependyma with a intraparenchymal haemorrhage (*large arrow*). A thrombus is still present in the ventricle

Thereafter, numerous correlation studies between US abnormalities and neuropathologic findings were performed with a great deal of perseverance, energy and controversy, giving rise to a large debate in the literature. Nevertheless, an overall agreement has progressively arisen to define a spectrum of US changes that refer to the broad variety of PVL lesions. Once more, one wishes to emphasize that the accurate ultrasonographic diagnosis of PVL can only be achieved if scannings are performed regularly in the neonatal period in order to obtain a precise description of the localization, extent and type of PVL.

3.6.4.1 US Features of Classic PVL

PVL is an ischaemic lesion which occurs more commonly in premature infants, although it has occasionally been reported in full-term babies. In 1962, Banker and Laroche described, for the first time, this clinicopathologic condition and the term "periventricular leucomalacia" was introduced. On US two stages can be distinguished.

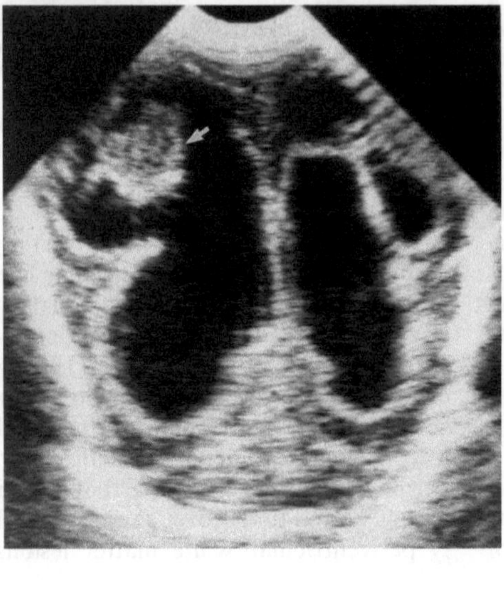

Fig. 3.22. Coronal scan showing the presence of a large porencephalic cyst opening into the ventricular cavity and replacing the parenchymal haematoma. A thrombus is still present in the ventricle (*arrow*)

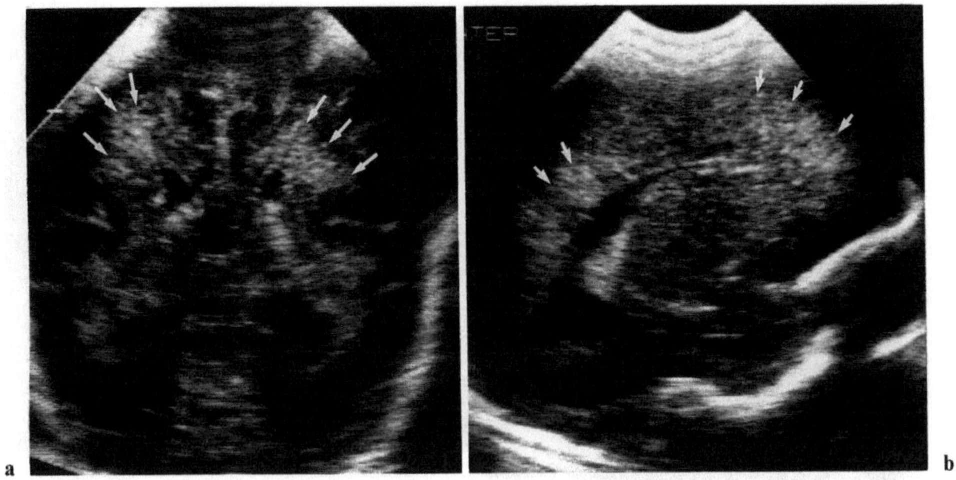

Fig. 3.23. Early stage of periventricular leucomalacia: bilateral, triangular increased echogenicities (*arrows*) visible on both coronal (**a**) and parasagittal (**b**) scans

1. The early stage of PVL is characterized by areas of increased echogenicities localized in the periventricular white matter in the vicinity of the external angle of the lateral ventricles. These areas have a characteristic triangular shape with the apex pointing towards the ventricle. These echogenicities should be demonstrated on both coronal and sagittal planes (Fig. 3.23). They may be focal or diffuse, and they occur more frequently at the outer borders of arterial territories, between the anterior and the middle cerebral arteries and middle and posterior cerebral arteries. On microscopic examination, these echogenic areas correspond to a fresh necrosis with pyknosis, sponginess and a marked vascular congestion. Secondary bleeding due to venous congestion may appear within the focus of necrosis, resulting in scattered areas of higher level echogenicity. Within a few days, these areas of increased echogenicities become well defined and circumscribed. Therefore, when the lesion is extensive, its ultrasonographic diagnosis, in our opinion, is straightforward.

2. In the late stage of PVL, areas of increased echogenicity resolve in 1–3 weeks into echo-free areas which progressively increase in size. The final stage is a cyst which, in most patients, does not communicate with the ventricular system (Figs. 3.24, 3.25). Cystic formations vary in diameter from 1–2 mm to over 1 cm. On microscopy, there is a liquefaction necrosis surrounded by an astrocytic reaction and microglia proliferation (Figs. 3.26, 3.27). The development of cysts will confirm the initial diagnosis of early stage PVL. These cysts remain visible for several weeks and then gradually diminish in size. They are usually no longer visible by 3–4 months of age. As cysts disappear, an enlargement of the ipsilateral ventricle and a widening of the interhemispheric fissure occur, attesting to a loss of tissue. Severe PVL will result in subsequent cerebral atrophy.

Other patterns of PVL changes include:

1. transient increased echogenicities or periventricular flares: In the early neonatal period, PVL changes may be subtle and less delineated. They appear on US as "flares", visible on both coronal and parasagittal planes, and usually disappear within the first week of life. These minimal changes in periventricular white

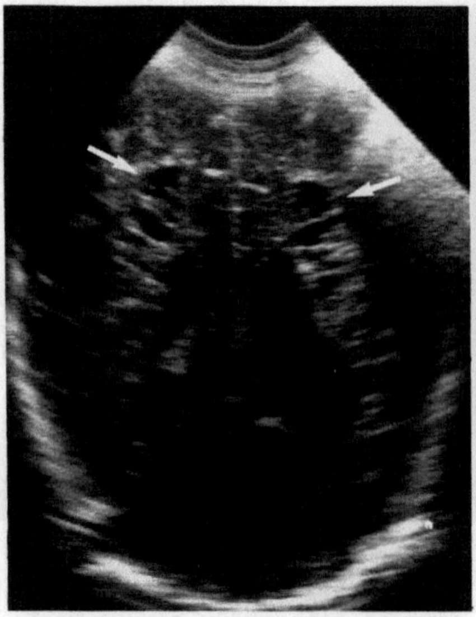

3.24

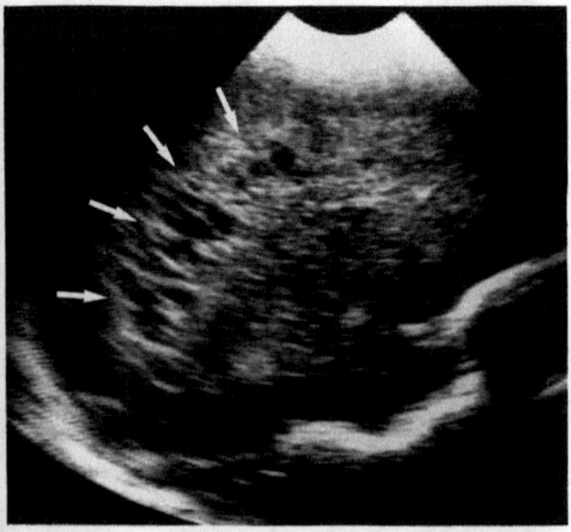

3.25

Fig. 3.24. Coronal scan showing late cystic stage of periventricular leucomalacia with multiple echo-free areas (*arrows*) in the periventricular white matter, variable in size

Fig. 3.25. Parasagittal scan. Cyst (*arrows*) are clearly visible in this plane

matter may represent transient and reversible ischaemic injury. There is some neuropathologic evidence that these slight alterations in echogenicity could be related to perivascular oedema altering the acoustic properties of cerebral tissue. However, the diagnosis of PVL at this stage of evolution is extremely difficult. Further histological investigations are warranted although unlikely to be performed, as most infants with such US abnormalities will survive.

2. Persistent Increased Echogenicities: This entity refers to the appearance of relatively increased echogenicity in the periventricular region demonstrated in both coronal and parasagittal sections and lasting more than 2 weeks without the development of cystic degeneration (Fig. 3.28). On histology, echogenicities correspond to microcalcifications and glial scars. The ultrasonographic evolution is characterized by progressive irregularity in the size and shape of the ventricular walls with rounded configurations of the external angles of the ventricles.

3.6.4.2 Small and Focal Changes in PVL

Careful and sequential scannings allow the identification of both small or focal areas of increased echogenicity and tiny cysts (1–2 mm in diameter) in the frontal, parietal or occipital periventricular regions, most often associated with a slight enlargement of the ventricles (Fig. 3.29). These minimal subacute or chronic changes may be present without any preexisting increased echogenicities. On microscopy, they correspond either to small cavitations or focal areas of gliosis and microcalcification (Fig. 3.30). Detection and recognition of the precise topography of these subtle changes are essential, as they represent markers of more diffuse parenchymal injury likely to result in later neurodevelopmental disorders.

3.26
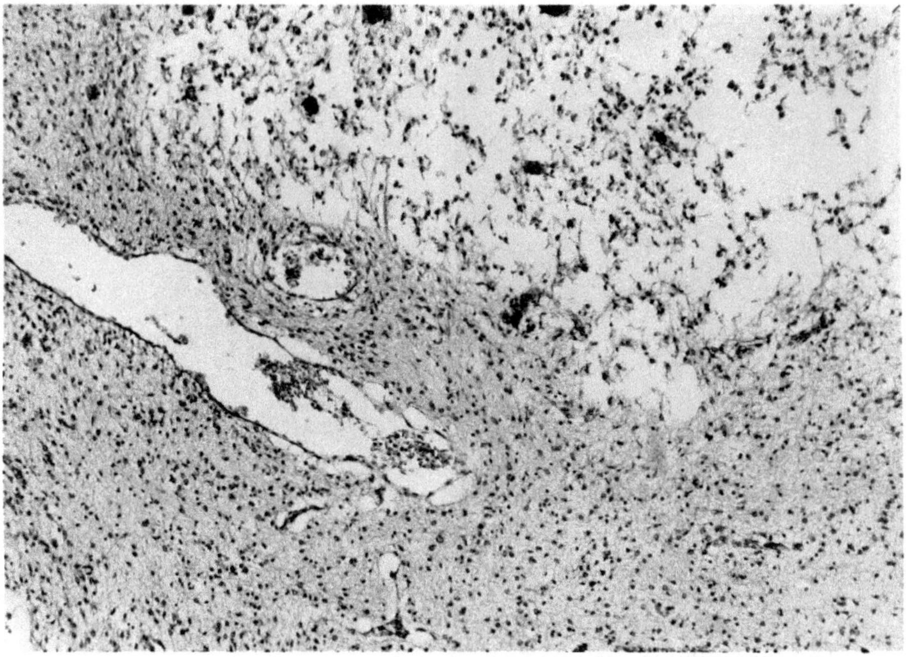

3.27
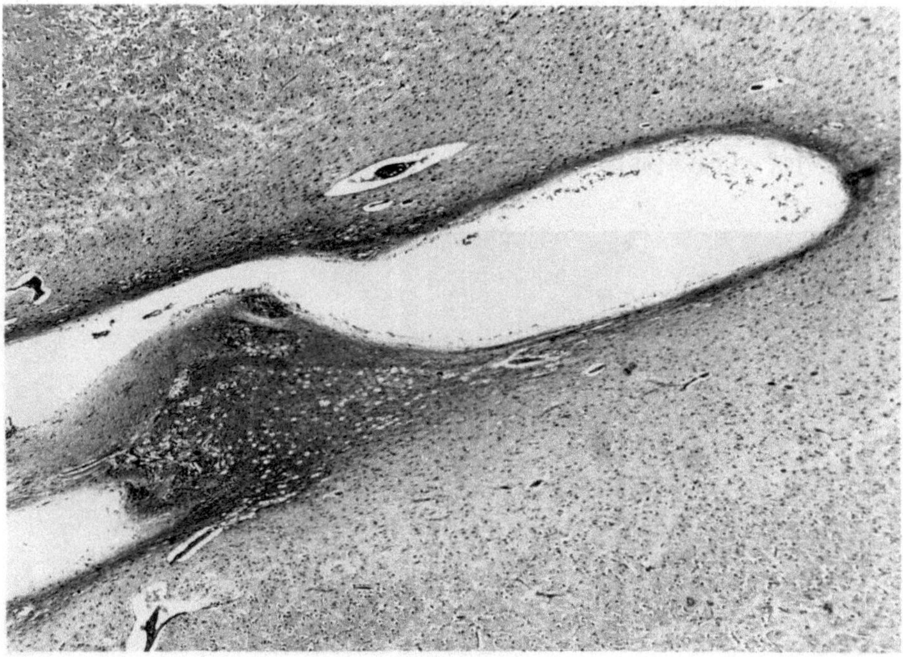

Fig. 3.26. Light microscopy. Liquefaction necrosis with vascular congestion and microcalcifications

Fig. 3.27. Light microscopy. Development of a cyst delineated by a marked gliosis

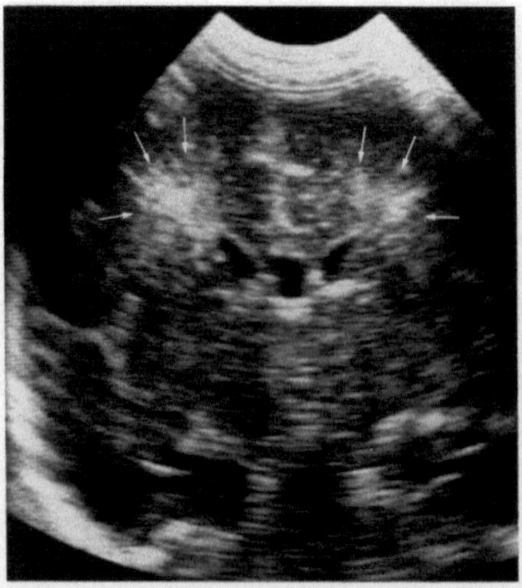

3.28

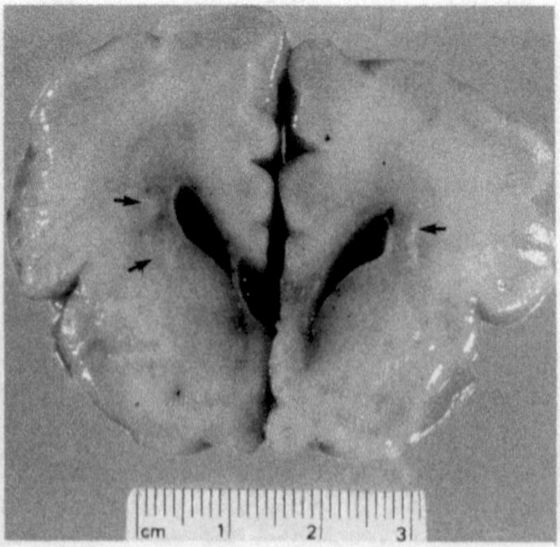

3.30

3.6.5 Sensitivity and Specificity of US

A few studies have explored the validity of ultrasonography in the diagnosis of white matter injury (Table 3.2). Although the investigators referred to different ultrasonographic definitions and histological terminology, the specificity of US appeared, in these studies, to be fairly high, whereas sensitivity ranged from 50%–90% (Pape et al. 1983; Szymonowicz

Fig. 3.28. Marked, persistent increased echogenicities lasting more than 2 weeks (*arrows*). This infant developed a moderate diplegia

Fig. 3.29 a, b. Small focal changes of PVL appearing in this patient as **a** focal areas of increased echogenicities lasting more than 2 weeks and **b** as a tiny cyst

Fig. 3.30. Post-mortem. Small focal PVL corresponding to focal areas of microcalcification and gliosis (*arrows*)

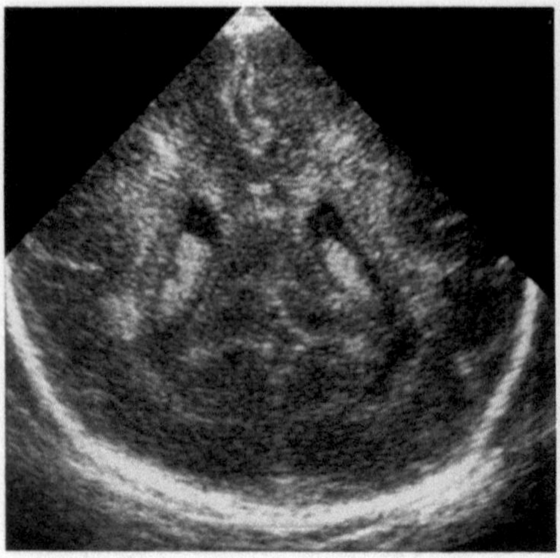

3.29 a

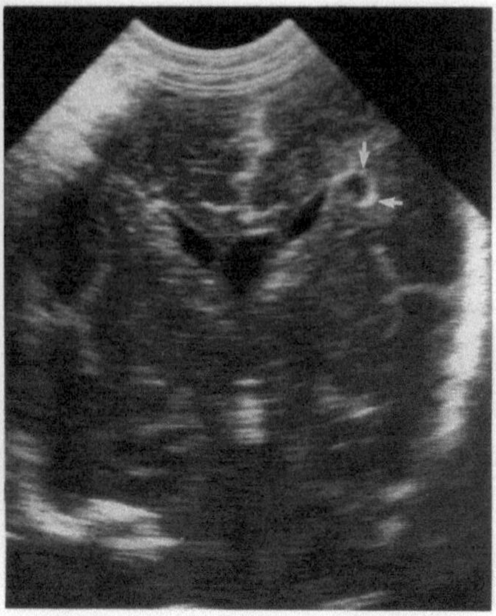

b

Table 3.2. US changes and neuropathology

Authors	US changes	Sensitivity (%)	Specificity (%)
Pape et al. 1983	Haemorrhage	50	100
Szymonowicz et al. 1984	Haemorrhage	85	100
	PVL	63	64
Nwaesei et al. 1984	White matter infarct	75	82
Trounce et al. 1986	Hypoxic-ischaemic lesions	85	93
Hope et al. 1988	Haemorrhage	82	97
	Hypoxic-ischaemic lesions	28	86
De Vries et al. 1988	PVL	72	98
Paneth et al. 1990	Increased echogenicities and ventricular enlargement	67	92

et al. 1984; Nwaesei et al. 1984; Trounce et al. 1986; Hope et al. 1988; De Vries et al. 1988; Paneth et al. 1990). The presence of haemorrhagic parenchymal involvement or ventricular enlargement in association with white matter US abnormalities correlated better with white matter neuropathologic findings.

In our opinion, regular scannings up to the 40th post-conceptional week, a meticulous description of all abnormal ultrasonographic findings of the periventricular and peripheral regions of the brain and the use of up-to-date equipment should improve the diagnostic validity of ultrasonography.

3.7 Haemorrhagic and Hypoxic-Ischaemic Lesions in Term Infants

Despite new imaging techniques, early evaluation of the consequences of perinatal asphyxia in term infants remains one of the most difficult challenges in neonatology. A wide and heterogeneous spectrum of cerebral lesions has been reported: focal or diffuse increased echogenicity, arterial boundary zone infarctions, PVL and subcortical leucomalacia, lesions in the basal ganglia, thrombosis of one or more major cerebral arteries and cerebral oedema (Figs. 3.31–3.33). A mixed pattern of lesions is most often noted; however, there is usually a predominance of one or two. Furthermore, these lesions are unpredictable, may appear several days after the insult and are not always directly related to the severity of the clinical course. An apparently normal brain at ultrasonography does not preclude a neurodevelopmental impairment and, vice versa, increased echogenicities may appear at a given stage of the clinical course, yet without apparent macroscopic abnormalities at postmortem. Therefore, prognostic criteria have not yet entirely been established. Repeated neurologic examinations, early EEGs, Doppler patterns, and brain imaging are necessary for the assignment of prognosis.

3.8 Ventricular Dilatation

Ultrasonography accurately delineates ventricular morphology and size. It represents therefore the first imaging procedure to evaluate many conditions related to ventricular dilatation. It also allows one to determine whether ventricular dilatation is progressive or stable. Quantitative measurements of normal ventricu-

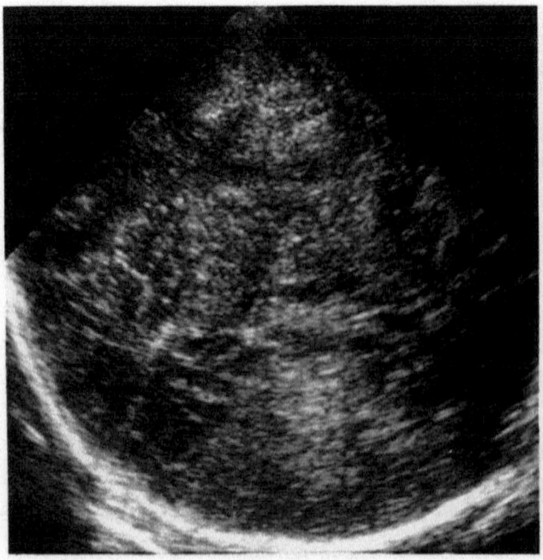

3.31 a

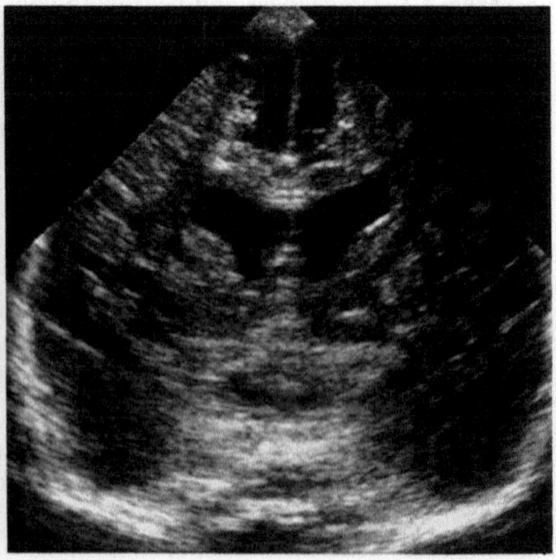

b

lar size from the fontanelle access have been reported. The width and the depth of the lateral ventricles are the most currently used reference measurements (Fig. 3.34). In practice, additional qualitative appreciation helps detect early ventricular dilatation, i.e. an enlargement of the occipital horns and, on coronal view, a progressive rounded configuration of the external angles of the frontal horns and bodies of both lateral ventricles. A dilatation of the third and fourth ventricles can also be recognized on coronal and sagittal scannings.

Fig. 3.31. **a** Coronal scan at 3 days of life showing diffuse increased echogenicities and loos of the main structural landmarks following a severe perinatal asphyxia. These echogenicities evolved into leucoencephalomacia. **b** After 2 months, a marked cerebral atrophy was noted with ventricular dilatation and enlarged pericerebral spaces

Fig. 3.32. Thrombosis of the left middle cerebral artery (*arrows*). The left Sylvian fissure is no longer visible

Fig. 3.33. Subcortical leucomalacia and cerebral atrophy occurring after a severe birth asphyxia

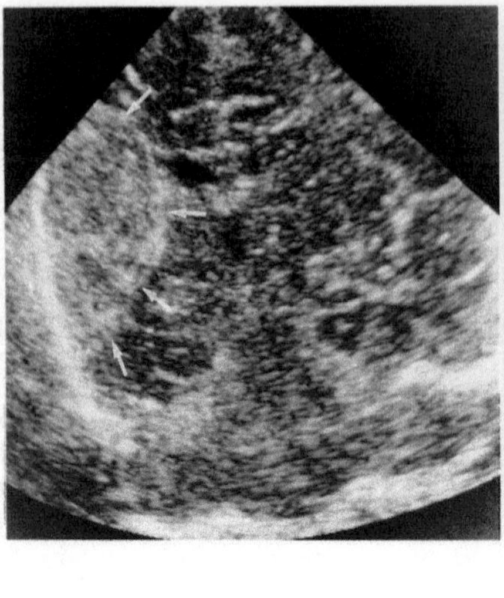

3.32

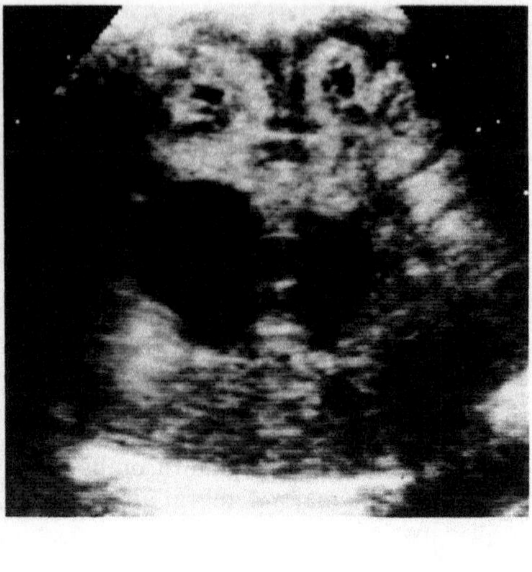

3.33

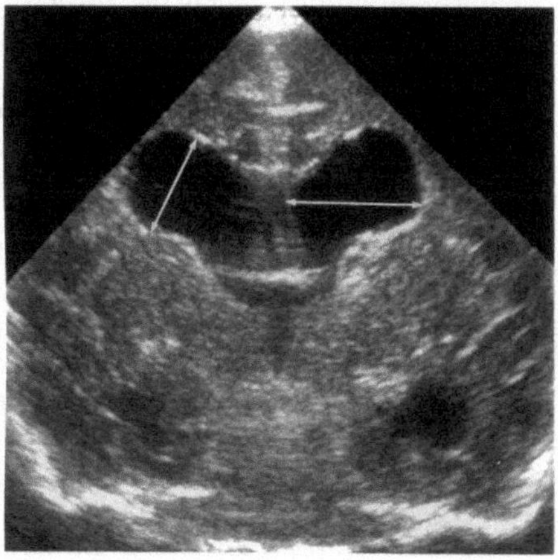

Fig. 3.34. Width and depth (*arrows*) of the lateral ventricles at the level of the bodies are the most currently used reference measurements

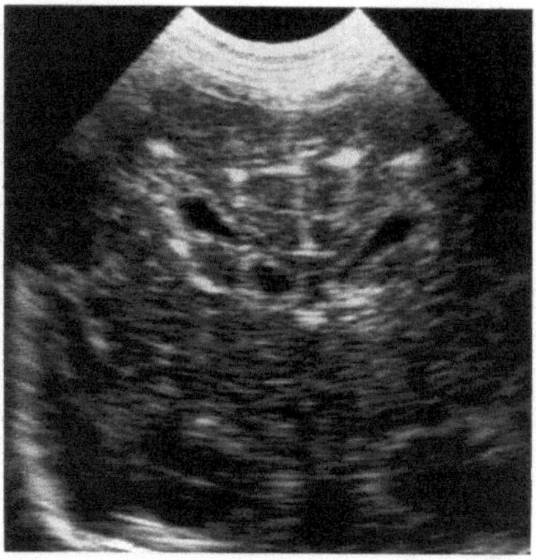

Fig. 3.35. Congenital cytomegalovirus infection. Multiple calcifications are visualized. A subependymal cyst is also noted in the floor of the left ventricle

Sonography also permits visualization of the extracerebral spaces and assessment of their size. Their access, however, can be limited by a small fontanelle. Ultrasonography will also aid in establishing the cause of ventriculomegaly or hydrocephalus. Finally, medical treatment, i.e. serial lumbar puncture or surgical interventions, can also be monitored by US.

3.9 Infections

In congenital, perinatal and postnatal infections, US appearances will depend on the timing of injury, with regard to brain development, and the type and virulence of the microorganism. Thus, an early intrauterine infection may lead to an impairment of organogenesis that might mimic a cerebral malformation, whereas a late infection may cause no detectable cerebral lesions.

Nowadays, ultrasonographic features of congenital rubella, toxoplasmosis and cytomegalovirus are well established (Fig. 3.35). Microcalcifications are a good marker of CNS infectious involvement and are easily detectable on US.

Bacterial meningitis and sepsis are associated with various cerebral complications depending mainly on the microorganism's etiopathogenic mechanism. Vascular injury and/or inflammatory processes may occur. In our experience, preterm infants will more likely develop early haemorrhagic and ischaemic lesions because of the high incidence of circulatory disturbances. Term infants will frequently present with ventriculitis, echogenic sulci, enlargement of CSF spaces, parenchymal increased echogenicities and abcesses (Naidich and Quencer 1986; Fawer 1990). However, not rarely no ultrasonographic abnormality is detected.

3.10 Congenital Malformations and Various Prenatal Disorders

US of the neonatal brain also provides the clinician with a very useful diagnostic tool for the detection of cerebral malformations. A wide variety of prenatal, structural, CNS anomalies can be diagnosed by US, i.e. malformations of the midline (agenesis of corpus callosum, holoprosencephaly, lipoma of corpus callosum), malformations of the posterior fossa (Dandy-Walker, megacisterna, cerebellar hypoplasia), hydrocephalus and external hydrocephalus, ventricular dilatation associated with meningocoele, arachnoid cysts, prenatal vascular anomalies (hydraencephaly, porencephaly, subependymal pseudocysts) and US appearances in some metabolic disorders. Exhaustive descriptions of congenital anomalies and their ultrasonographic diagnostic criteria have been extensively reported (Naidich and Quencer 1986; Fawer 1990). In addition, a good correlation with other brain imaging techniques and autopsy findings has been established. In the neonatal period, US should therefore be performed as a screening procedure in all clinical conditions in which a congenital malformation, is suspected in order to allow an early diagnosis, better management, better prognosis and, when necessary, genetic counselling.

3.11 The Limits of US

Like other imaging techniques, US has some limitations that should be recognized:

1. Pericerebral CSF spaces and cortex. Until recently, the peripheral regions of the brain, especially the *pericerebral CSF spaces and cortex,* were difficult to explore. Large subdural and subarachnoid haemorrhages, located on the convexity or in the parietal region, are readily identified on US. However, small haemorrhages are more difficult to detect on US and, furthermore, if recent, they are anechoic and indistinguishable from prominent normal CSF spaces. CT scannings should therefore be performed in critical clinical situations, when the formal exclusion of any of the above lesions cannot be ascertained by US. In addition, US does not differentiate subarachnoid from subdural haemorrhages and it is also unlikely that a small cortical haemorrhage will be detected.

Nowadays, sulci and gyri may be satisfactorily imaged with a high frequency transducer and sector scan, but magnetic resonance imaging is superior for detecting and defining abnormal gyration and myelination.

2. Posterior fossa: The investigation of the *posterior fossa* poses a few ultrasonographic limitations. A huge cisterna magna may be difficult to distinguish from a cyst of the posterior fossa, unless there is an association with a cerebellar hypoplasia.

Tentorium tear and a haematoma of the posterior fossa are also difficult to diagnose. The cerebellar tentorium is not directly visualized on US, as the beam is parallel to this structure.

3. Hypoxic-ischaemic lesions in the term asphyxiated infant. Ultrasonography, by itself, is of limited value in the acute management of infants with *hypoxic-ischaemic injuries.* Disturbances of brain metabolism and circulation are most commonly present well before the occurrence of morphological changes. CT scanning or US appear to have a better predictive value only after the first week of life. The prognosis of severely asphyxiated term infants or the decision to withdraw or continue intensive care should be therefore based on the global appreciation of the following methods: brain imaging, clinical examinations, Doppler and EEG.

4. Intraparenchymal increased echogenicities. Haematoma, thrombosis, venous infarction, tumor and lipoma appear on US as *heterogeneous increased echogenicities.* It is the infant's clinical condition that often offers some clue to the diagnosis. For precise diagnosis, CT scannings or magnetic resonance imaging is preferred.

3.12 The Prognosis Based on Ultrasonographic Appearances

The predictive value of US has been extensively investigated (Graham et al. 1987; Cooke 1987; Nwaesei et al. 1988; Bozynski et al. 1988; Calame and Fawer 1990). Despite the well-known "semantic ultrasonographic divergence" between investigators, reasonable conclusions can be drawn from these studies (Table 3.3). The most powerful US predictors for the development of major handicaps were found to be cystic PVL, late major haemorrhagic and ischaemic lesions and persistent increased echogenicities (Fawer et al. 1987). By contrast, a favourable scan and a normal neurologic examination near term were reported to be good predictors for normal developmental progress (Stewart et al. 1988). Very recently, Levene reviewed the current understanding of the significance of cerebral US abnormalities (Levene 1990).

In our experience, the timing of the scanning and a rigorous description of the lesions, with regard to the site, size and extent, are essential to achieve the most accurate ultrasonographic diagnosis. They are also necessary to establish a classification of US abnormalities based on explicit criteria, with special emphasis on white matter involvement, whatever the underlying pathologic condition. Our currently used US classification is illustrated in Fig. 3.6.

In the developmental unit of the paediatrics department in Lausanne, 132 children, born at 34 weeks gestation or less, were examined at 3½ years of age. Their neurodevelopmental outcome is shown in Fig. 3.7. The vertical axis represents the intellectual general index, obtained by the McCarthy children's abilities scale. The normal mean index is 100. There were 28 term infants in the control group. Preterm infants with normal scans, isolated haemorrhage and hydrocephalus had a good neurologic prognosis, whereas children with PVL had a variable outcome. In the latter group, 18 major handicaps were diagnosed.

Figure 3.38 shows the relationship which could be established between the

Table 3.3. US changes and prediction of outcome

Authors	Sensitivity (%)	Specificity (%)	Most powerful US predictor of handicaps	Most powerful predictor of normal neurodevelopmental progress
Graham et al. 1987	67	96	Cystic PVL Prolonged flare	
Cooke 1987	56	95	Late cystic PVL	
Nwaesei et al. 1988	58	100	Late major haemorrhagic and ischaemic lesions	
Bozynski et al. 1988	70	100	Late haemorrhagic and PVL lesions	
Calame and Fawer 1990	80	100	Cystic PVL, persistent increased echogenicity	
Stewart et al. 1988	62	100		Favourable scan and normal neurological examination near term

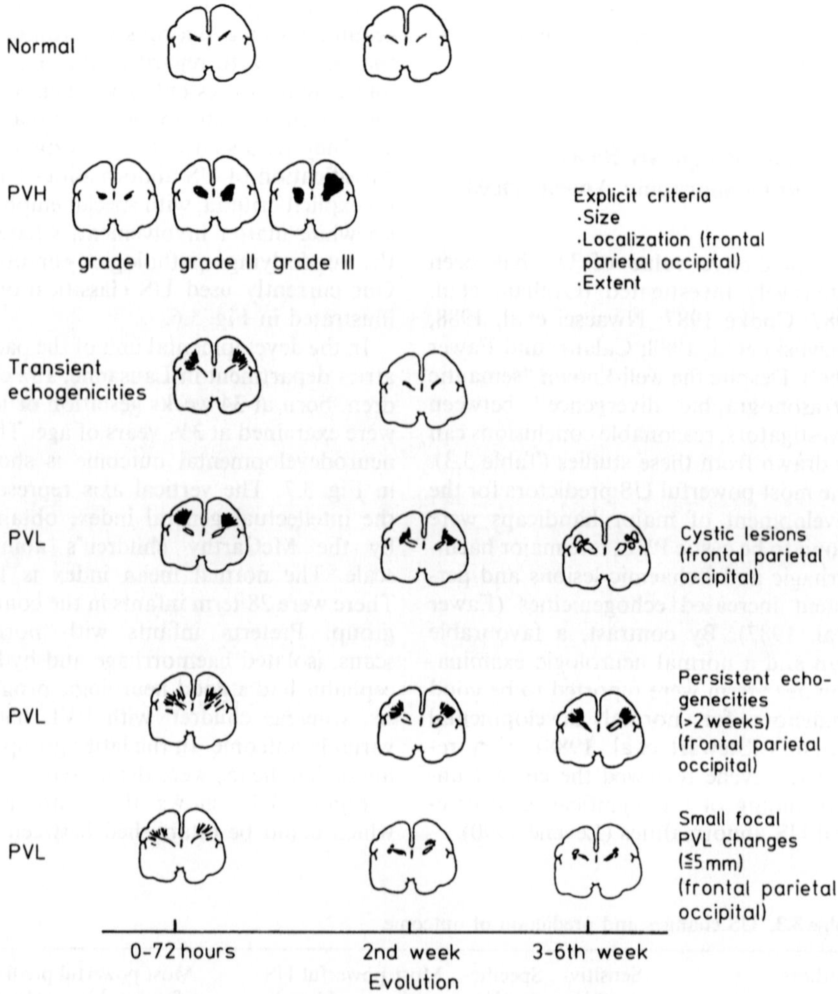

Fig. 3.36. Classification of US findings with criteria regarding size, extent, localization and evolution of the lesion

size and extent of the PVL lesions and the type and severity of the handicaps. All children with isolated PVL changes in the frontal areas developed normally. Among children with frontal and parietal lesions, seven had a major handicap. Children with extensive lesions in the frontal, parietal and occipital regions had a poor prognosis, as most of them developed a multiple handicap (cerebral palsy, visual impairment and mental retardation).

A further study was undertaken to determine whether small, focal PVL changes had any effect on late cognitive function at 5 years of age. Fine psychometric abilities measured in the PVL group were compared with those of children with normal scans and isolated haemorrhage (Fig. 3.39). Mean scores of verbal, perceptual performance quantitative, memory and motor subscales were lower in the small, focal PVL group. This

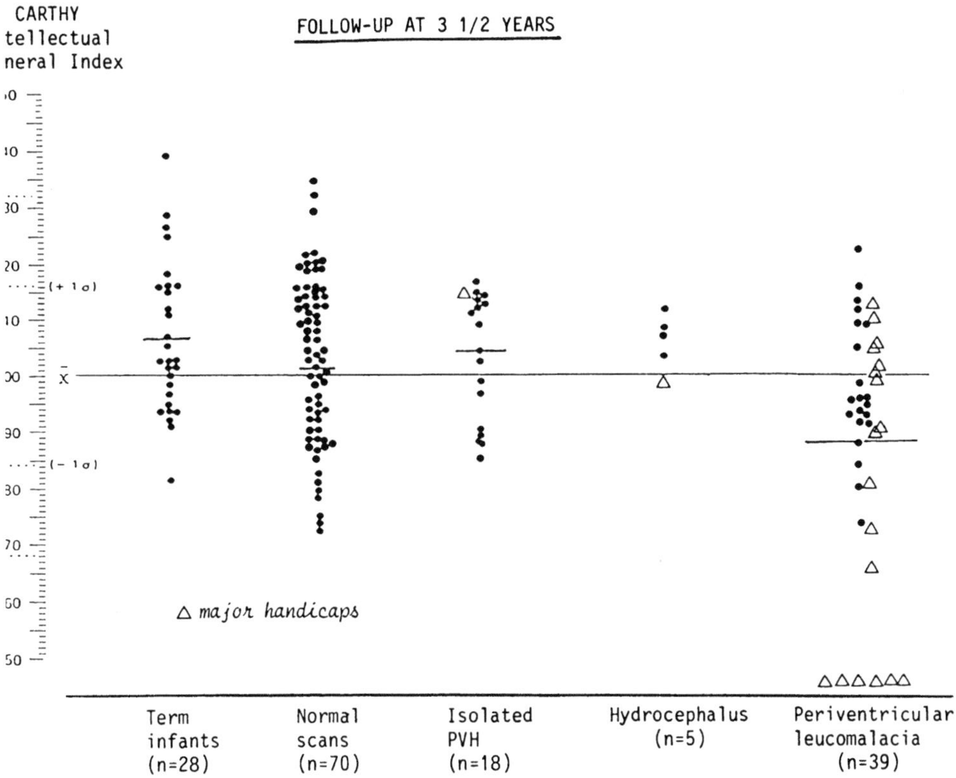

Fig. 3.37. Outcome at 3½ years of age: US changes, general intellectual index and major handicap

difference did reach statistical significance for the motor subscale. Moreover, the children with small changes of PVL were also noted to present with more abnormal neuromotor signs and more attention deficit. Minor US changes in the periventricular white matter therefore cannot be ignored, as they might represent a morphological marker of a more diffuse brain injury. A few post-mortem neuropathologic reports have already demonstrated diffuse gliosis and other various hypoxic-ischaemic microscopic changes in brains of preterm infants. This recent work (Fawer and Calame 1991) indicates that small, focal PVL lesions seem to interfere with cognitive development at 5 years of age, suggesting that the later learning disorders and school problems described in very low birthweight children might have this morphological substrate. Further studies are warranted to confirm this hypothesis and to assess the importance of environment on outcome.

3.13 Conclusions and Perspectives

Improvements in both obstetrics and neonatal intensive care have accounted for a reduction in perinatal mortality over the last 20 years. At present, most neonatologists have adopted a dynamic approach including full resuscitation and artificial ventilation for even the smallest infants. With the advent of noninvasive

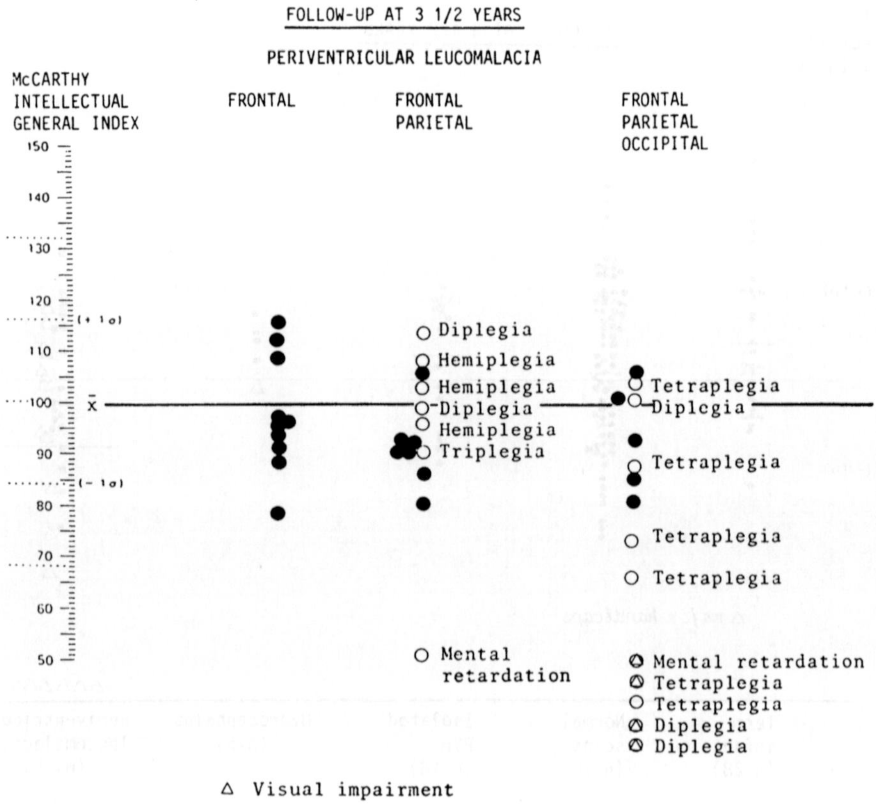

Fig. 3.38. Relationship between size and extent of PVL lesions and type and severity of handicap

imaging techniques, neonatal intensive care has become "brain-oriented". The task of the neonatologist encompasses regular reappraisals of quality of care, diagnosis and prognosis. Over the last decade, the practice of regular scanning, the correlation with neuropathology and the experience of long-term follow-up studies have allowed us to believe that recognition of brain lesions in the neonatal period by US enables the identification of infants at highest risk for subsequent major neurodevelopmental impairments. Although any prediction of the future is difficult, we are nevertheless now in a better position than 15 years ago to make some prognosis for the neonates who come under our care.

Although there are constant technolocial advances in exploring the perinatal brain, US imaging is still the first choice because it is a well established investigative procedure and its advantages are widely recognized. With further application of current ultrasonography, both fetal and neonatal brains will be evaluated accurately. With optimal spatial resolution, we can expect the display of almost all important anatomic features of the CNS and the detection of structural anomalies and cerebral lesions which may develop prenatally or perina-

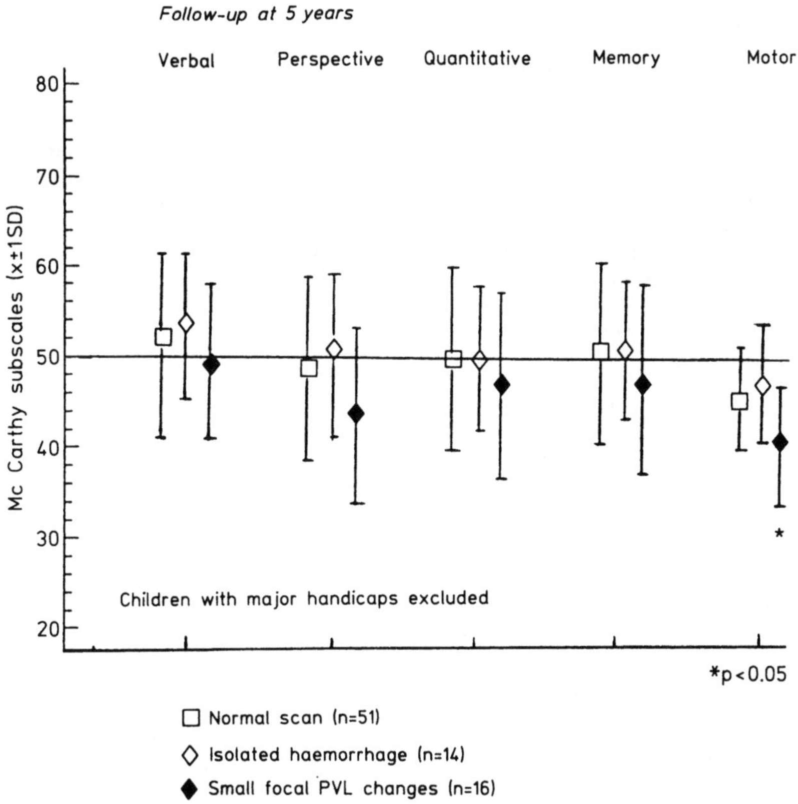

Fig. 3.39. Fine psychometric abilities at 5 years of age of children with normal scans, isolated haemorrhage and small focal PVL changes

tally. Their detection will be extremely helpful in providing the clinician with information regarding the type and timing of the insult. This is an essential issue when attempting to achieve the best possible outcome for the fetus and for the premature infant. The sequential application of US throughout fetal and neonatal development and the exploitation of the full potentials of this technique should also enlighten epidemiological studies which investigate the etiological causes of major handicaps and which question the role of intensive care in the changing panorama of cerebral palsy.

Further correlation studies based on imaging techniques and other modalities, neuropathology and long-term neurodevelopmental data will help in the diagnosis, assessment and prognosis of brain lesions. Better knowledge of neuroanatomy and of pathogenesis will also help define guidelines for better neonatal care and for a rational health policy.

Acknowledgements. We wish to thank Dr. K. Schisler for help in preparing the manuscript and M. Marion for secretarial assistance. We also thank Prof. R. Laurini for the neuropathological illustrations. This work was supported by the Swiss National Science Foundation No 32-25474.88.

References

Banker BW, Larroche JC (1962) Periventricular leukomalacia of infancy: a form of neonatal anoxic encephelopathy. Arch Neurol 7:386–410

Bozynski MEA, Nelson MN, Genaze D et al. (1988) Cranial ultrasonography and the prediction of cerebral palsy in infants weighing <1200 grams at birth. Dev Med Child Neurol 30:342–348

Calame A, Fawer CL (1990) Prognostic value of cerebral ultrasound and Doppler during the first weeks of life. In: Duc G, Huch A, Huch R (eds) The very low birthweight infant: a challenge to neonatology and obstetrics. Thieme, Stuttgart, pp 14–24

Cooke RWI (1987) Early and late cranial ultrasonographic appearances and outcome in very low birthweight infants. Arch Dis Child 62:931–937

DeVries LS, Wigglesworth JS, Regev R, Dubowitz LMS (1988) Evolution of periventricular leukomalacia during the neonatal period and infancy: correlation of imaging and postmortem findings. Early Hum Dev 17:205–219

Fawer CL (1990) Transfontanelläre Hirnuntersuchung. In: Schulz RD, Willi UV (eds) Atlas der Ultraschalldiagnostik beim Kind. Thieme, Stuttgart, pp 1–23

Fawer CL, Calame A (1991) Significance of ultrasound appearances in the neurological development and cognitive abilities of preterm infants at five years. Eur J Pediatr 150:512–520

Fawer CL, Diebold P, Calame A (1987) Periventricular leucomalacia and neurodevelopmental outcome in preterm infants. Arch Dis Child 62:30–36

Graham M, Levene MI, Trounce JQ, Rutter N (1987) Prediction of cerebral palsy in very low birthweight infants: prospective ultrasound study. Lancet ii:593–596

Hope PL, Gould SJ, Howard S, Hamilton PA, Costello AML, Reynolds EOR (1988) Precision of ultrasound diagnosis of pathologically verified lesions in the brains of very preterm infants. Dev Med Child Neurol 30:457–471

Levene MI (1990) Cerebral ultrasound and neurological impairment: telling the future. Arch Dis Child 65:469–471

Naidich TP, Quencer RMJ (1986) Clinical neurosonography. Neuroradiology 28:379–640

Nwaesei CG, Pape KE, Martin DJ et al. (1984) Periventricular infarction diagnosis by ultrasound: a post-mortem correlation. J Pediatr 105:106–110

Nwaesei CG, Allen AC, Vineer MJ, Brown SJ, Stinson DA, Evans JR, Byrne JM (1988) Effect of timing of cerebral ultrasound on the prediction of later neurodevelopmental outcome in high-risk preterm infants. J Pediatr 112:970–975

Paneth N, Rudelli R, Monte W, Rodriguez E, Pinto J, Kairam R, Kazam E (1990) White matter necrosis in very low birth weight infants: neuropathologic and ultrasonographic findings in infants surviving six days or longer. J Pediatr 116:975–984

Pape KE, Bennett-Britton S, Szymonowicz W, Martin DJ, Fitz CR, Becker L (1983) Diagnostic accuracy of neonatal brain imaging: a postmortem correlation of computed tomography and ultrasound scans. J Pediatr 275–280

Stewart A, Hope PL, Hamilton P et al. (1988) Prediction in very preterm infants of satisfactory neurodevelopmental progress at 12 months. Dev Med Child Neurol 30:53–63

Szymonowicz W, Schafler K, Cussen LJ (1984) Ultrasound and necropsy study of periventricular haemorrhage in preterm infants. Arch Dis Child 59:637–642

Trounce JQ, Fagan D, Levene MI (1986) Intraventricular haemorrhage and periventricular leukomalacia: ultrasound and autopsy correlation. Arch Dis Child 61:1203–1207

4 Cerebral Doppler in the Neonate

J. MESSER

CONTENTS

4.1 Introduction

The pathogenesis of most brain disorders encountered in the neonatal brain is related to altered cerebral blood flow (CBF). This fact concerns the full-term newborn, and especially the premature baby. For that reason, neonatologists have long been interested in evaluating the cerebral perfusion of their patients. However, the study of neonatal cerebral circulation has been difficult due to a lack of suitable techniques. Xenon clearance, jugular venous occlusion plethysmography and, more recently, positron emission tomography have all drawbacks. They are more or less invasive, expensive, and not available in all neonatal units and, in any case, give only instantaneous information. Consequently, the Doppler ultrasound technique, which is noninvasive and can be repeated at the bedside, has provoked considerable interest and encouraged several studies by pediatricians since the pioneering work of Bada et al. in 1979.

4.2 Principles and Method

4.2.1 The Doppler Effect

The frequency of sound waves reflected from a moving object is shifted by an amount proportional to the velocity of the object. Thus, ultrasound waves emitted by a transducer are reflected by moving red blood cells and their frequency is shifted proportional to the blood velocity.

The Doppler shift is expressed by the following formula:

$$F = 2 \times F_0 \times v \cos \alpha / c$$

where F = Doppler shift (Hz); F_0 = mean frequency of the emitted ultrasound; v = blood flow velocity (cm/s); α = angle between the direction of the sound beam and the axis of the blood flow and c = velocity of sound in tissue (1.550 m/s).

If angle α and the emitting frequency remain constant, the Doppler shift is proportional to the blood velocity; a maximum shift value is obtained if the angle α is near 0°.

4.2.2 Techniques

There are different technique modalities which use the Doppler effect:

1. Continuous wave technique: The ultrasound beam is continuously transmitted by an oscillatory piezo element. Signals from the whole penetration depth of the ultrasonic waves are measured.

2. Pulsed (or range gated) technique: Only pulses of millisecond duration are transmitted intermittently. By varying the receiving time, one can record the signals reflected from a defined area at a determined depth (sample volume).

3. Duplex scan technique: This is a combination of the two-dimensional ultrasonic technique with pulsed Doppler sonography. Under visual control, a sample volume in the region of interest can be chosen.

4. Transcranial Doppler (TCD) sonography (pulsed technique): This technique uses low emitting frequencies (2 MHz), so that ultrasonic beams can penetrate through thin "windows" of the skull, such as the thin temporal bone. This technique allows studies of the intracranial vessels. Higher emitting frequencies do not easily cross bone so that the open fontanelle has to be used as a window.

4.2.3 Doppler Parameters

Doppler signal contains a spectrum of frequencies corresponding to the parabolic velocity profile of red cells in the vessels. Velocities are calculated according to the equation:

$$V = F \times c/(2 \times F_0 \times \cos \alpha)$$

Different parameters can be defined: the systolic peak flow velocity (v_s), the mean peak flow velocity (v_m) and the diastolic peak flow velocity (v_d).

They are obtained from the envelope curve of the Doppler frequency spectra: (a) the resistance index (RI) of Pourcelot

$$= \frac{(v_s - v_d)}{v_s}$$

(b) the pulsatility index (PI) of Gosling

$$= \frac{(v_s - v_d)}{v_m}$$

and (c) the area under the Doppler curve (AUC)

$$= v_m \times (t_2 - t_1)$$

where t_1 is the beginning of the wave and t_2 the end.

4.3 Neonatal Applications

4.3.1 Method

The open anterior fontanelle of the newborn represents a unique "window" allowing studies of intracranial vessels using relatively high frequencies (4–8 MHz). The arteries which can be investigated are the anterior cerebral artery, at a depth of 25 mm from the skin, and the internal carotid artery, at a depth of 50–70 mm.

With TCD one can record velocities of the middle cerebral artery, through the temporal bone with an angle of nearly 0°, and of the posterior cerebral artery.

Parameters which influence velocities and which have to be considered in Doppler data interpretation are: (a) Postnatal and gestational age (GA), birthweight, blood pressure (velocities increase); (b) hematocrit (velocities inversely related) and (c) blood gases (high PCO_2 increases velocities, low PCO_2 decreases).

4.3.2 Normal Results

The recording is best performed during quiet sleep. As many parameters can influence the Doppler signal, one always has to know the clinical and biological condition of the patient in order to interpret correctly Doppler curves of the neonate: arterial blood pressure, blood gases, hematocrit, blood sugar, spontaneous or artificial ventilation, presence of a patent ductus arteriosus, different medications.

We show here results obtained during the first and third days after birth of 30 full-term healthy neonates examined with TCD sonography using a 2 MHz frequency transducer (Table 4.1; Grojean-Gibondi 1988). Bode has shown that the values obtained by TCD correlate well with duplex scan sonography (Bode 1988).

Table 4.1. Velocities (cm/s) recorded in 30 full-term healthy neonates on the first and third day (from Grojean-Gibondi 1988)

	Day 1	Day 3
RMCA		
V_s	45.46±8.62	54.33±8.59
V_d	16.28±3.47	19.39±3.22
V_m	22.86±4.56	28.6 ±5.01
ACA		
V_s	36.26±6.25	42.46±9.4
V_d	13.22±2.75	15.55±4.04
V_m	19.4 ±3.32	22.53±5.06
RICA		
V_s	43.53±8.49	48.4 ±8.34
V_d	15.07±3.79	17.42±4.14
V_m	23.2 ±4.62	26.26±5.16

RMCA, right middle cerebral artery; ACA, anterior cerebral artery; RICA, right internal carotid artery

4.3.2.1 Physiological Variations

The velocities of all cerebral arteries correlate with postnatal age. They increase regularly during the first month of life (Fig. 4.1). Values of RI decrease between birth and the third day of life (RI at 0.64 the 3rd day). Velocities are also correlated with GA (lower with low GA) and birthweight (lower with low birthweight). In premature and low birthweight infants, diastolic velocities are low and often near zero.

Velocities are inversely correlated with hematocrit. There is a parallel increase, during the first days of life, in both blood pressure and cerebral arterial velocities.

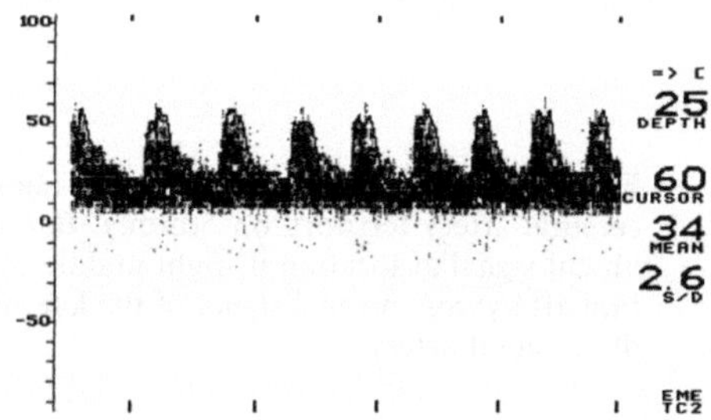

Fig. 4.1. Doppler recording of right middle cerebral artery in a full-term newborn on the 5th day of life; V_s, 60 cm/s; V_m, 34 cm/s; V_d, 20 cm/s

4.3.3 Abnormalities

4.3.3.1 Perinatal Asphyxia

Most studies have found an increase in diastolic velocities in full-term infants with severe birth asphyxia (Fig. 4.2); consequently, there is a decrease in the RI (Archer et al. 1986; Levene et al. 1989). These modifications could be the result of a decrease in arteriolar vascular resistance, i.e. a maximal arteriolar dilatation resulting from liberation of local metabolites. Archer et al. (1986), found that a decrease in RI in the first days of life carried a poor long-term neurologic prognosis. However, it should be noted

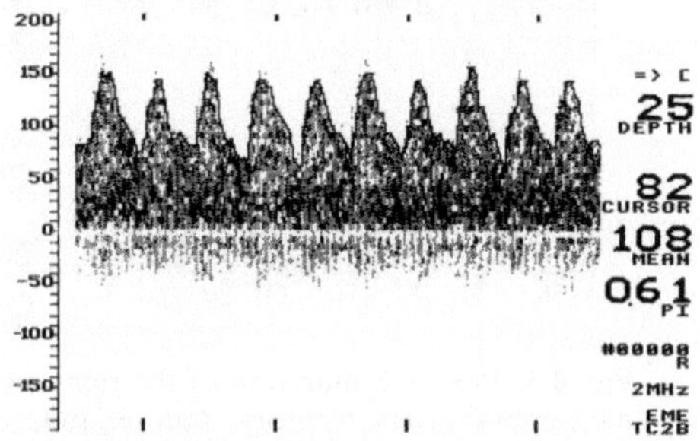

Fig. 4.2. Perinatal asphyxia on 2nd day of life; high velocities, RI = 0.22

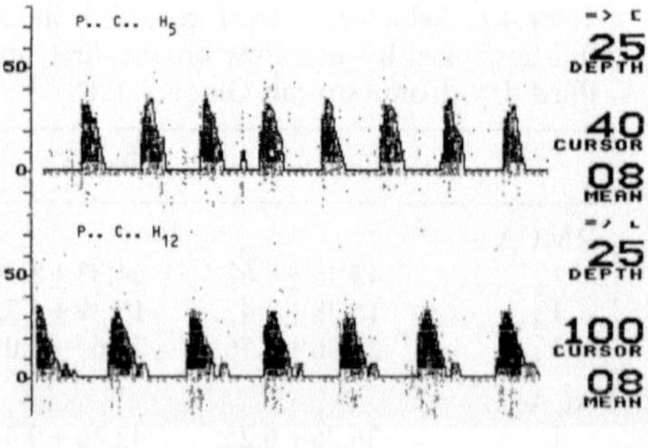

Fig. 4.3. Perinatal asphyxia. Low velocities in this first hours of life

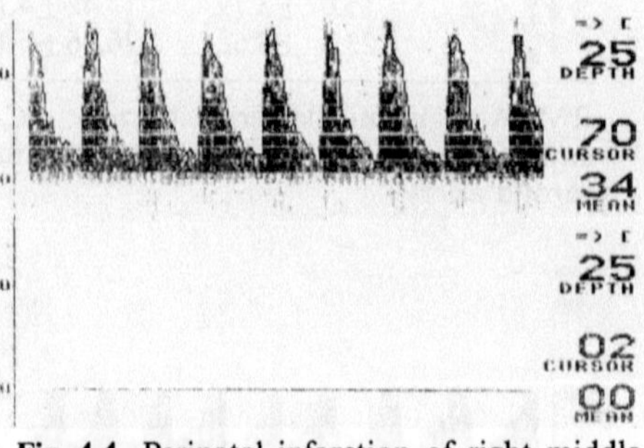

Fig. 4.4. Perinatal infarction of right middle cerebral artery territory on 5th day. *Bottom*, absent signal at location of right middle cerebral artery; *top*, normal signal of the left middle cerebral artery

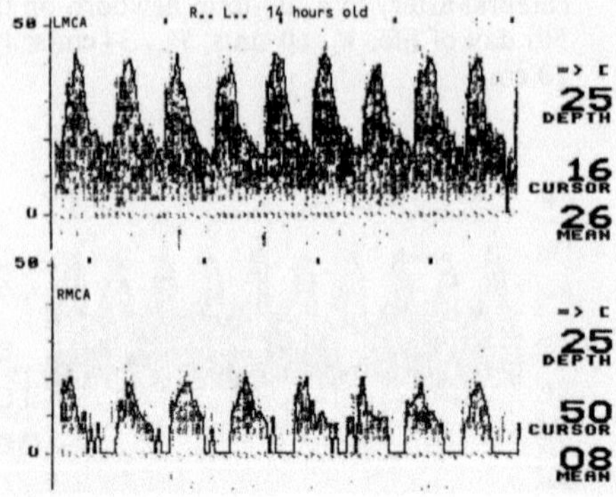

Fig. 4.5. Prenatal infarction of the right middle cerebral artery territory. *Bottom*, reduced signal of right middle cerebral artery (*RMCA*); *top*, normal signal of the left middle cerebral artery (LMCA)

that some babies show low CBF velocities in the first hours after birth (Fig. 4.3) which could be caused by an arteriolar vasospasm (Levene et al. 1989).

4.3.3.2 Intracranial Hemorrhages or Cerebral Ischemia of Premature Babies

Many investigators hoped that using Doppler technique immediately after birth would allow better understanding of the pathogenesis of cerebral hemorrhages and ischaemic brain insults in premature babies. These studies have not succeeded and data obtained are conflicting. Nonetheless, high velocities have been recorded on the side of the injury at the time of occurrence of intraventricular hemorrhage (IVH). During the following days, velocities were reduced on both sides (Ment et al. 1984).

4.3.3.3 Cerebral Infarction

The middle cerebral artery (MCA) is the most frequent site of obstruction in neonatal cerebral infarction. In such instances, we observed an absence of signal or diminished flow velocities of the MCA on the side of the infarction. In one cerebral infarction, which occurred near birth, the signal was absent during the first few days (Fig. 4.4) and reappeared on the tenth day, corresponding to recanalization. In another infarction, which occurred in utero, signal was present at birth but markedly reduced (Fig. 4.5). In all patients with cerebral infarction, low velocities persisted during the first months of life (Messer et al. 1991).

4.3.3.4 Polycythemia

Polycythemia increases blood viscosity and the Doppler signal is generally reduced. By contrast, during marked anemia, one can record high velocities. This is well illustrated in patients with twin

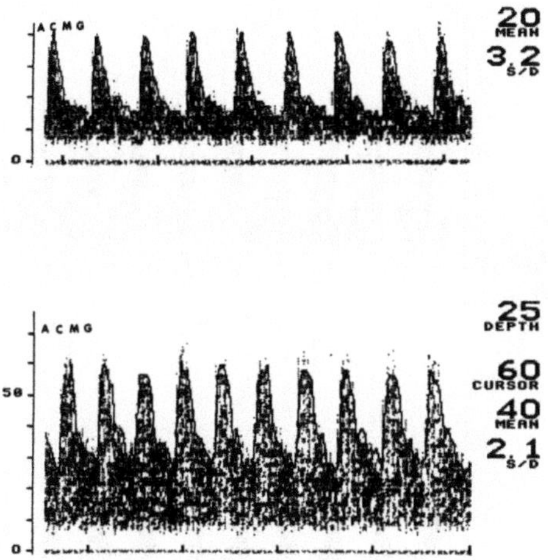

Fig. 4.6. Neonatal polycythemia. *Top*, before partial exchange transfusion; *bottom*, afterward

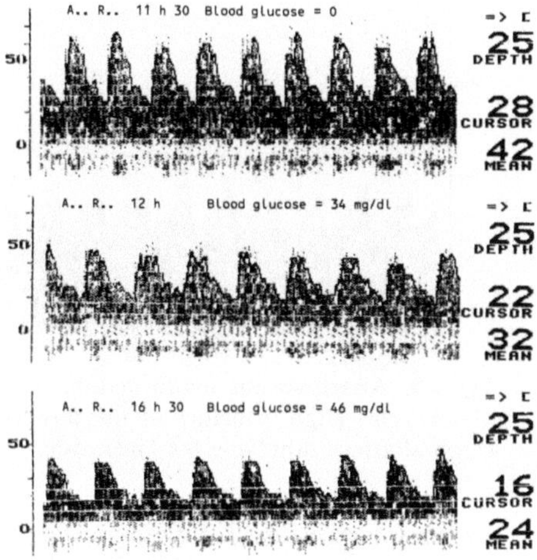

Fig. 4.7. High velocities during hypoglycemia. Velocities decrease after correction

fetofetal transfusion syndrome. The effect of partial exchange transfusion in polycythemia can be noted by a restoration of higher velocities (Fig. 4.6) (Maertzdorf et al. 1989).

4.3.3.5 Hypoglycemia

During hypoglycemia occurring in small for GA infants, we recorded high velocities, which decreased slowly to the normal range after IV glucose perfusion (Fig. 4.7). This observation is in accordance with Pryds' data showing an increase of CBF during hypoglycemia in preterm babies (Pryds et al. 1990a).

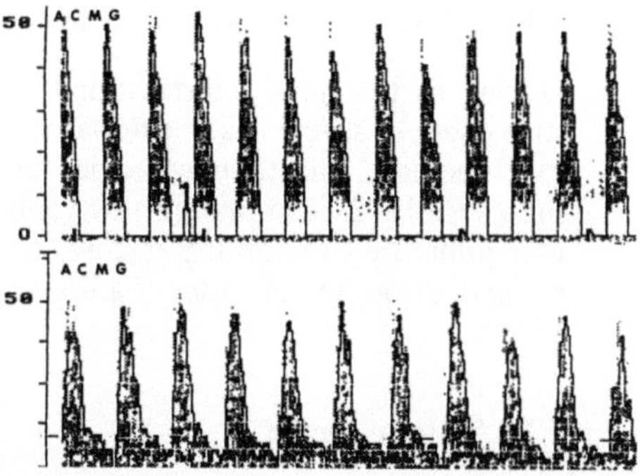

Fig. 4.8. Patent ductus arteriosus in a premature baby. *Top*, absent diastolic signal; *bottom*, after indomethacin therapy, restoration of a positive diastolic velocity

4.3.3.6 Vascular Abnormalities

Patent ductus arteriosus is frequent among prematures. One observes a reduction of diastolic velocity or even its abolition and, if the left to right shunt is significant, a negative diastolic velocity in relation to diastolic flow from the aorta to the pulmonary artery through the ductus. This abnormal pattern disappears after medical treatment (indomethacin) or surgical closure (Fig. 4.8). The same recordings are obtained in heart defects with dependence on a left to right shunt through the ductus. Recordings do not show such abnormalities when the ductus is shunting from right to left, such as in persistent fetal circulation or pulmonary hypertension of the neonate.

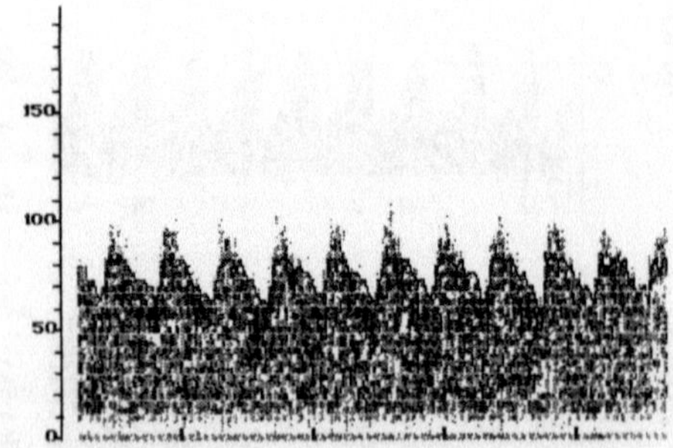

Fig. 4.9. Arteriovenous malformation of the Galen vein. High velocities in the posterior cerebral artery supplying the Galen vein

In arteriovenous malformation of the Galen vein, one records a high diastolic velocity in the arteries supplying the Galen vein, which represents a low resistance vessel (Fig. 4.9).

4.3.3.7 Increased Intracranial Pressure

During hydrocephaly, intracranial pressure rises. In severe cases, arterial velocities decrease, diastolic velocities more than systolic. Decompression by ventricular puncture or shunting restores more normal diastolic velocities (Saliba et al. 1985).

4.3.3.8 Brain Death

One can observe a characteristic sequence of deterioration of the flow velocities during evolution to brain death: reduction followed by abolition of diastolic velocities, appearance of diastolic retrograde flow, reduction of systolic velocities and, last, no detectable signal in the cerebral circulation (Fig. 4.10). Doppler technique appears as a useful noninvasive complement to other methods in the determination of brain death in the newborn.

4.3.3.9 Therapy

Doppler technique has been successfully used to acquire information about the

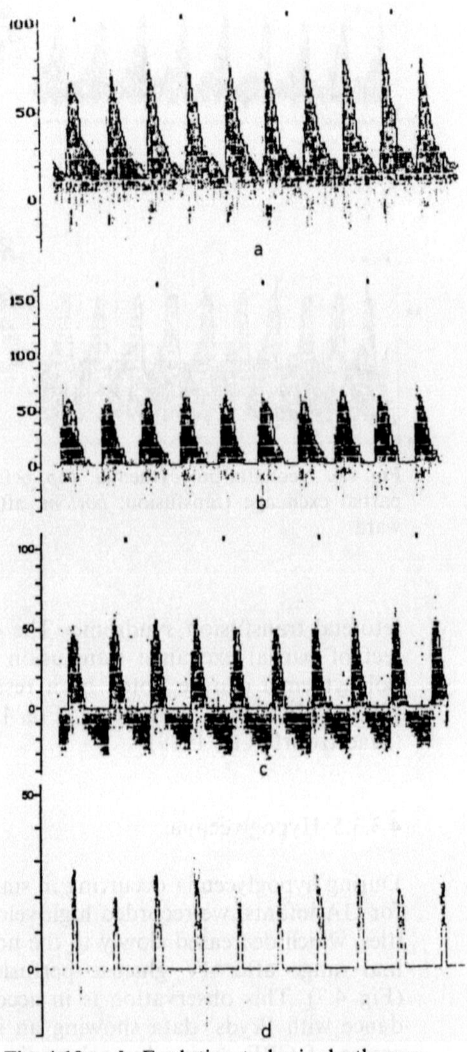

Fig. 4.10 a–d. Evolution to brain death: **a** reduced diastolic velocities; **b** absent diastolic velocity; **c** diastolic retrograde flow; **d** reduction of systolic velocities

effects of different treatments on the cerebral circulation:

1. *Artificial ventilation:* During hyperventilation with hypocapnia, one records a reduction of the Doppler signal. If the baby is hypoventilated and hypercapnic there is an increase. Thus, the vasodilator

effect of hypercapnia and vasoconstrictor effect of hypocapnia can be illustrated. Vasoreactivity to CO_2 can be evaluated, thereby providing prognostic information (Pryds et al. 1990b). Hyperoxia can reduce flow velocities (Nijima et al. 1988). During tracheal suctioning, pneumothorax or seizures, cerebral artery velocities increase. Perlman and Volpe showed, in premature babies on ventilators, fluctuating velocities in the anterior cerebral arteries associated with a high incidence of IVH. They could abolish these fluctuations with administration of curare and noted a decrease of intracranial hemorrhages (Perlman et al. 1983).

The administration of surfactant improves hematosis and can influence cerebral arterial velocities by changes in blood gases, so that the ventilation settings have to be adjusted carefully (Jorch et al. 1989).

2. *Drugs:* Indomethacin and barbiturates decrease the Doppler signal (Fig. 4.11). Halothane decreases flow velocities and seems to impair CBF autoregulation (Messer et al. 1989) (Fig. 4.12). Curare and caffeine have little effect.

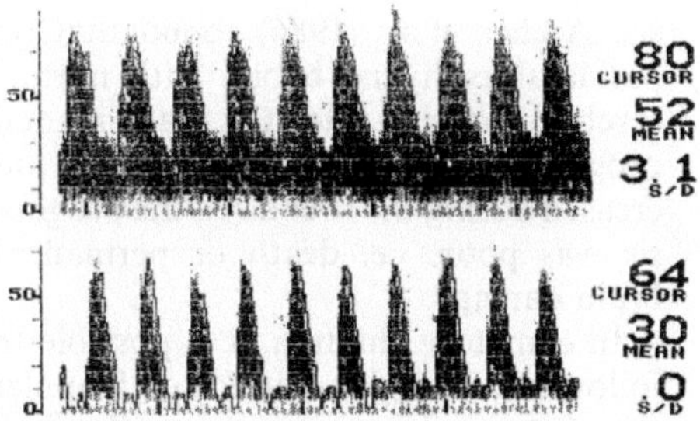

Fig. 4.11. Effect of thiopental anesthesia on CBFV of right middle cerebral artery in an infant. *Top*, before anesthesia, *Bottom*, during anesthesia

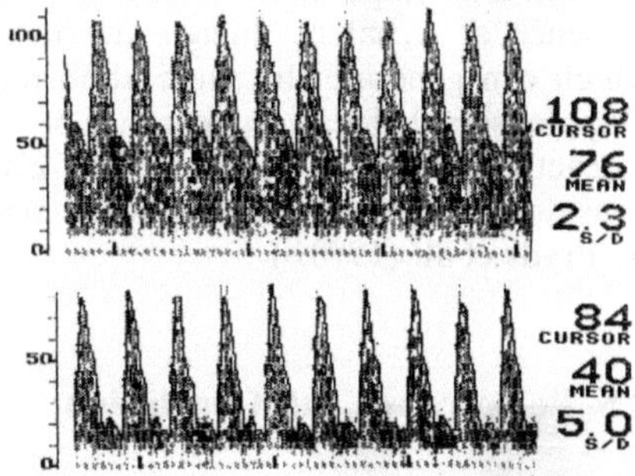

Fig. 4.12. Effect of halothane anesthesia on CBFV of right middle cerebral artery in an infant. *Top*, before anesthesia; *bottom*, during anesthesia

4.3.4 Limits of the Technique

It is the estimation of CBF which interests the neonatologist, not the velocity by itself. Do Doppler measurements of CBF velocity actually reflect changes in CBF? Different studies comparing Doppler to microspheres in animals (Hansen et al. 1983) and to radioactive xenon in humans (Greisen et al. 1984) have reported good correlations between Doppler data and CBF estimated by these other techniques. The correlation was closer with the pulsed technique using the AUC as the compared parameter.

A prerequisite for validating Doppler measurements for estimation of CBF is that the diameter of the vessel studied does not change: it is well known that vasoactivity occurs essentially in cerebral arterioles and is limited in the proximal part of basal cerebral arteries. The major changes therefore occur at a level distal to the site of insonation. Thus, most often, high velocities, especially high diastolic velocities, are related to high CBF. We obtain, of course, only relative values of CBF; to obtain absolute values would require simultaneous measurement of the diameter of the vessel, which is not possible now.

4.4 Prognosis

At the present time, some Doppler aspects have been related to a poor prognosis. Archer et al. (1986) found that, in perinatal asphyxia, babies with normal cerebral arterial velocities had a good prognosis; however, if these were increased during the first days, the prognosis was poor, i.e. death or permanent brain damage.

In comatose children, it is possible to follow the changing pattern of Doppler signals towards a progressive reduction, suggesting evolution to brain death. In our experience, when one records a Doppler signal with a retrograde flow during the entire diastole in all cerebral arteries, the evolution is irreversible. Of course, it is imperative to exclude the presence of a patent ductus arteriosus which can generate the same abnormal Doppler signal. The disappearance of vasoreactivity to PCO_2 changes was also considered to be a poor prognostic sign by Pryds et al. (1990b).

4.5 Perspectives and Conclusion

At the moment, the Doppler technique, as applied to cerebral arteries, has markedly improved our knowledge about the cerebral circulation in both physiologic and pathologic conditions. However, we gain information only about changes in CBF and not about absolute values. If, in the future, it is possible to measure the diameter of the vessel insonated, we will be able to determinate absolute values of blood flow. Another perspective is the use of continuous recordings allowing monitoring of cerebral hemodynamics. The problems of fixing the probe are currently being resolved (the ultrasonic power must be limited to avoid deleterious effects of long-term insonation). At the present time, clinical applications include perinatal asphyxia, patent ductus arteriosus, hydrocephaly, brain death and drug effects on CBF.

References

Archer LNJ, Levene MI, Evans DH (1986) Cerebral artery Doppler ultrasonography for prediction of outcome after perinatal asphyxia. Lancet ii:1116–1118

Bada HSA, Hajjar W, Chua C, Summer DS (1979) Noninvasive diagnosis of neonatal asphyxia and intra-ventricular hemorrhage by Doppler ultrasound. J Pediatr 95:775–779

Bode H (1988) Pediatric applications of transcranial Doppler sonography. Springer, Berlin Heidelberg New York

Greisen G, Johansen K, Ellison PH, Fredriksen PS, Mali J, Friis-Hansen B (1984) Cerebral blood flow in the newborn infant: comparison of Doppler ultrasound and [133]xenon clearance. J Pediatr 104:411–418

Grojean-Gibondi F (1988) Etude de la vélocimétrie artérielle intracérébrale chez le nouveau-né normal, à terme, à J1 et J3. Thesis, Louis Pasteur University, Strasbourg

Hansen NB, Stonestreet BS, Rosenkrantz TS, Oh W (1983) Validity of Doppler measurements of anterior cerebral artery blood velocity: correlation with brain blood flow in piglets. Pediatrics 72:526–531

Jorch G, Rabe H, Garbe M, Michel E, Gortner L (1989) Acute and protracted effects of intratracheal surfactant application on internal carotid blood flow velocity, blood pressure and carbon dioxide tension in very low birth weight infants. Eur J Pediatr 148:770–773

Levene MI, Fenton AC, Evans DH, Archer LNJ, Shortland DB, Gibson NA (1989) Severe birth asphyxia and abnormal cerebral blood flow velocity. Dev Med Child Neurol 31:427–434

Maertzdorf WJ, Tangelder GJ, Slaaf DW, Blanco CE (1989) Effects of partial plasma exchange transfusion on cerebral blood flow velocity in polycythaemic preterm, term and small for date newborn infants. Eur J Pediatr 148:774–778

Ment IR, Duncan CC, Ehrenkranz RA, Lange RC, Taylor KJ, Kleinman CS, Scott DT, Sivo J, Gettner P (1984) Intraventricular hemorrhage in the preterm neonate: timing and cerebral blood flow changes. J Pediatr 104:419–425

Messer J, Haddad J, Bientz J, Jochum D (1989) Influence of anesthetics on cerebral blood flow velocity in infancy. Dev Pharmacol Ther 13:145–149

Messer J, Haddad J, Casanova R (1991) Transcranial Doppler evaluation of cerebral infarction in the neonate. Neuropediatrics (in press)

Nijima S, Shortland DB, Levene MI, Evans DH (1988) Transient hyperoxia and cerebral blood flow velocity in infants born prematurely and at full term. Arch Dis Child 63:1126–1130

Perlman JM, McMenamin JB, Volpe JJ (1983) Fluctuating cerebral blood flow velocity in respiratory distress syndrome. N Engl J Med 309:203–209

Pryds O, Christensen NJ, Friis-Hansen B (1990a) Increased cerebral blood flow and plasma epinephrine in hypoglycemic preterm neonates. Pediatrics 85:172–176

Pryds O, Greisen G, Lou H, Friis-Hansen B (1990b) Vasoparalysis associated with brain damage in asphyxiated term infants. J Pediatr 117:119–125

Saliba E, Santini JJ, Arbeille P, Cherghi A, Gold F, Pourcelot L, Laugier J (1985) Mesure noninvasive du flux sanguin cérébral chez le nourrisson hydrocéphale. Arch Fr Pédiatr 42:97–102

5 Magnetic Resonance Spectroscopy

E. B. Cady, J. Hennig, and E. Martin

CONTENTS

5.1 Introduction

This chapter is devoted to magnetic resonance spectroscopy (MRS) of the brain in neonates and young infants. The application of MRS to the noninvasive assessment of cerebral metabolism in vivo is new in neuroscience and is certainly one of the most exciting recent developments in paediatric research. Information available to date on the safety of magnetic resonance (MR) gives strong indication that there are no health risks involved and long-term sequelae are not to be expected when present safety recommendations are adhered to (Shellock 1989).

In order to be detectable, the molecules of the chemical species under investigation have to carry suitable isotopes (see Sect. 5.2). In addition, they have to be mobile – preferably in solution (in order to obtain well-resolved resonances) – and in a sufficiently high concentration. The latter is one of the major limiting factors of in vivo MRS. Minimum detectable concentrations depend on the particular nucleus (via both the relative MR sensitivity and the natural abundance of the MR visible isotope), the magnetic field strength (B_0) and its homogeneity, the size of the observed volume and the examination time available. In order to obtain adequate spectral resolution (i.e. good frequency separation of the resonances), a B_0 of 1.5 T or higher is required normally, whereas magnetic resonance imaging (MRI) can be performed with B_0 as low as 0.02 T. As a general rule, concentrations must be above 0.5 mmol/kg wet weight for a given substance to be detected. To improve the signal to noise ratio (SNR) for a given B_0, the number of measurements averaged has to be high, which leads to long examination times – often as much as 1 h. Newer and more sophisticated MR methods (e.g. spectral editing or heteronuclear experiments, see Sect. 5.2) can potentially increase the SNR under certain circumstances. The ^1H nucleus is the most intrinsically sensitive and also the most abundant nucleus in living tissues, hence the ^1H water signal is used for clinical applications of MRI. Considering equal concentrations, the ^{31}P nucleus has a sensitivity of about 7% of that of ^1H. Furthermore, the concentrations of mobile phosphates in brain are low (a few mmol/kg wet weight), further reducing the signal obtained. The low natural abundance, low signal strength and low concentrations of ^{13}C metabolites give rise to even weaker signals. ^{19}F has almost the same sensitivity as ^1H, but is practically absent in living tissue, unless administered through, e.g. fluorinated anaesthetics. Generally, a lack in sensitivity has to be compensated for by lower spatial or time resolution, i.e. increased sensitive volume (voxel) size or longer data collections. Minimal voxel size for ^{31}P is around 27 cc at present field strengths.

The first horizontal-bore superconducting magnet MR systems available for clinical spectroscopy had narrow apertures. Therefore, studies of cerebral metabolism in neonates and infants (being small enough to insert with their heads at the centre of the magnet) provided some of the earliest available MRS data from humans (Cady et al. 1983; Younkin et al. 1984; Martin et al. 1988). These early results suggested that, by using MRS, important information about normal and pathologic metabolic processes could be obtained from the infant brain. However, technical and methodological feasibility in a clinical environment, complexity of the spectroscopic information, difficulty in quantifying the data and the exact spatial localisation of the volume of interest within the body have delayed the general acceptance of in vivo MRS in medicine. The eventual application of MRS for diagnosis and prognosis to the benefit of the patient remains a matter of research.

The adaptation of high technology (such as MR) for application to the paediatric patient is a prerequisite for obtaining optimal results. It is necessary to take into account the infant's psyche, the great variations in body size during development, the infant's fears and parent's fears and expectations. A friendly and agreeable situation calms the subject and makes the examination easier for all involved. Besides MR system optimisation and maintenance, patient management and physiological monitoring during the examination are crucial determinants of the spectrum quality obtainable from the infant brain. Continuous surveillance of vital signs, such as heart rate (stethoscope, ECG, or a Doppler flow meter), oxygen saturation by pulse oximetry and body temperature (skin and/or rectal sensors) must be available at all times. For the safe examination of sick and unstable newborn babies and infants (e.g. from the intensive care unit), respiration (end tidal CO_2) and blood pressure have to be monitored continuously. In addition, noninvasive measurements of blood gases, i.e. transcutaneous pO_2 and pCO_2, are essential (Boesch and Martin 1988). However, these procedures are not without problems. There are many interactions between the monitoring equipment and the MR system. Sensors and associated cables may contain ferromagnetic material which can distort the local static magnetic field. Cables may also act as antennae and pick up radio frequency (RF) interference thereby decreasing SNR. The pulsed RF from the transmitter may also interfere with monitoring equipment. Electrocardiographic or blood gas monitors may malfunction in the presence of changing magnetic or RF fields. Furthermore, the microprocessors of newer monitors can emit RF interference detectable by the MR spectrometer. Hence, special RF Faraday shields and high frequency filters are often required (Boesch and Martin 1988). Recently delivered full-term and premature infants have to be studied in a temperature controlled incubator equipped with all necessary life support and monitoring systems, including the possibility of artificial ventilation (Boesch et al. 1988). While lying in the magnet, there is only limited access to the child who has to be completely immobilised during the whole examination time. Although many neonates can be examined during their natural sleep (e.g. postprandial sleep), infants and older children have often to be sedated. With unstable patients or patients with certain major cerebral illnesses, there are situations where more elaborate MR examinations, predominantly imaging, can only be carried out under general anaesthesia. The equipment for monitoring vital signs and performing general anaesthesia has often to be placed next to the patient in the magnet room for optimal conditions of safety.

All these constraints make the use of MR in paediatrics cumbersome, and sometimes almost impossible, so that many centres hesitate to examine small children. Neonates and infants should, however, not become diagnostic orphans.

5.2 Principles and Methods

Atomic nuclei make up more than 99.9% of all matter and certain nuclei have been known, since the early days of quantum theory, to possess a magnetic moment. This nuclear magnetic moment is, however, exceedingly difficult to measure, since the elementary magnetic moments of each nucleus tend to be randomly oriented in bulk matter, which contains billions and billions of nuclei, and the tiny residual magnetism is dominated by the far greater magnetic moment of the electrons – the other principal constituents of matter. Although an ingenious laboratory experiment using extremely inhomogeneous magnetic fields demonstrated the nuclear magnetic moment in 1939, it took 7 more years until a practical method for its measurement was found by Purcell. The insight, which led him to his experiment, was the recognition that the nuclear magnetic moment is not static as in a compass needle, but the consequence of what could be understood, in classical terms, as a rotation of the electrically charged nucleus around its axis. If such a magnetic "top" is brought into a magnetic field, its axis will start to precess around the direction of the main field, just as the axis of rotation of a child's toy top rotates around the earth's gravitational field. The frequency of this so-called Larmor precession is directly proportional to both the magnetic moment and the strength of the external magnetic field. The net nuclear magnetisation in a sample can be measured by first disturbing the equilibrium of the magnetic moments by a short RF pulse exactly in resonance with this precession and then observing the resonant signal.

Soon after the first experimental verification of this phenomenon, a number of other groups found slight differences in the observed resonant frequencies of nuclei in different chemical substances. Since the nuclear magnetic moment of each isotope is a fundamental and invariable constant, this could only mean that the magnetic fluxes at the locations of the nuclei must be slightly different from the external field. This modification is caused by the electrons in the observed molecules, which create their own magnetic response to the outer field and consequently reduce or – more seldom – increase the magnetic flux at the nuclei. This response of the electron depends on the exact electronic structure of the molecule and can therefore be used to characterise different chemical substances. The size of this change in frequency (called the chemical shift) depends on the strength of the interaction between the nucleus and the electronic cloud. It is of the order of only a few parts per million (ppm) for hydrogen (^{1}H) but up to several hundreds of ppm for both carbon-13 (^{13}C) and fluorine-19 (^{19}F).

MRS, based on this principle, is nowadays an indispensable tool in analytical laboratories. It can be used to study all molecules containing nuclei with a non-zero magnetic moment. For the examination of organic molecules, this condition is fulfilled by ^{1}H, ^{31}P, ^{23}Na and ^{19}F amongst others, while the normal isotopes of carbon, nitrogen and oxygen possess no nuclear magnetism. For each of the latter, however, less abundant isotopes exist which do have magnetic moments. The natural abundance of ^{13}C for example is about 1%.

Since MRS uses only magnetic fields and RF waves for the creation of a spectrum, it can be used – at least in principle – for the noninvasive monitoring of biochemistry in living tissues. For many reasons, the practical realisation of such an experiment is, however, quite a formidable task even with today's most sophisticated apparatus. The major problem of in vivo MRS is the exceedingly low intensity of the signals to be detected. Technical advances during the last few years have led to very good signal quality for MRI. It has to be borne in mind, however, that MRI is performed by observing primarily protons in water (and some lipid) molecules. The concentration of hydrogen nuclei in pure water is roughly 110 *M*. The concentrations of the metabolites that we may wish to observe in order to study biochemistry are tiny in comparison. The most abundant metabolites have concentrations of a few millimoles and many typical concentrations lie in the micromolar range. Figure 5.1 displays comparative volume sizes for different nuclei that will produce the same signal intensity as that given by one pixel of a conventional MR image. It is easy to see that, for example, ^{13}C spectroscopy with a spatial resolution of $1\ mm^3$ is infeasible.

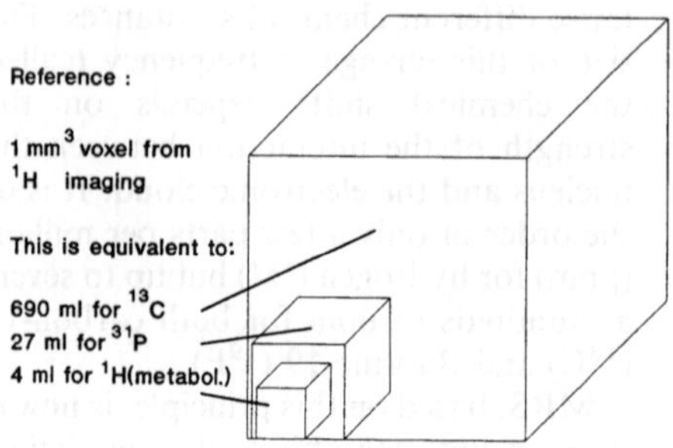

Fig. 5.1. Comparative volumes delivering isointense signals for different MRS applications

5.2.1 Pulse Fourier Transform MRS

Figure 5.2 shows the basic outline of a MR spectrometer. It consists of a computer which controls the MR experiment and collects and processes the incoming data, a RF transmitter tuned to the Larmor frequency of the nuclei under study, a main magnet with a constant field strength over the whole sample volume, a power supply and appropriate coils for the generation of time-dependent magnetic field gradients, and a RF receiver system which detects the MR signals and sends them to the computer for storage and processing. The main magnetic field for MRS is generated normally by a superconductive magnet. For field strengths considerably below 0.5 T (about 10,000 times the earth's magnetic field), magnets using resistive windings or permanent magnets are also available. Since the resonant frequency increases in proportion to the field strength, spectroscopic discrimination of different chemical compounds becomes easier with increasing field strength. For in vivo applications on whole body systems, 1.5 T is regarded as the minimum requirement, although some spectroscopic results have been obtained at lower field strength.

All components of the MR system are computer controlled. The RF transmitter sends a short pulse with a duration of typically up to 5 ms to a RF coil, which, in the simplest case, consists of a loop of copper wire. During the excitation pulse, the net magnetisation of the atomic nuclei, which was initially oriented parallel to the main field, is rotated by an angle called the "flip angle" (often about 90°) and then precesses at the Larmor frequency around the main field. The rota-

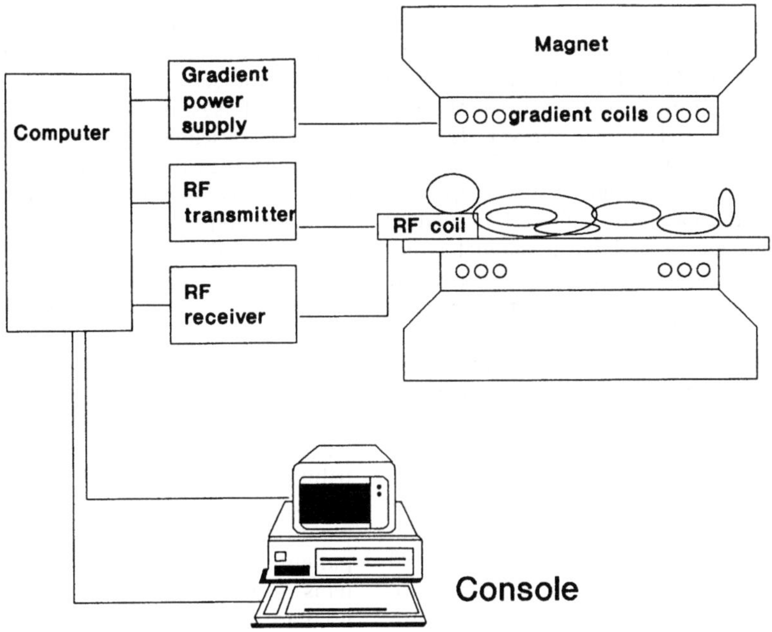

Fig. 5.2. A whole body MR spectrometer

tion of this transverse magnetisation inside of the RF coil leads to the generation of a time-dependent alternating current in the RF coil via inductance (the same principle is used in a bicycle dynamo). This signal is called the free induction decay (FID). Sometimes two different coils are used – one for excitation and one for signal detection. Since the magnetic moments of the nuclei are very small, the induced voltage is of the order of only a few millivolts, even if all the nuclei in a human body are thus excited. The time-dependent voltage is converted into numbers (digitised) and sent to the computer for further analysis. The most fundamental processing step is frequency analysis, which converts the time-dependent signal intensity (the FID) into its frequency components (a spectrum) by an algorithm called Fourier transformation.

There are several factors which determine the decay of the signal. Since it is technically impossible to make the magnetic field totally homogeneous over the whole sample volume, the Larmor frequencies of the observed nuclei will not be identical. The slight differences in frequency cause incoherence of the magnetisation vectors. This means that, after a certain time, the magnetisations at different locations will point in different directions and tend to cancel each other. The time required for loss of coherence depends, of course, on the size of the field inhomogeneities. A characteristic time of this mechanism for signal loss is that taken to bring two parallel magnetisation vectors into the antiparallel position. For example, if this happens within 10 ms, we can easily calculate that the difference in frequency between the two vectors must be $1/(2 \times 10\ \text{ms})$ or 50 Hz. Considering a Larmor frequency of, for example, approximately 40 MHz, a field inhomogeneity of only 1.25 ppm will lead to this signal loss. As a consequence, it is not surprising that the design and construction of a magnet with an extremely homogeneous magnetic field is the most challenging (and cost-intensive) technical problem in MRS. However, even with an infinitely homogeneous magnet the signal would not persist forever. Interactions at the molecular level also lead to loss of coherence and, as a consequence, to signal decay, although each individual nucleus may still have a magnetisation component in the plane transverse to the static magnetic field. There are numerous mechanisms for this so-called spin-spin (or transverse) relaxation. The relaxation time (T_2) can be as short as a few microseconds for large macromolecules or solids or up to several seconds in pure liquids like water. While such T_2 processes lead to signal loss, other mechanisms bring the magnetisation back to its equilibrium state parallel to the main field with a characteristic time T_1. These processes are called spin-lattice (or longitudinal) relaxation. Since the equilibrium state is energetically favoured compared to transverse magnetisation, such T_1 processes are always accompanied by energy exchange of the nuclear magnetisation with the surrounding environment. It is a fundamental fact that, as a consequence of this, T_1 will always be longer than T_2. The difference is very small in pure liquids, where T_1 and T_2 are approximately equal. Under the conditions encountered in an in vivo MRS experiment, for medium sized molecules (e.g. nucleoside phosphates), T_2 of ^{31}P can be of the order of a few milliseconds, while T_1 exceeds 1 s.

The decay time of the FID signal determines the accuracy with which resonance frequencies can be measured. The faster the decay, the greater the uncertainty. This uncertainty can be characterised by the width of the line in the spectrum generated by Fourier transformation of the FID. Broad lines will make signals with Larmor frequencies which are close together impossible to resolve.

Part of the sensitivity problem mentioned above is due to the imperfect experimental apparatus which can be built with today's technology. One has, however, to bear in mind that there are some principal limitations set by nature which restrict the sensitivity even of an "ultimate" MR system. The thermal motion of the (electrically charged or at least polar) molecules in the human body produces a noise signal which will be invariably detected whenever a MR measurement is being made. The noise level depends on the actual measurement frequency. For the human body, the maximum noise intensity lies at about 100 MHz. The amount of noise contamination of a measurement depends on the spectral width – the broader the detected frequency range, the more noise will contribute to the spectrum. For MRI, where typical bandwidths of about 20–50 kHz are used, the image noise is dominated by patient noise even on today's MR systems. For MRS, where the bandwidths used are much smaller, this limit has not yet been reached. Another point of consideration is the relation of the coil size to the volume under observation. A larger coil is not only inherently more insensitive to a small volume than a smaller coil, it also picks up more patient noise. Taking these and other arguments together, one can expect an increase in the SNR for MRS examinations of one to (optimistically) two orders of magnitude in the next few years. This falls, however, still short by several orders of magnitude from the sensitivity one needs for the direct observation of most metabolically active substances.

A considerable part of the skill needed for the successful execution of a biologically or clinically sensible experiment is therefore the translation of the biochemistry of the metabolism under study into terms of MR observable substances. The direct observation of the relevant part of a metabolic pathway is possible only in a few instances – most notably the metabolism of high-energy phosphates. A further problem of MRS is related to its ability to identify and distinguish different metabolites. In general, a large chemical shift range and narrow spec-

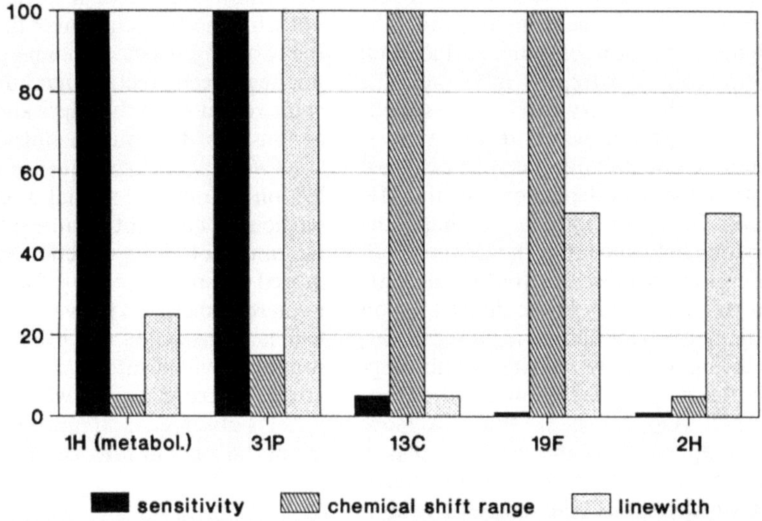

Fig. 5.3. A qualitative comparison of different spectroscopic parameters for a number of nuclei commonly used for in vivo MRS. The *vertical scale* is in arbitrary units. The parameters for this graph are those for typical spectroscopic examinations using each nucleus. The proton parameters are valid for the spectroscopy of metabolites occurring in millimolar concentrations. For the detection of the water signal, the sensitivity would be about 10^4-10^5 times higher due to the higher concentration. The ^{31}P values correspond to spectroscopic examinations of high-energy phosphates. For ^{13}C and ^{19}F, tracer experiments were taken as representative. The deuterium (^2H) parameters illustrate that the low sensitivity, the narrow chemical shift range and the broad linewidth make this nucleus especially unsuitable for spectroscopy. Non-spectroscopy measurements of ^2H in macroscopic concentrations might, however, be useful for the observation of, for example, lipid metabolism

tral lines allow better resolution of different substances than a narrow shift range and broad and overlapping lines. The aliphatic groups of lipid molecules produce, for example, one broad more or less featureless hump when observed in vivo with proton spectroscopy. A ^{13}C spectrum of the same material shows a pattern of many lines, most of which can be attributed unambiguously to the multitude of different lipids occurring in living tissue. A purely qualitative comparative diagram of the fundamental spectroscopic parameters for a number of biologically and clinically interesting nuclei is shown in Fig. 5.3.

After these more fundamental reflections on the basics of MRS, we will turn to experimental problems of measuring a spectrum from a well-defined volume of the body. Two problems have to be solved before such an experiment can be performed: First, the problem of spectrum localisation. Second, it is sometimes required to select only parts of the spectrum for observation, which is especially the case when some unwanted signal – like that of water in proton spectroscopy – becomes exceedingly large compared to the signal from the metabolites of interest.

5.2.2 Spectrum Localisation

The simplest approach to spectrum localisation is the use of a surface coil with a sensitive volume that coincides approximately with the desired volume under study. For a circular coil the sensitive volume corresponds roughly to a sphere with the same diameter as the coil. The volume definition of pure surface coil spectroscopy is extremely inflexible. The selected volume very rarely corresponds to the object one wants to examine. A better volume definition can be achieved by using the field dependence of the MR signal. One possibility is to shape the magnetic field such that the frequency of the excitation pulse is equal to the Larmor frequency only in the desired region of the body. This can be achieved by introducing spatially varying static magnetic fields, as in the technique called topical MR (Gordon et al. 1980). A more simple approach is the use of a plastic sheet dotted with ferromagnetic particles, which "spoils" the magnetic field in its immediate surroundings and consequently allows the measurement of spectra from deeper lying tissue without contamination from surface material. Apart from alterations in the static magnetic field, changes in the strength of the excitation pulse can also be used for spatial selection (Hoult 1979). The amplitude and phase of the signal depends on the strength of the magnetic component (B_1) of the RF field and the distance to the coil. Consecutive measurements with different B_1 and subsequent two-dimensional Fourier transformation gives spectra at increasing distances from the coil. It should be noted, however, that although this gives some kind of depth selection to the spectra, the voxels are by no means well-defined especially parallel to the plane of the coil.

A much superior strategy for spatial selection is the use of linear magnetic field gradients in combination with frequency selective pulses. It is easy to see that a pulse with a narrow excitation bandwidth excites only those spins with Larmor frequencies within the selected bandwidth. If such a pulse is applied under a constant magnetic field gradient, only spins lying in a narrow plane (sometimes called a slice) orthogonal to the gradient will "see" this pulse. Since the frequency content of a finite pulse has not an exactly rectangular distribution, the resulting selected volume profile will not be perfectly rectangular but will show some rounding at the edges and will have a non-zero distribution outside the desired volume. A consequence of this selection of only one spatial direction by a particular constant gradient is that a minimum of three selection steps is required for the selection of a voxel. The numerous methods for volume selection, which are based on this principle, can be roughly divided into two groups: single voxel experiments, in which only one voxel is observed, and multi-voxel experiments. Both will now be discussed.

5.2.2.1 Single Voxel Techniques

Single voxel techniques can again be subdivided into two groups: those which use predominantly *z*-magnetisation for the volume selection step and those which use transverse magnetisation for that purpose. T_1 relaxation is the dominant mechanism during the volume selection step which leads to selection imperfections. Since T_1 is long in high-energy phosphates while T_2 is short, ^{31}P MRS has been performed more or less exclusively with *z*-magnetisation techniques. Since the first such technique, Aue's VSE method, numerous similar techniques have been proposed with acronyms like SPARS, ISIS, OSIRIS, etc. The most simple and most frequently used approach is taken by the ISIS technique (Ordidge et al. 1986), which uses three inversion pulses in order to label different regions with positive or negative *z*-magnetisation. After this labelling, signal is read out by a simple excitation pulse just as in non-volume selective MRS. As demonstrated in Table 5.1, a sequence of eight such experiments with subsequent linear combination of the signals will give the desired spectrum of the selected voxel. The fact that volume selection requires more than one experiment is a serious disadvantage of the ISIS technique, since nonreproducibilities in the execution of the measurement will invariably lead to contamination of the resultant spectrum with signal from outside of the required voxel. Since the voxel volume can be smaller, by several orders of magnitude, than the surrounding tissue, even slight variations from one excitation to the next can lead to considerable extravoxel contamination. There are other methods using z-magnetisation which work as single shot methods. However, these need considerably more RF pulses and more gradient switching steps, which in themselves lead to further imperfections and have caused limited success for these alternative approaches.

Methods using transverse magnetisation are much more straightforward. As Fig. 5.4 shows, only three RF pulses are required in order to select a voxel in one step (Frahm et al. 1987). Since T_2 is always involved during at least parts of the selection step, these methods are most successfully used for proton spectroscopy, where the T_2s of the observed metabolites are sufficiently long. (It was recently demonstrated that, using state-of-the-art equipment, ^{31}P spectroscopy can also be performed with this approach by making the experiment sufficiently fast, e.g. an echo time; T_E, of 20 ms.) The main difference between the spin echo method (PRESS) and the stimulated echo method (STEAM) lies in the fact that the stimulated echo sequence produces intrinsically only half of the signal amplitude of the spin echo sequence. This theoretical signal loss is somewhat compensated, in practice, by the fact that magnetisation is lost with T_1 rather than T_2 during the time interval between the second and third RF pulse. Using the capabilities of today's MR equipment, this compensates the intrinsic signal loss with T_2s of about 20 ms for nuclei with long T_1s. So the stimulated echo technique might be advantageous for ^{31}P spectroscopy. For protons, however, the spin echo sequence is definitely to be preferred.

A curiosity of the spin echo localisation technique is that it really has no predecessor. The possibility of doing such an experiment was proposed by Bottomley (1984) in a patent concerning the much simpler DRESS sequence, but its practical application was never really demonstrated. Ordidge (1985) published a paper using this sequence but the technical

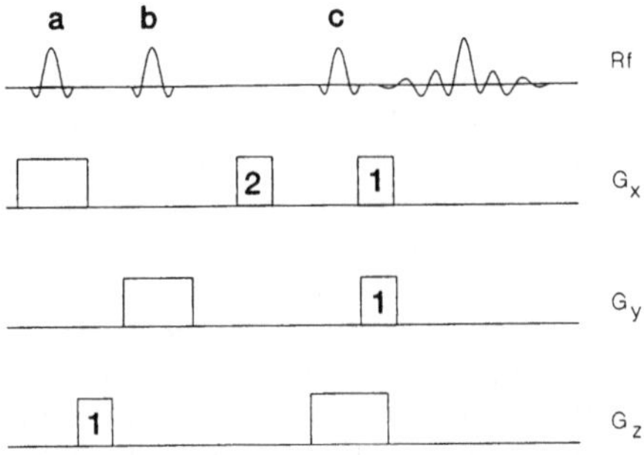

Fig. 5.4. Volume selective spectroscopy with selective pulses. *Rf*, pulses *a*, *b* and *c* and the subsequent signal; G_x, G_y, and G_z switched gradients in three orthogonal directions. If the flip angles of *a*, *b* and *c* are all 90° and the gradients labelled *1* are added to three unlabelled gradients, a stimulated echo is created. Alternatively, if $a=90°$ and *b* and $c=180°$ and gradient pulse *2* is used instead of gradients *1* a spin echo is formed

Table 5.1. Sequence of selective pulses for volume selection by ISIS

Experiment number	Pulse flip angle (°) x	y	z	Phase Receiver	Signal
1	0	0	0	+	+
2	180	0	0	−	+
3	0	180	0	−	+
4	180	180	0	+	+
5	0	0	180	−	+
6	180	0	180	+	+
7	0	180	180	+	+
8	180	180	180	−	+

performance of the MR system was such that the idea was not pursued any further. Quite a number of groups have recently published results using this technique, some mainly using it, others "re-inventing" it. The most generally used acronym for this sequence is PRESS, as proposed by Bottomley (1984).

Comparing localisation via *z*-magnetisation with techniques utilising transverse magnetisation, some principal differences can be observed which are independent of the implementation of these methods. It has already been mentioned that localisation errors in methods using *z*-magnetisation lead to contamination of the spectrum. Errors in methods using transverse magnetisation, by contrast, will lead only to reduced signal in the spectrum, but not to contamination. This fact, together with the straightforward selection in one excitation, has made these experiments the method of choice whenever relaxation times allow. It should not be forgotten, however, that *z* methods have their own distinct advantages. A point, which may be of considerable interest when more intricate MR experiments than simple spectrum acquisition are performed, is that the *z* methods clearly separate the volume selection from the spectrum acquisition. As a consequence, these methods can be used to apply any of the more complicated methods known from analytical MRS by the simple addition of the volume selection step. STEAM and PRESS do not possess a similar flexibility and, since the time required for volume selection intrinsically serves also as evolution time for processes like J-coupling, care has to be taken in the interpretation of spectra. The most prominent example is the measurement of lactate in proton spectroscopy. It is not widely known that lactate does not give any stimulated echo signal when measured with STEAM and a T_E of 135 ms.

5.2.2.2 Multi-voxel Techniques

The simplest approach to obtaining signal from more than one voxel during one acquisition cycle is to extend the idea of multi-slice imaging to spectroscopy (i.e. to measure more than one spectrum during one acquisition cycle in an interleaved manner). This approach restricts the number of voxels to only a few. However, it does maintain all the advantages of single voxel methods such as, for example, the possibility of voxel selective optimisation of the magnetic field in each voxel. For application to more voxels, the single voxel techniques can be extended by using RF pulses with frequency distributions that lead to the excitation of more than one voxel at a time. Labelling the different voxels with different signal phases can then be used to extract the spectrum from each voxel either by linear combination according to a Hadamard scheme (similar to the principle of ISIS) or by using a different phase label and simple Fourier transformation. These approaches can be used to excite many voxels at a time and allow free choice of the placement of each voxel. The complexity of the pulse shapes and the high peak RF power of the pulses for a large number of simultaneously excited voxels limit their practical application to the simultaneous measurement of some tens or at most hundreds of voxels at a time.

A truly contiguous acquisition of spectra over a large volume of the human body can be achieved using the chemical shift imaging (CSI) method (Brown et al. 1982). This technique can be used either without any additional volume selection or in combination with any of the selection techniques discussed above, preferably single-shot techniques. After selection of a fairly large region of interest, spatial resolution can be increased by adding an additional phase-encoding gradient, as in MRI. This additional phase-encoding can be done in one, two or three dimensions. The minimum number of excitations is given by the number of voxels in the resulting chemical shift image. An image resolution of 32×32 voxels needs at least 1024 excitations, not counting signal averaging, and consequently requires a long acquisition time. The time required for three-dimensional spatial resolution is prohibitive for most practical purposes, unless very small matrix sizes are used. A chemical shift image can be presented either as a matrix of spectra or the data can be processed to give metabolite maps showing the spatial distribution of different compounds on a grey scale image. The strength of CSI lies in such qualitative maps, which can demonstrate the spatial extent of metabolically affected tissue, e.g. in ischaemic or other diseases. The disadvantages of CSI are, firstly, that the field homogeneity can be optimised only for the total volume. This means that the homogeneity inside various voxels will be different and can be very bad for voxels which are located near interfaces of tissues with differing magnetic susceptibilities. If this is not corrected for properly, a presumed metabolite map might easily turn out to be a simple magnetic field map. Secondly, an additional problem of CSI is the rather poor voxel definition afforded by the Fourier transformation process. This can be described by the so-called point-spread function, which defines the way signal from a single voxel will appear after the imaging process. This function is a $\sin(x)/x$ function for the Fourier transformation. Integration reveals that, even for one-dimensional CSI, less than 60% of the signal from a voxel will appear at the proper location in the CSI image. The rest is smeared out over neighbouring voxels. More than 40% of the signal which appears in the CSI image is, in reality, contamination from outside. Since the exact amount of contamination depends also on geometrical factors, like the spatial distribution of the substances leading to contamination with respect to the image matrix, extreme care should be taken not to over interpret quantitative results in CSI. In the worst case, a simple shift of the image matrix by one half of the voxel size will lead to an increase in the contamination from zero to more than 50% of the total signal.

5.2.3 Chemical Shift Selection

The selection of the chemical shift range to be observed (also known as spectral editing) is normally performed by the addition of chemical shift selective RF pulses to any of the localisation techniques described above. These pulses are identical in principle to volume selection pulses in that they have a narrow frequency bandwidth. Such pulses can either be used to selectively excite the wanted section of the spectrum or to selectively suppress unwanted parts. In addition, parts of the spectrum can be selectively inverted in successive scans and retained or suppressed by linear combination. There is no technique which is optimal for all cases. In general, if a large signal is to be suppressed, only those approaches should be used which do not excite this resonance at all. Otherwise, even small errors can lead to large residual spectral contamination. Techniques using linear combinations of differently labelled spectra are, however, quite useful to edit signals of comparable intensity.

Apart from editing according to chemical shift, other parameters can also be used for signal suppression or selection. A simple technique is the use of an inversion pulse prior to excitation such that the excitation pulse occurs exactly at the zero-crossing of the T_1 relaxation. Other more elaborate selection schemes, which can only be mentioned here briefly, use editing sequences based on MR specific parameters, like J-coupling, the nuclear Overhauser effect or polarisation transfer, in order to selectively enhance particular signals and distinguish them from other substances, even if the chemical shifts of the spectral lines are identical.

5.2.4 Limitations of the Technique

MR offers quite a large repertoire of methods and strategies for in vivo spectroscopy. Unfortunately, for clinical applications, only a limited range of such techniques is installed on any single MR scanner. Thus, the choice of spectroscopic techniques is often determined by availability rather than by rational decision. The increased flexibility of MR systems gives hope that better techniques will become available at more and more sites. The most severe current technical limitations are finite gradient switching times and eddy current problems caused by switching magnetic fields inside the magnets, the cryostats (needed for maintaining the superconductivity of the main magnet coils) of which are made of electrically conductive stainles steel. Despite the optimism about further technical developments at all levels of MR technology, it should not be forgotten that MRS has some significant limitations regarding sensitivity. MRS will, consequently, never replace many existing techniques, but will rather be an extremely useful modality in addition to the existing range of investigative technologies.

5.3 Studies of Neonatal Brain Metabolism

Neurons have a poor ability to regenerate, thus continuous provision of an energy supply is essential for the function and integrity of the brain (Siesjö 1978). Mitochondrial oxidative phosphorylation is the principal energy source of neurons (Fig. 5.5). A major part of the free energy, derived predominantly from the oxidation of glucose, is supplied by the blood and is transformed into a special energy form, i.e. adenosine triphosphate (ATP). In addition, the neonatal brain seems to be able to use lactate, β-hydroxybutyrate and other alternative fuels which are able to cross the blood-brain barrier in order to meet its energy requirements. ATP is then transported out of the mitochondrion into the cytosol where it drives chemical reactions for biosynthesis and is also used for molecular and ion transport. ATP is the principal carrier of free energy in the brain because of its three phosphate groups and plays a central role as an energy coupling agent in transferring high-energy phosphoryl groups between substrates and products. When ATP is hydrolysed to adenosine diphosphate (ADP) and inorganic orthophosphate (Pi), a large amount of free energy is liberated:

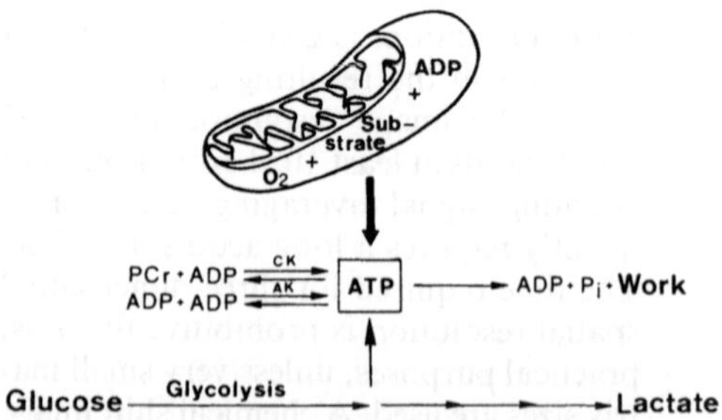

Fig. 5.5. A mitochondrion with the major pathways of endo-mitochondrial and exo-mitochondrial ATP synthesis and turnover

$$[ATP^{4-}] + [H_2O] \rightarrow [ADP^{3-}] + [HPO_4{}^{2-}] + [H^+] + \Delta G^{0\prime} \quad (5.1)$$

where $\Delta G^{0\prime} \cong -30.5$ kJ/mol. The ATP-ADP cycle is the fundamental cellular energy exchange system. The direction and the rate of the reaction in this cycle is controlled by the respective substrate concentrations. Increased ATP breakdown would lead to an accumulation of ADP and Pi, which stimulate mitochondrial ATP synthesis and vice versa. In this context, [ADP] is the principal controller of cellular respiration. Since its turnover rate is fast, the continuous and rapid generation of ATP is, therefore, of vital importance for cells and tissues in order to maintain a rather high and constant ATP concentration. A fall in [ATP] is immediately followed by breakdown of cellular homeostasis, and both ion transport and biosynthesis no longer occur. Creatine is phosphorylated by the action of the enzyme creatine kinase to produce phosphocreatine (PCr, the storage form of high-energy phosphates) from which ATP can be mobilised very rapidly. Thus, besides the efficient mitochondrial ATP synthesis, there are two important extramitochondrial sources for ATP production – the creatine kinase reaction and the adenylate kinase reaction (Fig. 5.5).

[ATP]/([ADP] × [Pi]) is an index of the energy reserve of the cell, called the 'phosphorylation potential' (Siesjö 1978), and this is derived from Eq. (5.1). It expresses the balance between energy production and consumption and is largely independent both of variations in the size of the adenine nucleotide pool and of pH. Due to the cellular concentration ratios [ATP]:[ADP]:[AMP] of roughly 100:10:1, and because AMP is mainly structurally bound, the latter two metabolites are not directly visible by in vivo ^{31}P spectroscopy. If oxidative phosphorylation is impaired, [ATP] decreases because its synthesis does not match its consumption. In the healthy brain, where the creatine kinase reaction is in equilibrium, a drop in [ATP] is buffered immediately, maintaining [ATP] close to normal. A fall in [ATP] would, therefore, signal the end of the steady state of the creatine kinase equilibrium. On the other hand, [PCr] can fall and this will be associated with a concomitant [Pi] increase. Therefore, the ratio [PCr]/[Pi] can change rapidly during situations of physiological stress. Since this ratio is proportional to the phosphorylation potential, it is often used to express the (thermodynamic) energy potential of the cell.

5.3.1 ^{31}P MRS of High-Energy Phosphates: The Normal Neonatal Brain

In the ^{31}P in vivo spectrum, the high-energy phosphates ATP and PCr, and also Pi, are easily detected. Phosphorus atoms from other nucleotides are either present in only small concentrations or are tightly bound to proteins giving rise to low or very broad signals, respectively, and these often underlie the ATP resonances. However, [ADP] can be calculated from the equilibrium equation of the creatine phosphokinase (CPK) reaction. From Pi only a single ^{31}P resonance is observed in the spectrum, although the chemical shifts of $H_2PO_4^-$ (acid) and HPO_4^{2-} (base) differ by 2.4 ppm, because there is a rapid chemical exchange between these acid and base forms of Pi, resulting in one averaged peak. The equilibrium of this reaction, and thus the resonant frequency of the Pi peak in the spectrum, depends on the ratio of the concentrations of the two species ($pK_a \cong 6.8$) which is modified by the intracellular $[H^+]$ and hence by the intracellular pH (pH_i). From the chemical shift difference (δ) between PCr and Pi in the phosphorus spectrum, pH_i can be estimated to an accuracy of about 0.1 pH units according to the Henderson-Hasselbalch equation (Petroff et al. 1985):

$$pH_i = 6.75 + \log_{10} \cdot [(\delta - 3.72)/(5.69 - \delta)] \qquad (5.2)$$

The extracellular concentrations of phosphorus metabolites are negligible.

In 1978, Chance et al. (amongst others) pioneered in vivo phosphorus MRS by obtaining the first ^{31}P spectrum from an animal brain. They demonstrated that acute hypoxia was followed by a fall in PCr and a rise in Pi in combination with tissue acidosis. Subsequent work has shown that relative, and recently also absolute, concentrations of these metabolites can be measured in chemical equilibrium and these concentrations yield important information about the energy status of the part of the brain examined. In vivo MRS can detect acute metabolic changes rapidly, often within minutes, when appropriate methods are applied.

Figure 5.6 illustrates typical ^{31}P brain spectra from a neonate and a 15 month

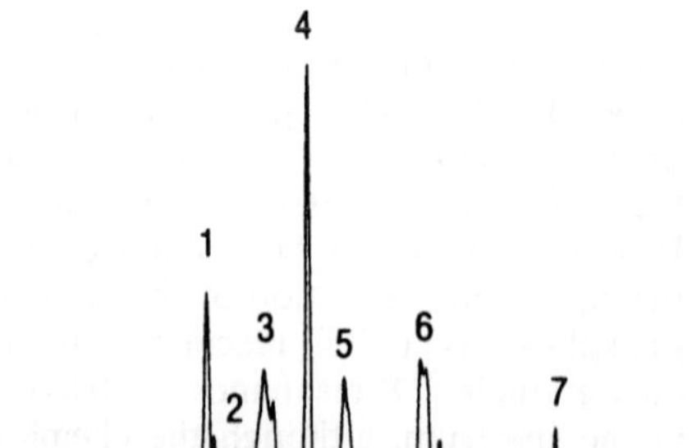

Fig. 5.6. ^{31}P brain spectra obtained with a surface coil, of two children, at 43 weeks PCA (*lower spectrum*) and at 98 weeks PCA (*upper spectrum*). The *abscissa* displays the chemical shift of the various phosphorus metabolites expressed in ppm. Peak assignments and approximate chemical shifts: *1*, PME (6.8 ppm); *2*, Pi (4.9 ppm); *3*, PDE (2.9 ppm); *4*, PCr (0 ppm); *5*, γ-NTP (−2.5 ppm); *6*, α-NTP (−7.6 ppm); *7*, β-NTP (16.2 ppm). The shoulder at −8.3 ppm (*arrow*) is probably due to NAD+NADH. The individual peak areas are proportional to the metabolite concentrations but, due to differential saturation effects, only in a fully relaxed spectrum will relative areas correspond directly with concentration ratios. The narrow PCr resonance peak serves as a chemical shift reference and is conventionally set to 0 ppm. (Reprinted from Boesch et al. 1989)

old infant. The spectra were obtained with a surface coil placed over the parietotemporal region. Signals from superficial tissues (muscle, scalp) have been eliminated. Phosphates from structural tissue components, e.g. bone, have very short relaxation times and lead to broad signals which underlie the peaks due to mobile metabolites in the spectrum. The γ-nucleoside triphosphate (NTP) resonance represents predominantly the γ-phosphate group of ATP, but has a small contribution from other NTPs and from the β-phosphate of ADP (Cady et al. 1983; Hope et al. 1984). At about −8.3 ppm, a shoulder on the right hand side of the α-NTP signal is frequently observed (Boesch et al. 1989) and originates from a nicotinamide adenine dinucleotide pool (mainly NAD+NADH) which has been identified in studies of brain extracts. (α-ADP, resonating at about the same chemical shift, has a concentration far below the detection limit.) Finally, the resonance labelled β-NTP only contains signals from the β-phosphate groups of NTPs (predominantly ATP) and is often used as a reference for concentration ratio calculations. The phospho-monoesters (PME) and phospho-diesters (PDE) will be discussed in Sect. 5.3.2.

5.3.1.1 ^{31}P MRS of High-Energy Phosphates: Variations with Age

In recent years, distinct differences between neonatal and adult in vivo ^{31}P brain spectra have been observed. PCr and Pi have been used to describe the energy status both of the normal neonatal brain and of the brains of infants who have suffered perinatal hypoxia-ischaemia (Hope et al. 1984; Hamilton et al. 1986; Azzopardi et al. 1989 a, b) and also to measure pH_i (Petroff et al. 1985). However, slow age-dependent changes of these metabolites during postnatal brain development have to be distinguished from acute and rapid alter-

Table 5.2. Values of the longitudinal relaxation time (T_1) of brain phosphorus metabolites

T_1 (s)[a]	PME	Pi	PDE	PCr	γ-NTP	α-NTP	β-NTP
Neonates ($n=10$)	5.1 ± 1.0	2.0 ± 0.7	1.7 ± 0.4	4.5 ± 1.1	1.3 ± 0.3	1.6 ± 0.4	1.6 ± 0.5
Infants[b] ($n=10$)	3.4 ± 1.3	1.8 ± 0.6	1.6 ± 0.2	3.5 ± 1.0	1.6 ± 0.3	1.8 ± 0.3	1.3 ± 0.4

There is a significant difference in the T_1 relaxation time of the PME resonance between the two groups, which signifies age-dependent changes in the relaxation of the monoesters.
[a] Mean$\pm$SD
[b] Age around 1 year

ations resulting from diseases. An age-dependent increase of PCr/ATP and PCr/Pi has been demonstrated in normal mammalian brain, and also in newborn human infants by comparing results from preterm and term infants (Azzopardi et al. 1989a). For the quantitative analysis of brain spectra during the first year of life, age-related changes of longitudinal relaxation times (T_1) of the various metabolite resonances have to be taken into account. In particular, partial saturation of the signals may occur when repetition times (T_R) are short compared to the T_1s of the various phosphorus metabolites, i.e. $T_R < 5\,T_1$. To assess these saturation effects and their changes during brain development, measurements of the T_1s of the various resonances visible in ^{31}P brain spectra were recently carried out on two groups of children (Gruetter et al. 1990a). The first group consisted of ten healthy neonates, postconceptional age (PCA) range 37–45 weeks (median PCA 41 weeks), and the second group contained nine infants, age around 1 year (median PCA 99 weeks). Table 5.2 summarises the T_1 values found for these two groups.

When ^{31}P brain spectra from neonates are compared with those from older infants, the PME signal is relatively larger and the PDE and PCr peaks are smaller in neonates (see Fig. 5.6). To illustrate these age-dependent variations, representative brain spectra from four infants of increasing ages (37, 47, 69 and 340 weeks PCA, respectively) are displayed in a stacked plot in Fig. 5.7. Again, the most striking changes can be observed in the PCr, PME and PDE signals. During the period that the PCr and PDE appear

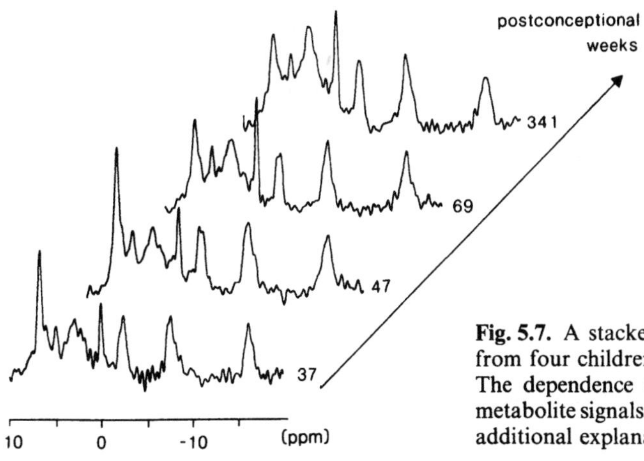

Fig. 5.7. A stacked plot of ^{31}P brain spectra from four children at various postnatal ages. The dependence of the various phosphorus metabolite signals on age is demonstrated. For additional explanation, see text

to increase with age, the PME decreases. The three NTP signals in Fig. 5.7, however, do not seem to vary appreciably with age, although the data have not been evaluated quantitatively. Differences in spectra were analysed by comparing the peak areas relative to the β-NTP signal area. β-NTP was chosen for two reasons:

1. The ATP concentration in the brain is generally believed to be rather constant at about 3 mmol/litre wet, although available literature data on absolute nucleoside triphosphate concentrations differ slightly and may depend on the method used, the anatomical location and possibly also on the stage of development (Cady and Azzopardi 1989). Acute changes in [ATP] are buffered by the CK reaction (Fig. 5.5).
2. The β-NTP resonance at −16.2 ppm largely originates from ATP (mostly magnesium complexed) and no other metabolite with a significant concentration contributes to it apart from other low concentration NTPs (mainly cytidine-TP, uridine-TP and guanosine-TP).

The approximate chemical shifts of the various high-energy phosphorus metabolites are given in the legend of Fig. 5.6. Table 5.3 summarises the mean peak area ratios of PCr/β-NTP and PCr/Pi from ten newborn infants and also from ten infants of age about 1 year. T_R/T_1 was large enough to ensure that the high-energy metabolite ratios were not significantly affected by saturation effects. The analyses of 48 brain spectra acquired from 40 neonates and infants (Boesch et al. 1989) revealed sharp increases in PCr/β-NTP (Fig. 5.8a), α-NTP/β-NTP (related to [NAD + NADH], Fig. 5.8b) and PCr/Pi (Fig. 5.8c) during early postnatal life. The changes may be related to an increase in the phosphorylation potential and an indication that the free energy change of ATP hydrolysis is raised compared to the brain metabolism of older infants (see Table 5.3) or adults. Another explanation could be that there is more energy released for storage after the completion of major membrane phospholipid synthesis implying an increase in phosphorylation potential (Azzopardi et al. 1989a). The scatter in the plots in Fig. 5.8 is most probably due to the heterogeneous population, with respect to perinatal medical histories, and also to varying rates of postnatal development. Only 12 children could be classed as normal controls as judged by their clinical history. Some 36 spectra in the study were potentially abnormal, because they included children recovering from infections and mild perinatal asphyxia or with medically controlled seizure disorders or mild neurologic symptoms. As mentioned above, under situations of physiological stress, PCr may change rapidly. Hence, the correlations with age shown in Fig. 5.8 must be interpreted with caution because of the possibility of short-term physiological and pathologic changes that are not age-dependent. Similar observations have been reported also in a group of 41 children (age up to 16.5 years) indicating that major changes in high-energy phosphorus metabolites take place within the first 1–2 years of life (van der Knaap et al. 1990).

The peak area between −6.5 and −9.5 ppm appears to be consistently greater than that of the β-NTP resonance. This may be explained by an addi-

Table 5.3. Peak area ratios of PCr/β-NTP and PCr/Pi

	PCr/β-NTP (mean ± SD)	PCr/Pi (mean ± SD)
Neonates [a] (n = 10)	0.73 ± 0.12	0.94 ± 0.18
Infants [b] (n = 10)	1.34 ± 0.11	1.28 ± 0.17

[a] PCA range 38–40 weeks
[b] Age around 1 year; PCA range 85–112 weeks

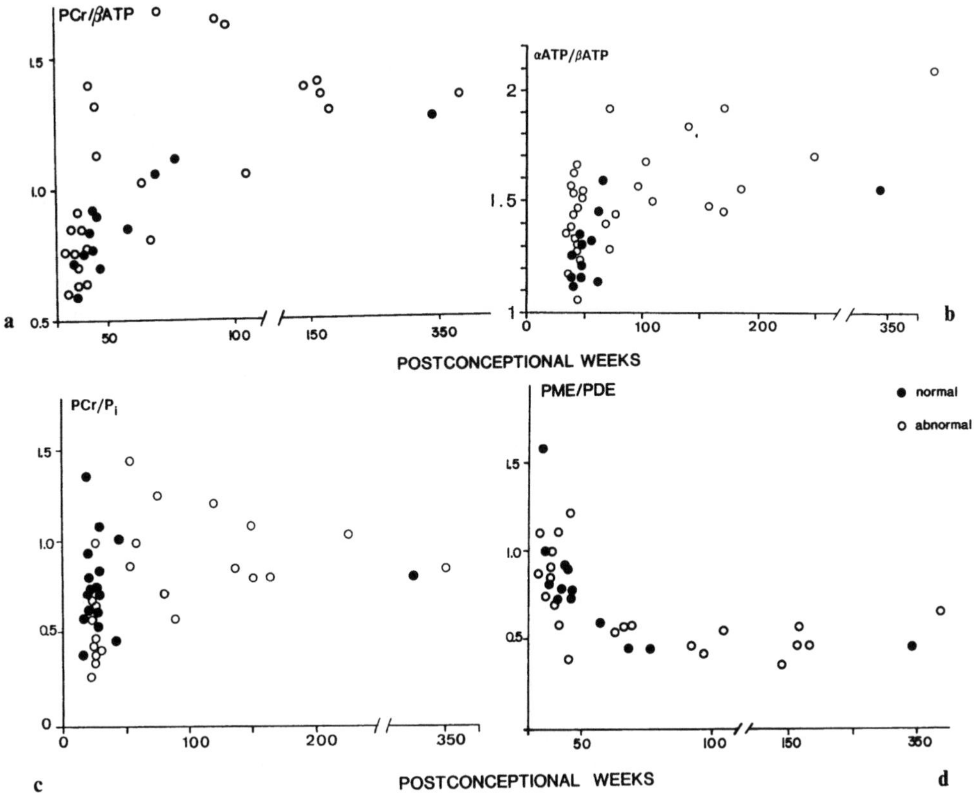

Fig. 5.8 a–d. Ratios of ^{31}P signal intensities as a function of PCA from birth up to 360 weeks. ●, healthy children; ○, children with potentially abnormal ^{31}P spectra. **a** PCr/β-NTP ratio; **b** ratio of the peak at -7.6 ppm (assigned as α-NTP) to the area of the β-NTP peak; **c** PCr/Pi ratio; **d** PME/PDE ratio. The distinctly higher values of the α-NTP peak can be explained by the NAD signal at -8.3 ppm. Although the ordinate axes in **a** and **b** are labelled ATP, the peak areas include contributions from other NTPs with lower concentrations

tional resonance, which is frequently observed at about -8.3 ppm and probably originates from the NAD + NADH pool. It seems reasonable to interpret the initial age-dependent increase of the integral ratio α-NTP/β-NTP (Fig. 5.8 b) as an indicator of change in the NAD/NADH redox system. Since the oxidative phosphorylation and cytochrome oxidase kinetics are biochemically related to the bioenergetic reserve (e.g. PCr), it is not surprising that a linear relationship may exist between the ratios α-NTP/β-NTP (related to [NAD + NADH]) and PCr/β-NTP (Fig. 5.9). An increase in the NAD + NADH pool can be explained by the increased glucose and oxygen consumption of the mature brain. More than two-thirds of the energy gained by glycolysis is temporarily stored in the redox system NAD/NADH (Siesjö 1978). The respiratory chain converts the energy into the more usable form of ATP. A higher tissue NAD content and higher oxygen and glucose consumption would result in a higher rate of production of ATP. The increase of PCr/β-NTP in the normoxic resting brain is presumably a conse-

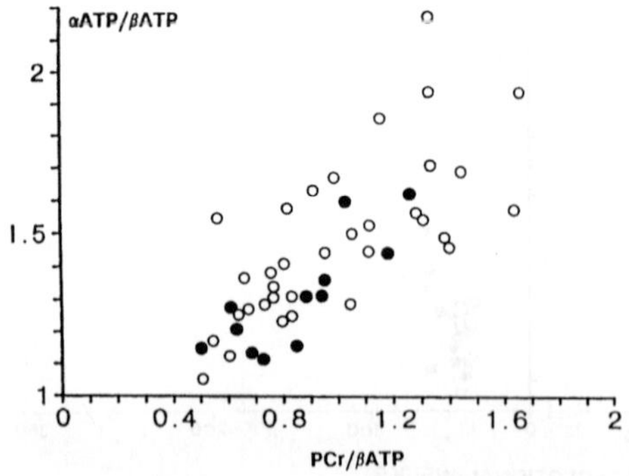

Fig. 5.9. Relationship between the ratios α-NTP/β-NTP (related to [NAD + NADH]) and PCr/β-NTP. Although the ordinate axis is labelled ATP, the peak areas include contributions from other NTPs with lower concentrations

quence of an increased NAD + NADH content. At present no statements can be made concerning the compartmentation of NAD + NADH, i.e. as to whether the concentration increases in the cytosol or mitochondria, or whether the number of mitochondria per cell increase. More research is needed to resolve these questions.

The pH_i, as estimated from the PCr to Pi chemical shift difference (see Eq. 5.2), remains fairly constant at 7.12 ± 0.15 (mean ± SD) over this age range for all 40 children in the study mentioned previously (Boesch et al. 1989) and is in good agreement with results from previous neonatal studies (7.14 ± 0.10) (Hope et al. 1984). The pH_i is slightly lower, 7.08 ± 0.10, for the 12 normal infants.

5.3.2 ^{31}P MRS of Phospholipid Metabolism

The biosynthesis of macromolecular precursors, such as the phospholipids, is another metabolic pathway that can be elucidated with in vivo ^{31}P MRS. Phosphoglycerides, e.g. glycerol phosphorylethanolamine (GPE) and glycerol phosphorylcholine (GPC), are the main constituents of membrane phospholipids and, together with sphingomyelin, are important components of myelin sheaths in the CNS. In animals and humans, the phospholipids are synthesised by a pathway that utilises the amino-alcohols choline and ethanolamine from an internal pool and from the diet, which are phosphorylated to form phosphorylcholine (PCh) and phosphorylethanolamine (PEt). The phospholipids, e.g. the phosphoglycerides, are characterised by phosphorus containing polar head groups. They are synthesised by PCh and PEt reacting with cytidine-TP and diacylglycerol, a common intermediate metabolite. Sphingomyelin, a major component of myelin, does not contain glyceride, however, and the amino-alcohols are esterified with sphingosine instead. As membrane constituents, the brain phospholipids have a diester structure and are highly organized and structurally bound.

5.3.2.1 PME and PDE: Two Characteristic ^{31}P Brain Resonances

The ^{31}P brain spectrum exhibits two, strong characteristic resonances, which are far less prominent in the skeletal muscle spectrum: the PME peak, at about 6.7 ppm, and the broader PDE peak, at about 2.9 ppm (see Figs. 5.6, 5.7, 5.10 and 5.11). PEt is now commonly assumed to be the major constituent of the PME signal in neonatal brain spectra but this peak also contains contributions from PCh and α-glycerophosphate (the common anabolic precursor of the phospholipids). Only minor contributions to the PME signal stem from phosphoserine and phosphoinositol. The PDE resonance contains contributions from mobile brain phosphoglycerides, non-glycerol containing sphingomyelin and the phospholipid degradation products GPE and GPC. Therefore, the PME resonances are found predominantly in anabolic pathways of brain membrane phospholipids, e.g. in myelin synthesis and glial and neuronal proliferations, whereas the PDE (GPE, GPC and to a minor extent GP-serine and GP-inositol) generally reflect catabolic activity representing phospholipid breakdown products. However, only a small fraction of the total phospholipid pool, containing signals from relatively mobile components of membranes, produces relatively narrow lines in the MR spectrum. Variations in the relative concentrations of PME and PDE (e.g. higher relative PME concentrations) have been observed in brain tumours (den Hollander et al. 1989) indicating altered metabolic turnover in brain cell membrane and myelin synthesis and degradation (van der Knaap et al. 1990).

5.3.2.2 PME and PDE: Developmental Changes

The PME resonance at about 6.7 ppm is very strong in ^{31}P spectra obtained from newborn infants, but is much lower in spectra acquired from the brains of older children and adults (see Figs. 5.6 and 5.7). In the 1 year old infant the PME signal is lower, whereas the PDE resonance is relatively larger (Fig. 5.7). The chemical shift of the PME peak does not appear to vary with age, indicating that PEt and PCh are still the major compounds of PME in older children. Bearing in mind that the PME resonances originate from the phospholipid precursors, these findings may be related metabolically to an increased synthesis rate of the membrane phospholipids and of myelin, e.g. in glial and neuronal membranes in neural tumors or in brain development during early postnatal life. However, it is important to note that the majority of phospholipids are structurally bound in membrane phospholipid bilayers and just yield a very broad ^{31}P MR signal which contributes to the background hump underlying unedited ^{31}P spectra. In surface coil spectra, this hump may also include a contribution from immobile phosphorus in cranial bone.

The analysis of brain spectra acquired from 40 newborn and older infants (Boesch et al. 1989) revealed a significant decrease in the PME/PDE ratio during the first 6 months of life (Fig. 5.8 d). The decline of PME and the increase of PDE with age probably reflect not only a higher phospholipid content, but also increasing membrane activity, e.g. of neurotransmitter containing mobile transsynaptic vesicles. The PME/PDE plateau at about 70 weeks PCA, after a decrease during early postnatal life, can be interpreted as an indication that phospholipid synthesis has reached a steady state. Since the PME peak was still prominent several hours after the death of a newborn child (Younkin et al. 1984), the compounds giving rise to the PME signal (i.e. phospholipid precursors) do not appear to be metabolically active and are not affected by acute insults. Therefore, the observed changes in PME/PDE over the first 20 months of life (Fig. 5.8 d) are most probably related to age-dependent changes in phospholipid metabolism and may serve as a maturation index for the developing human brain. It should be remembered that recent studies of PME saturation showed that not only was the T_1 relatively long, but that, for this peak only, the T_1 was also age-dependent (Gruetter et al. 1990 a). The T_1 of the PME resonance decreased from 5.1 ± 1.0 s (mean ± SD) in the neonates (first group) to 3.4 ± 1.3 s in the 1 year old infants (second group).

In conclusion, these results indicate that variations in ^{31}P peak area ratios with PCA can be related to changes in metabolite concentrations during development of the human brain. However, alterations in saturation effects have to be taken into account when considering the PME resonance.

Clinical Studies
ain Abnormalities

ɔdevelopmental impairment or in newborn infants is often d by cellular hypoxia due to either ɛmia related to cerebral haemor- or to arterial hypoxaemia. Ultra- l, MRI or X-ray computerised to- aphy can visualise changes due to orrhage. However, the occurrence ochemical effects due to hypoxia ɔt be detected by these modalities ross structural changes are only ob- l when loss of brain tissue has taken ^{31}P MRS has the capability to :or the levels of high-energy phos- s, such as PCr, ATP and Pi, and ɔolites related to membrane me- .sm (PMEs and PDEs), pH_i and ytosolic magnesium concentration $^{+}$]). Thus MRS provides a nonin- ɛ clinical method whereby, in addi- o the investigation of other disor- the biochemical response of brain to hypoxia-ischaemia can be evalu- ınd sequentially monitored.

ɛ results described here and in Sect. ıve all been obtained using simple :e coil methods. The localisation herefore, been relatively crude and nsitive volume from which spectro- ɛ information was obtained was ap- mately the same as a hemisphere of s equal to that of the coil. The sur- oils used in these studies depended e size of the infant's head and had ɛters of 5 cm or 7 cm. Hence, the ɔolite signals originated from a su- ial layer of brain extending in depth ɛw centimetres only; thus the infor- ɪn obtained relates mainly to corti- sue. This provides a possible expla- ı why lesions restricted to close to id-line (e.g. periventricular haemor-) need not necessarily produce ob- ɔle changes in relative metabolite .

nical studies have shown that ^{31}P is sensitive to abnormalities of oxi- ɛ phosphorylation in the neonatal brain (Azzopardi et al. 1989 b; Delivoria-Papadopoulos and Chance 1988; Hamilton et al. 1986; Hope et al. 1984, 1986). Changes in relative metabolite concentrations, as determined from spectra, have been found following birth asphyxia, postnatal asphyxia, after the observation of abnormal cerebral echodensities on ultrasound scans (Azzopardi et al. 1989 b; Hamilton et al. 1986; Hope et al. 1984, 1986), following focal seizures and stroke (Delivoria-Papadopoulos and Chance 1988; Hamilton et al. 1986) and in infants with inborn errors of metabolism (Hope et al. 1986).

5.3.3.1 Relative Concentrations and pH_i

On the first day of life, infants who have suffered birth asphyxia often, but not always, exhibit spectra similar to those obtained from normal infants of comparable PCA (Fig. 5.10) (Azzopardi et al. 1989 b; Hope et al. 1984, 1986). In severely affected infants subsequent studies showed the development of abnormalities in the spectra. PCr/Pi was observed to fall and occasionally pH_i indicated a slight alkalosis. In some of these infants NTP/total mobile phosphate (P_{tot}) may fall also (P_{tot} is defined as PME + Pi + PDE + PCr + 3 × β-NTP). The ratios PCr/Pi and NTP/P_{tot} have been shown to be useful prognostic indicators (see Sect. 5.4. Eventually the Pi peak may dominate the spectrum and, in occasional extreme cases, PCr and NTP may become undetectable. Similar low or undetectable PCr and NTP levels have also been found in spectra acquired from infants with inborn errors of metabolism such as propionic acidaemia and arginosuccinic aciduria (Hope et al. 1986). In observations on surviving infants, the metabolite ratios measured from the spectra often return to normal values over a period of weeks, but the overall signal strength may be reduced (Azzopardi et al. 1989 b; Delivoria-Papadopoulos and Chance 1988). This decrease in signal is support-

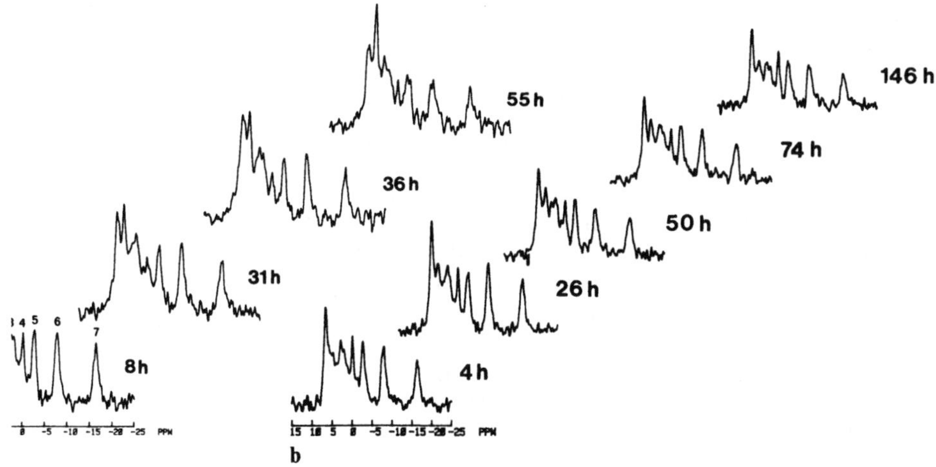

10 a, b. Two series of ^{31}P spectra ob- from the cerebral cortex of birth as- ıted infants born at 37 weeks (**a**) and 36 (**b**) gestation. The postnatal ages at the of study are indicated. Peak assign- : *1*, PME; *2*, Pi; *3*, PDE; *4*, PCr; *5*, *6* and γ, α and β resonances of NTP. **a** At age Cr/Pi was 0.99, NTP/P_{tot} 0.09 and pH_i ›H_i rose to a maximum of 7.28 at 36 h. ıinimum value for PCr/Pi was 0.32 at 55 :n NTP/P_{tot} was 0.04 and pH_i was 6.99. fant died aged 60 h. **b** At age 4 h, PCr/Pi 97, NTP/P_{tot} 0.09 and pH_i 7.08; pH_i rose ıaximum of 7.23 at 26 h. The minimum for PCr/Pi was 0.65 at 50 h, but by 146 h normal, 0.93. NTP/P_{tot} never fell below ıl. The infant died aged 27 days with al atrophy. (From Azzopardi et al. ')

results from absolute quantitation :s (Cady and Azzopardi 1989; Cady which will be described in Sect. 2. These time-dependent changes an important implication for clini- :udies. Obviously, the results ob- ı will depend on when a study is . In birth asphyxia, studies per- :d on the first day of life or when the t is more than 1 week old may not a true indication of the degree of ge when assessed on the basis of ve concentrations and pH_i alone. In to obtain a realistic estimate of the severity of the injury it is preferable to perform sequential studies on a daily basis.

Results from studies both on normal infants and on infants suspected of hypoxic-ischaemic brain injury, who were investigated because of evidence of birth asphyxia, postnatal asphyxia or increased echodensities on ultrasound scans, are presented in Tables 5.4 and 5.5. The metabolite ratios were determined from the spectra using integration to obtain peak areas and hence may be subject to systematic, but consistent, errors due to the effects of peak overlap. The values given are those which were measured when PCr/Pi was at its lowest observed value. In Table 5.4, the infants are grouped according to clinical classification but without regard to developmental changes related to PCA. Table 5.5 compares the results from abnormal infants with those from normal infants by presenting the results as standard deviation scores (SDS) corrected for PCA. The results given in Table 5.5 show that several metabolite ratios, including PCr/Pi, PCr/P_{tot} and NTP/P_{tot}, were significantly less (Mann-Whitney test) in the abnormal infants and that Pi/P_{tot} and Pi/NTP were significantly higher. No statistically significant dependence of pH_i on clinical classification was found.

Table 5.4. Phosphorus metabolite ratios[a] and pH_i[b] in normal infants with suspected hypoxic-ischaemic brain injury

	Normal infants	Infants suspected of hypoxic-ischaemic brain injury			
		All infants	Birth asphyxia	Postnatal asphyxia	Increased echodensities
Gestation (weeks)	33 (26–42)	38 (27–42)	41 (31–42)	33 (31–38)	33 (27–41)
Age (days)	5 (1–96)	3 (1–23)	3 (1–10)	5 (4–23)	9 (3–16)
PCr/Pi	0.99±0.18	0.69±0.35	0.67±0.35	1.04±0.20	0.61±0.32
NTP/P_{tot}	0.09±0.01	0.08±0.03	0.08±0.03	0.10±0.02	0.08±0.03
PCr/P_{tot}	0.09±0.01	0.08±0.02	0.08±0.02	0.10±0.01	0.07±0.03
Pi/P_{tot}	0.10±0.01	0.15±0.09	0.16±0.10	0.10±0.01	0.16±0.10
PME/P_{tot}	0.29±0.03	0.29±0.04	0.29±0.04	0.27±0.02	0.31±0.05
PDE/P_{tot}	0.20±0.02	0.20±0.03	0.20±0.03	0.22±0.01	0.19±0.03
PCr/NTP	1.02±0.20	1.16±0.63	1.21±0.68	1.06±0.18	1.07±0.03
Pi/NTP	1.05±0.23	5.22±18.75	3.28±4.48	1.05±0.29	11.36±36.44
PME/NTP	3.18±0.61	6.60±17.90	4.62±2.89	2.97±0.68	12.96±34.73
PDE/NTP	2.21±0.48	3.87±7.27	3.26±2.38	2.35±0.47	5.89±13.81
pH_i[c]	7.11±0.13	7.14±0.27	7.16±0.19	7.09±0.14	7.13±0.45

[a] For normal infants, $n=30$; all infants, $n=61$; birth asphyxia, $n=40$; postnatal asphyxia, $n=5$; increased echodensities, $n=16$

[b] For normal infants, $n=22$; all infants, $n=55$; birth asphyxia, $n=36$; postnatal asphyxia, $n=5$; increased echodensities, $n=14$

[c] pH_i was not calculated when the Pi peak resolution was inadequate

Table 5.5. Age-dependent standard deviation score (SDS) for phosphorus metabolite ratios[a] and pH_i[b] in infants with suspected hypoxic-ischaemic brain injury. (From Azzopardi et al. 1989 b)

	All infants	Birth asphyxia	Postnatal asphyxia	Increased echodensities
PCr/Pi	−2.14±2.10*	−2.14±2.19*	−0.03±0.76	−2.04±1.78*
NTP/P_{tot}	−0.98±1.86**	−1.17±1.82**	−0.01±1.03	−0.83±1.99
PCr/P_{tot}	−1.72±2.58*	−1.79±2.59*	0.33±1.04	−2.19±2.52*
Pi/P_{tot}	5.40±8.77*	5.97±8.91*	0.69±0.99	5.51±9.06**
PME/P_{tot}	0.42±1.69	0.63±1.58	−0.79±1.26	0.30±1.83
PDE/P_{tot}	0.44±1.43	−0.60±1.44***	0.39±0.50	−0.32±1.47
PCr/NTP	0.52±2.98	0.65±3.14	0.15±0.66	0.31±2.91
Pi/NTP	7.21±16.41*	8.96±17.94*	0.35±1.06	4.94±13.27**
PME/NTP	1.94±4.40***	2.49±4.71**	−0.26±1.11	1.25±3.72
PDE/NTP	1.02±3.84	1.43±4.48	0.17±0.77	0.23±1.81
pH_i	0.05±1.47	0.23±0.97	−0.28±0.22	0.00±2.21

Values are those obtained when PCr/Pi was at its lowest; mean values for SDS±SD vs the normal control infants are given

* $p<0.001$; ** $p<0.01$; *** $p<0.05$

[a] For n values see Table 5.4

[b] For n values see Table 5.4

5.3.3.2 Absolute Concentrations

Absolute concentrations of metabolites in the brains of newborn human infants have recently been estimated using a technique in which the ^1H MRS signal from brain water protons was used as an endogenous internal concentration reference (Cady and Azzopardi 1989; Cady 1990, 1991). The absolute concentration estimates obtained by MRS from normal human infants agree well with values obtained from neonatal mammalian brain using other invasive techniques. The agreement is improved if a rigorous spectrum analysis method is used, such as fitting Lorentzian profiles to the peaks using χ^2 minimisation (Cady 1991) (Fig. 5.11). Table 5.6 gives the estimated absolute concentrations for normal infants and compares these values with those obtained from a birth asphyxiated infant of similar PCA. There is evidence that absolute concentrations may increase with PCA in premature infants and hence it is important to take this into account (Cady and Azzopardi 1989). In Table 5.6, both sets of data from the birth asphyxiated infant show substantial reductions in all the metabolite concentrations, apart from that of Pi. At age 3 days, PCr/Pi was approximately 0.4 and this had doubled by age 6 days demonstrating recovery of normal metabolite ratios. However, the severity of the hypoxic-ischaemic insult is still indicated by the low absolute concentrations which were probably related to irreversible tissue damage. The normal [Pi] at age 3 days was probably related to hydrolysis of PCr and NTP. Figure 5.11 shows ^{31}P

Fig. 5.11 a, b. ^{31}P spectra from a fatally birth asphyxiated infant at ages 1 day (**a**) and 2 days (**b**). PCA at birth was 36 weeks. Both spectra are plotted on the same vertical scale and peak identifications are as in Fig. 5.10. The *dashed lines* are Lorentzian curves fitted to the spectrum using χ^2 minimisation (Cady 1991). The individual fitted components are shown also. The γ, α and β-NTP multiplets were fitted as doublets (γ and α) and a triplet (β) with J-coupling of 16 Hz. On both days, [PCr], [NTP] and [P_{tot}] were low and [Pi] was elevated. **a** Concentrations (mmol/l): Pi, 4.4; PCr, 0.7; NTP, 1.9; P_{tot}, 31.4. **b** Concentrations (mmol/l): Pi, 4.5; PCr, 0.4; NTP, 2.0; P_{tot}, 38.2. (Spectra collected in collaboration with D Azzopardi, DT Delpy, R Aldridge and EOR Reynolds)

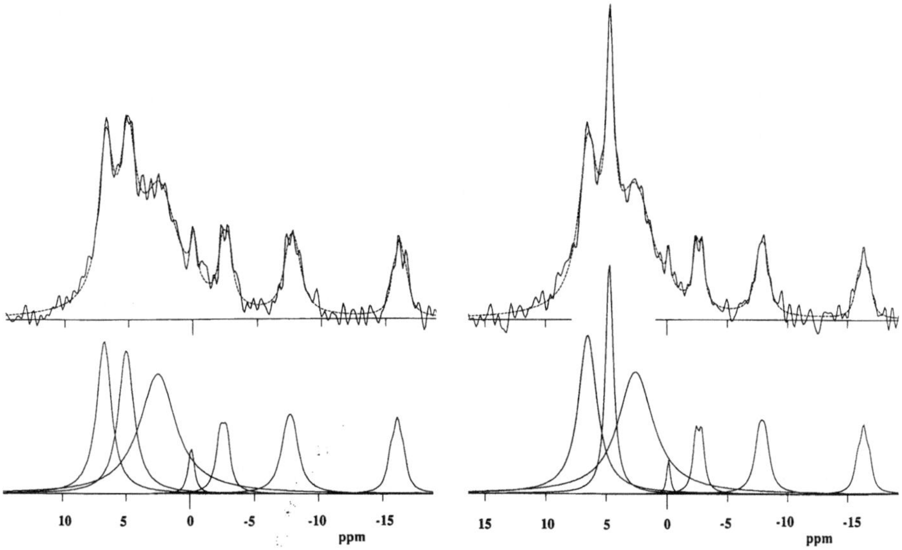

a **b**

Table 5.6. Absolute concentrations of phosphorus metabolites in the cerebral cortex of normal infants and a birth asphyxiated infant

	PME	Pi	PDE	PCr	NTP	P_{tot}
Normal infants (GPA 35–37 weeks; $n=7$)[a]	12.8 (2.5)	2.5 (0.7)	17.9 (4.8)	2.4 (0.6)	3.7 (0.6)	48.3 (7.4)
Birth asphyxia[b]						
age 3 days	5.8	2.6	10.2	1.1	1.9	26.7
age 6 days	2.8	1.7	6.5	1.3	1.3	17.1

Concentrations of metabolites in mmol/l; mean (SD).
Peak areas were measured from the spectra by fitting Lorentzian profiles to the resonances using χ^2 minimisation.
[a] Data for normal infants from Cady (1991)
[b] Both sets of data were obtained from the same infant who had major neurodevelopmental impairments at independent assessment at age 1 year

spectra obtained from another patient with severe birth asphyxia. The [Pi]s estimated for this infant, age 1 day and 2 days, were both higher than the mean value for normal infants given in Table 5.6; most other concentrations were reduced.

The results presented in Table 5.6 and Fig. 5.11 indicate that the estimates of absolute concentrations give new information about the physiological state of brain tissue which is additional to that provided by relative concentrations and pH_i alone. The spectrum obtained at age 6 days from the birth asphyxiated infant whose results are presented in Table 5.6 could have been considered "normal" without the insight provided by absolute quantitation. Furthermore, the evidence provided by absolute concentrations indicates that low PCr/Pi values may, in some cases at least, be related to both reduced [PCr] and raised [Pi] (see also Table 5.7 which is discussed in Sect. 5.4). It is of interest to note also that reduced absolute concentrations are seen in severe birth asphyxia before imaging modalities (e.g. ultrasound) show the presence of space occupying lesions (e.g. porencephalic cysts).

5.4 Prognostic Sensitivity and Specificity

Enough data have now been acquired to relate relative concentrations, measured within a few days of birth, to neurodevelopmental outcome, as assessed independently at age 1 year. Preliminary results are also available which provide some idea of the potential prognostic value of absolute concentration measurements.

5.4.1 Relative Concentrations

Figures 5.12a–c show the relationships between the minimum observed values for PCr/Pi, survival and independently assessed neurodevelopmental outcome at age 1 year (Azzopardi et al. 1989b). Infants who were progressing normally or with only minor impairments had minimum PCr/Pi values which were within or close to the 95% confidence limits for normal controls (Fig. 5.12a). Minimum PCr/Pi values for infants with major neuromotor impairments were often low especially when these were multiple (Fig. 5.12b). A very large proportion of the

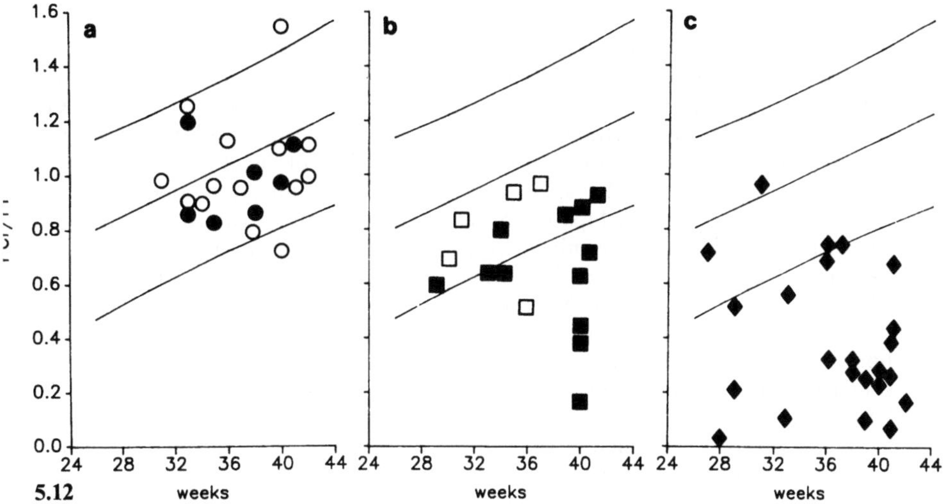

5.12

Fig. 5.12 a–c. The relationships between minimum values for PCr/Pi in the neonatal cerebral cortex, survival and neurodevelopmental outcome at age 1 year. The regression line and 95% confidence limits for normal values vs PCA are shown. **a** ○, normal progress: (standard deviation score vs normal infants (SDS) = -0.29 ± 1.21 (SD); not significant (ns); ●, minor impairments: SDS = -0.54 ± 0.52, ns. **b** □, major neuromotor impairment: SDS = -1.06 ± 1.22, $p < 0.05$; ■, multiple major impairments: SDS = -2.60 ± 1.44, $p < 0.001$. **c** ◆, died: SDS = -3.82 ± 1.89, $p < 0.001$. (From Azzopardi et al. 1989 b)

Fig. 5.13 a–c. Relationships between the values for NTP/P_{tot} (measured from the same spectra as the minimum PCr/Pi), survival and neurodevelopmental outcome at age 1 year. The linear regression and 95% confidence limits for normal values vs PCA are shown. **a** ○, normal progress: standard deviation score vs normal infants (SDS) = -0.22 ± 1.01 (SD), not significant (ns); ●, minor impairments: SDS = -0.03 ± 0.98, ns. **b** □, major neuromotor impairments: SDS = $+0.13 \pm 1.12$, ns; ■, multiple major impairments: SDS = -0.67 ± 0.74, $p < 0.05$. **c** ◆, died: SDS = -2.13 ± 2.45, $p < 0.002$. (From Azzopardi et al. 1989 b)

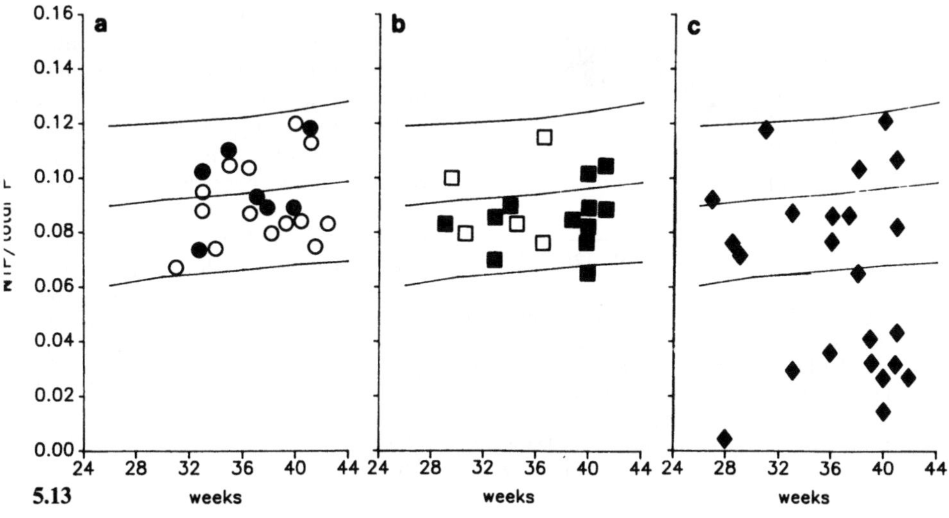

5.13

infants who died had minimum PCr/Pi values below 95% confidence limits (Fig. 5.12c). In this study, the minimum observed PCr/Pi value was found to have a sensitivity of 74%, a specificity of 92% and a positive predictive value for unfavourable outcome of 93%. Figures 5.13a–c give the relationships for measurements of NTP/P_{tot} determined from the same spectra on the occasion when PCr/Pi was at a minimum. Values for NTP/P_{tot} below the confidence limits for normal controls were almost always associated with a fatal outcome. NTP/P_{tot} had a sensitivity of 47%, a specificity of 97% and a positive predictive value for fatal outcome of 91%. Similar studies on infants with increased cerebral echodensities on ultrasound scans indicated that such infants were more likely to have low PCr/Pi and a poor prognosis if the echodensities were diffuse or consistent with intraparenchymal haemorrhage than when they were indicative of periventricular leucomalacia. Independent neurodevelopmental assessment of survivors at age 1 year also indicated a correlation between the Griffiths general quotient and the minimum PCr/Pi as shown in Fig. 5.14.

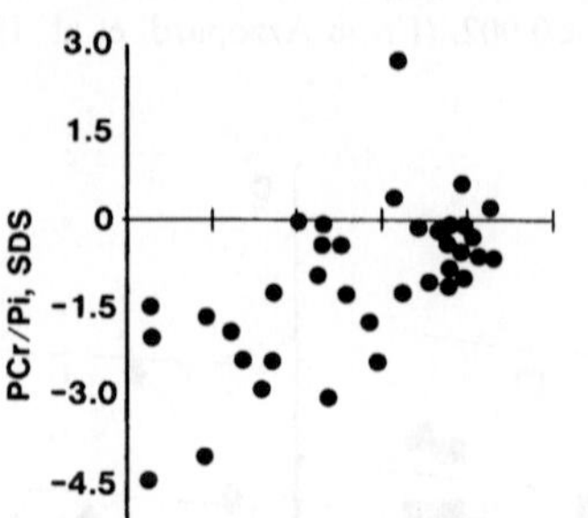

Fig. 5.14. The relationship between minimum observed values for PCr/Pi expressed as a standard deviation score (*SDS*) vs normal infants and Griffiths general quotient (*GQ*) assessed at age 1 year in 38 surviving infants. Scores of 50 or below are recorded as 50 ($r=0.67$, $p<0.001$). (From Azzopardi et al. 1989b)

5.4.2 Absolute Concentrations

At this time, it is only possible to discuss preliminary results concerning the prognostic value of absolute concentrations in studies of birth asphyxia. Table 5.7 gives mean absolute concentrations obtained from birth asphyxiated infants grouped according to neurodevelopmental outcome at age 1 year. Since the infants were all born at approximately full term it is appropriate to compare the absolute concentrations in Table 5.7 with those from normal infants given in Table 5.6. [Pi] was elevated in all groups but only significantly ($p<0.02$) when there was a fatal outcome. All other metabolite concentrations were similar to normal values apart from a reduced [PCr] in the group with fatal outcome ($p<0.01$). Due to the limited amount of data in Table 5.7 it is, as yet, difficult to anticipate the impact that absolute concentration estimates will have on the prognostic capability of ^{31}P MRS.

5.5 Perspectives and Conclusions

The capability to perform repeated metabolic analyses of living organs, such as the brain, noninvasively, in their natural environments and free of many of the artefacts which can affect results obtained using conventional biochemical methods, is an outstanding feature of MRS. This is of great importance, especially in paediatric medicine, and in the future might provide more detailed quantitative descriptions of organ functions than available at present. It must be emphasised that, although the central biochemical pathways are already generally established, understanding of the mechanisms of their regulation (i.e. enzyme concentrations, rate of synthesis, feedback inhibition, rate of degradation or catalytic activity) is still incomplete. Thus, comparing equilibrium concentrations of metabolites in health and disease

Table 5.7. Absolute concentrations of phosphorus metabolites in the cerebral cortex of birth asphyxiated infants and independent neurodevelopmental assessment at age 1 year (preliminary results)

Neurodevelopmental status	PME	Pi	PDE	PCr	NTP	P_{tot}
Normal progress ($n=5$)	10.4 (2.8)	3.6 (1.2)	15.0 (2.0)	2.4 (0.7)	3.1 (0.5)	42.4 (5.8)
Major/minor impairments ($n=5$)	9.4 (3.6)	3.6 (1.6)	15.0 (4.8)	2.3 (1.4)	3.3 (1.2)	41.9 (13.1)
Died ($n=4$)	13.0 (2.0)	4.7* (1.8)	16.0 (3.6)	1.1* (0.7)	3.1 (1.4)	44.2 (10.8)

Concentrations in mmol/l; mean (SD).
All spectra acquired from infants born at approximately full term and within 7 days of birth. Data collected in collaboration with D Azzopardi, S Roth, R Aldridge, DT Delpy and EOR Reynolds. Independent neurological assessments were carried out by AL Stewart and J Baudin
* $p<0.02$; ** $p<0.01$

and monitoring the effects of therapeutic interventions are major tasks of in vivo MRS. Even more interesting and important is the possibility of measuring the rates of in vivo enzymatic reactions that take place in a time scale of milli- and microseconds (e.g. the creatine kinase reaction) without disturbing the biochemical system by using special *magnetisation transfer* methods.

Many metabolites, e.g. PCr, ATP, PEt, PCh, GPE, GPC, glutamate and aspartate (both major excitatory neurotransmitters), together with other amino acids, like *N*-acetylaspartate (NAA), taurine and glycine, have assignable resonances in ^{31}P and ^{1}H spectra acquired from the human brain. The PCr/Pi ratio has been used to describe the energy status of the normal neonatal brain and following hypoxic-ischaemic injury. The chemical shift of Pi has been used to estimate pH_i. PEt has been identified as the major constituent of the PME peak and is a phospholipid precursor for membrane and myelin synthesis in the CNS. GPE and GPC, which are components of the PDE peak in the ^{31}P spectrum together with semi-mobile phospholipids, are thought to be primarily degradation products of these membrane constituents but also serve as precursors for synthesis de novo. Several brain metabolites show marked changes in concentration during normal ontogenesis. Age-dependent changes in phosphorus metabolites of the neonatal and infant brain have been observed in vivo by several investigators using ^{31}P MRS (Cady et al. 1983; Younkin et al. 1984; Hope et al. 1984; Boesch and Martin 1988; Boesch et al. 1989; Cady and Azzopardi 1989). Great interest centres on the lactate concentration in brain tissue and in the CSF both of normal children and of those suffering from birth asphyxia or hydrocephalus. Recent results from MRS studies on neonatal brain energy metabolism are promising and suggest that important information concerning normal and pathologic metabolic processes can be obtained. It is interesting to note also that ^{31}P spectroscopic results are beginning to be incorporated into the planning of paediatric patient management (Hamilton et al. 1986; Azzopardi et al. 1989b).

To achieve the final goal of incorporating this information into daily patient care (i.e. to improve the clinical understanding and management of diseases) many difficulties have yet to be solved. Apart from patient handling and physiological monitoring (see Sect. 5.1) there are three major problems which in vivo

MRS will have to deal with in the future: (1) sensitivity enhancement; (2) exact localisation of the anatomical source of the signals; and (3) the interpretation of spectra in the context of the pathophysiology of the patient. Thus, at the present, in vivo MRS is mainly a research tool and has not yet reached a well established position in clinical medicine. Spectrometer systems capable of performing both MRI and MRS in children will contribute to overcome these problems and will help to promote the future application of MRS in paediatrics. The eventual general clinical application of this important new information about cerebral metabolism to the benefit of the child will be our ultimate goal.

5.5.1 Sensitivity Enhancement and Multinuclear in vivo MRS of the Brain

Since the natural abundance of the ^{13}C isotope is only about 1%, the introduction of ^{13}C labelled metabolic precursors such as [^{13}C]glucose or [^{13}C]pyruvate into metabolic pathways opens up new fields for in vivo biochemistry studies under both physiological and pathologic conditions. Using this technique the metabolic fluxes of various substrates can be measured. Homonuclear and heteronuclear experiments for spin decoupling among protons or between protons and carbon nuclei result in spectrum simplification and can greatly increase the sensitivity of in vivo MRS to physiological change (Bottomley et al. 1989). Despite the promising possibility of using ^{1}H and ^{13}C MRS to obtain noninvasive insight into the glycolytic pathway, the citric acid cycle and even the turnover of certain amino acids, MR methods using these nuclei for studies of the brains of neonates and infants are still at a very early stage of research. Animal experiments and the first results from human multinuclear studies (e.g. using ^{1}H and ^{31}P, or ^{1}H and ^{13}C) promise significant insight into the relationships between high-energy phosphates, pH_i and lactate, or amino acid and carbohydrate metabolism, respectively (Bottomley 1989).

5.5.2 Improvements in Localisation and Quantification Techniques

Although localised ^{1}H and ^{31}P in vivo MRS of the adult human brain is an established technique for whole body systems in a few specialised centres worldwide (e.g. Bottomley et al. 1988; Luyten et al. 1989; Hubesch et al. 1990), volume-selected spectroscopic data from small children are still rare. To date, there is a large amount of information on cerebral metabolism from non-localised, surface coil ^{31}P MRS studies of neonates and infants in health and disease. Further technological developments using MR image-guided localisation methods with smaller voxels for infant brains (Gruetter et al. 1990b; van der Knaap et al. 1990) and methods for spectroscopic imaging (SI) and metabolite mapping (Maudsley et al. 1990) will allow the monitoring of regional brain metabolism during normal development and the comparison of metabolic processes in different brain regions during therapeutic intervention. Combining MRI and MRS will also improve the understanding of spectroscopic data, their acceptance by the clinical staff, their quantitative information content and hence their scientific value. The first in vivo image-guided localised ^{1}H spectra from normal infant brains have recently been published (van der Knaap et al. 1990). Absolute quantitation of cerebral metabolite concentrations is an important goal of in vivo MRS. Many different approaches exist for the establishment of internal or external concentration references. As emphasized in Sect. 5.3.2, such methods are urgently needed in order to detect subtle differences in brain metabolism during normal development and disease.

5.5.3 Interpretation of Data

Unlike the phosphorus metabolites, with biochemical functions which can be easily assigned to well established metabolic processes in the brain, the interpretation of resonances in the ^1H spectrum other than lactate, however, poses problems which have still to be solved. For example, signals from several acetyl residues contribute to the NAA CH_3 resonance (one of the most prominent peaks in ^1H brain spectra) and even the pathophysiological role of NAA itself is not at all clear. γ-Aminobutyrate (GABA), a major inhibitory neurotransmitter, although well assigned in ^1H spectra of acid extracts from animal brains, cannot, as yet, be identified with certainty in vivo. Furthermore, due to the study time available, it is difficult to obtain fully relaxed spectra in neonates and small children and hence apparent changes in relative and absolute concentrations during development or disease have to be interpreted with caution since they can also be caused by age- or pathology-dependent alterations in relaxation times without changes in real substrate concentrations.

References

Azzopardi D, Wyatt JS, Hamilton PA, Cady EB, Delpy DT, Hope PL, Reynolds EOR (1989a) Phosphorus metabolites and intracellular pH in the brains of normal and small for gestational age infants investigated by magnetic resonance spectroscopy. Pediatr Res 25:440–444

Azzopardi D, Wyatt JS, Cady EB, Delpy DT, Baudin J, Stewart AL, Hope PL, Hamilton PA, Reynolds EOR (1989b) Prognosis of newborn infants with hypoxic-ischemic brain injury assessed by phosphorus magnetic resonance spectroscopy. Pediatr Res 25:445–451

Boesch C, Martin E (1988) Combined application of MR imaging and spectroscopy in neonates and children: installation and operation of a 2.35-T system in a clinical setting. Radiology 168:481–488

Boesch C, Luescher K, Brunner P, Kewitz G, Martin E (1988) Monitoring and intensive care of premature neonates and children in a 2.35 T spectroscopy and imaging system. Proceedings of the Society of Magnetic Resonance in Medicine, 7th Annual Meeting, San Francisco, p 673

Boesch C, Gruetter R, Martin E, Duc G, Wüthrich K (1989) Variations in the in-vivo P-31 MR spectra of the developing human brain during postnatal life. Radiology 172:197–199

Bottomley PA (1984) Selective volume method for performing localized NMR spectroscopy. US Patent 4480228

Bottomley PA (1989) Human in vivo NMR spectroscopy in diagnostic medicine: clinical tool or research probe. Radiology 170:1–15

Bottomley PA, Charles HC, Roemer PB, Flamig D, Engeseth H, Edelstein WA, Mueller OM (1988) Human in vivo phosphate metabolite imaging with ^{31}P NMR. Magn Reson Med 7:319–336

Bottomley PA, Hardy CJ, Roemer PB, Mueller OM (1989) Proton-decoupled, Overhauser-enhanced, spatially localized carbon-13 spectroscopy in humans. Magn Reson Med 11:348–363

Brown TR, Kincaid BM, Ugurbil K (1982) NMR chemical shift imaging in three dimensions. Proc Natl Acad Sci USA 79:3523–3526

Cady EB (1990) Absolute quantitation of phosphorus metabolites in the cerebral cortex of the newborn human infant and in the forearm muscles of young adults using a double tuned surface coil. J Magn Reson 87:433–446

Cady EB (1991) A reappraisal of the absolute concentrations of phosphorylated metabolites in the human neonatal cerebral cortex obtained by fitting Lorentzian curves to the ^{31}P NMR spectrum. J Magn Reson 91:637–643

Cady EB, Azzopardi D (1989) Absolute quantitation of neonatal brain spectra acquired with surface coil localization. NMR Biomed 2:305–311

Cady EB, Costello AM de L, Dawson MJ, Delpy DT, Hope PL, Reynolds EOR, Tofts PS, Wilkie DR (1983) Non-invasive investigation of cerebral metabolism in newborn infants by phosphorus nuclear magnetic resonance spectroscopy. Lancet i:1059–1062

Chance B, Nakase Y, Bond M, Leigh JS, McDonald G (1978) Detection of ^{31}P nuclear magnetic resonance signals in brain by in vivo and freezed trapped assays. Proc Natl Acad Sci USA 75:4925–4929

Delivoria-Papadopolous M, Chance B (1988) ^{31}P NMR spectroscopy in the newborn. In: Guthrie RD (ed) Recent advances in neonatal intensive care. Churchill Livingstone, Edinburgh, pp 153–197

Den Hollander JA, Luyten PR, Marien AJH, Segebarth CM, Balériaux DF, de Beer R, van Ormondt D (1989) Potentials of quantitative image-localized human ^{31}P nuclear magnetic resonance spectroscopy in the clinical evaluation of intracranial tumors. Magn Reson Q 5:152–168

Frahm J, Merboldt KD, Hanicke W (1987) Localized proton spectroscopy using stimulated echoes. J Magn Reson 72:502–508

Gordon RE, Hanley PE, Shaw D, Gadian DG, Radda GK, Styles P, Bore PJ, Chan L (1980) Localization of metabolites in animals using ^{31}P topical magnetic resonance. Nature 287:736–738

Gruetter R, Fusch C, Martin E, Boesch C (1990a) Assessment of saturation effects in the in vivo P-31 NMR spectra of the normal human brain in the first year of life. Proceedings of the Society of Magnetic Resonance in Medicine, 9th Annual Meeting, New York, p 994

Gruetter R, Martin E, Boesch C (1990b) Gradient-localized in vivo P-31 NMR spectroscopy of infant brain on small-bore magnets. Proceedings of the Society of Magnetic Resonance in Medicine, 9th Annual Meeting, New York, p 1002

Hamilton PA, Hope PL, Cady EB, Delpy DT, Wyatt JS, Reynolds EOR (1986) Impaired energy metabolism in brains of newborn infants with increased cerebral echodensities. Lancet i:1242–1246

Hope PL, Costello AM de L, Cady EB, Delpy DT, Tofts PS, Chu A, Hamilton PA, Reynolds EOR (1984) Cerebral energy metabolism studied with phosphorus NMR spectroscopy in normal and birth-asphyxiated infants. Lancet ii:366–370

Hope PL, Costello AM de L, Cady EB, Delpy DT, Tofts PS, Chu A, Reynolds EOR (1986) Cerebral metabolism in newborn infants studied by phosphorus nuclear magnetic resonance spectroscopy. In: Rolfe P (ed) Neonatal physiological measurements. Butterworths, London, pp 382–389

Hoult DI (1979) Rotating frame zeugmatography. J Magn Reson 33:183–197

Hubesch B, Sappey-Marinier D, Roth K, Meyerhoff DJ, Matson GB, Weiner MW (1990) P-31 MR spectroscopy of normal human brain and brain tumors. Radiology 174:401–409

Luyten PR, Groen JP, Vermeulen JWAH, den Hollander JA (1989) Experimental approaches to image localized human ^{31}P NMR spectroscopy. Magn Reson Med 11:1–21

Martin E, Boesch C, Gruetter R, Kikinis R, Kewitz G, Boltshauser E, Werner B, Eich G (1988) Magnetresonanz in der paediatrischen Forschung und Klinik, Part II: Untersuchungen zur Entwicklung und Pathologie des Gehirns bei Neugeborenen, Säuglingen und Kleinkindern. Helv Paediatr Acta 43:75–86

Maudsley AA, Twieg DB, Sappey-Marinier D, Hubesch B, Hugg JW, Matson GB, Weiner MW (1990) Spin echo ^{31}P spectroscopic imaging in the human brain. Magn Reson Med 14:415–422

Ordidge RJ, Bendall MR, Gordon RE, Connelly A (1985) Volume selection for in-vivo biological spectroscopy. In: Govil G, Khetrapal CL, Saron A (eds) Magnetic resonance in biology and medicine. Tata – McGraw-Hill, New Delhi, p 387

Ordidge RJ, Connelly A, Lohman JAB (1986) Image-selected in vivo spectroscopy (ISIS). A new technique for spatially selective NMR spectroscopy. J Magn Reson 66:283–294

Petroff OAC, Prichard JW, Behar KL, Alger JR, den Hollander JA, Shulman RG (1985) Cerebral intracellular pH by ^{31}P nuclear magnetic resonance spectroscopy. Neurology 35:781–788

Shellock FG (1989) Biological effects and safety aspects of magnetic resonance imaging. Magn Reson Q 5:243–261

Siesjö BK (1978) Brain energy metabolism. Wiley, New York, pp 1–28, 151–209

Van der Knaap MS, van der Grond J, van Rijen PC, Faber JAJ, Valk J, Willemse K (1990) Age-dependent changes in localized proton and phosphorus MR spectroscopy of the brain. Radiology 176:509–515

Younkin DP, Delivoria-Papadopoulos M, Leonard JC, Subramanian H, Eleff S, Leigh JS, Chance B (1984) Unique aspects of human newborn cerebral metabolism evaluated with phosphorus nuclear magnetic resonance spectroscopy. Ann Neurol 16:581–586

6 Near Infrared Spectroscopy

J. S. Wyatt and D. T. Delpy

CONTENTS

6.1 Introduction

Near infrared spectroscopy (NIRS) involving transillumination of several centimetres of intact tissue was first described by Jobsis in 1977, although visible optical spectroscopy through thin tissue sections had long been employed (Matthes 1935; Millikan 1942; Brinkman et. al. 1950; Merrick 1975). NIRS when applied to the head can provide noninvasive quantification of a number of important indices of cerebral oxygenation and haemodynamics in sick newborn infants undergoing intensive care.

6.2 Principles

The technique depends on two fundamental physical properties: (a) the relative transparency of biological tissue to light in the near infrared region of the spectrum and (b) the existence within the tissues of a small number of chromophores (colour-bearing compounds) which are present in variable concentrations and whose light absorbing properties vary with oxygenation.

6.2.1 The Relative Transparency of Biological Tissue

The principle chromophore present in human tissue is water. However, in the region between 400 and 1000 nm, its optical absorption is low and there is thus a "window of transparency" which permits light penetration through several centimetres of tissue. Melanin in the surface layers of the skin is a powerful absorber of light in the UV and visible parts of the optical spectrum, but its absorption falls rapidly with increasing wavelength and is quite low in the near infrared (Boulnois 1986). The other major tissue chromophores are haemoglobin and myoglobin, which have intense absorption bands in the visible region of the spectrum, extending up to 650 nm. Light at visible wavelengths is therefore strongly attenuated in tissue and the maximum distance of penetration is about 1 cm. At near infrared wavelengths (700–1000 nm) the absorption coefficients of haemoglobin and myoglobin are about two orders of magnitude less than in the visible region and light attenuation is therefore greatly reduced. In this near infrared region, optical attenuation is dominated by light scattering in the tissues, and the fall in intensity is approximately one order of magnitude per centimetre of tissue thickness (this is usually expressed as one optical density per centimetre). Using modern light sources and detectors, it is possible to detect light across a total attenuation of ten optical densities, equivalent to about 8–9 cm of brain (Cope and Delpy 1988). It is therefore feasible to detect light that has traversed the infant head from one side to the other.

6.2.2 Chromophores in Brain Tissue

There are only three chromophores with significant absorption in the near infrared region that are also present in brain tissue in variable concentrations. These are oxyhaemoglobin (HbO_2), deoxyhaemoglobin (Hb) and oxidised cytochrome aa_3 (cyt aa_3), the terminal member of the mitochondrial respiratory chain. Detection of these chromophores allows the assessment of cerebral oxygenation and haemodynamics. Changes in cerebral [HbO_2] and [Hb] concentrations provide information about cerebral haemoglobin oxygenation, blood volume and whole brain oxygen delivery. Electrons passed down the respiratory chain are transferred by cyt aa_3 to molecular oxygen and protons producing water, a reaction which accounts for over 95% of oxygen consumption within the body (Fig. 6.1). Changes in the redox state of this enzyme, detected from changes in [cyt aa_3], may thus reflect changes in the adequacy of oxygen delivery at a mitochondrial level. All other absorbers present within brain tissue can be assumed to have a fixed concentration and will therefore not contribute to any changes in optical attenuation that are measured.

6.2.3 The Beer-Lambert Law

The relationship between optical absorption and chromophore concentration in a clear solution with a single chromophore is described by Beer-Lambert law:

$$\mathrm{Log}(I_0/I) = OD = a \times c \times L \qquad (6.1)$$

where *OD* (a dimensionless factor known as the optical density) is the logarithm of the ratio of the incident intensity (I_0) to

Fig. 6.1. Simplified outline of oxidative phosphorylation

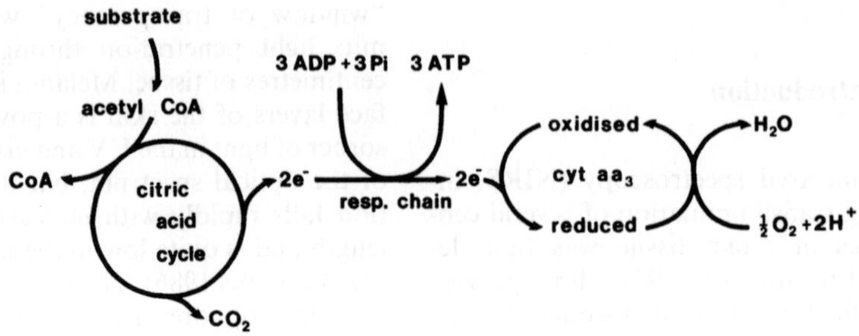

the transmitted intensity (I), a is the absorption coefficient of the chromophore ($mM^{-1} \times cm^{-1}$), c is concentration (mM) and L is the distance (cm) between light entry and exit points. The Beer-Lambert relationship was initially derived for nonscattering solutions in which photons travel in straight lines between the source and detector. Biological tissue, however, is a highly scattering medium and photons travel in an extended path with multiple reflections between the sites of light entry and exit. Nonetheless, the Beer-Lambert law can be applied to a scattering medium (Cope et al. 1988), but the relationship must be modified (Delpy et al. 1988):

$$OD = a \times c \times L \times B + G \qquad (6.2)$$

Here, B is a dimensionless "pathlength factor" which accounts for the increase in optical pathlength caused by scattering and G is a geometrical factor which accounts for loss of photons by scattering out of the line between the source and detector. If L, B and G remain constant, then changes in optical density may be converted into changes in chromophore concentration by the relationship:

$$\Delta c = \Delta OD / a \times L \times B \qquad (6.3)$$

If a, L and B are known it is then possible to convert changes in optical attenuation (measured in optical densities) into changes in concentration (in mmol $\times l^{-1}$). If more than one chromophore is present it is necessary to measure optical density changes at several wavelengths. A series of simultaneous equations are then obtained which can be solved to provide concentration changes for each chromophore. This series of equations is frequently called an "algorithm" (Wray et al. 1988). As there are four chromophores within brain tissue (HbO_2, Hb, oxidised Cyt aa_3, reduced Cyt aa_3), it is in theory necessary to make measurements at a minimum of four different wavelengths within the near infrared region. However, since the total concentration of cytochrome remains constant and only the ratio of the oxidised to reduced forms varies, in principle it is only necessary to measure at three wavelengths. If more than three wavelengths are employed, standard curve-fitting analysis may be used to increase the accuracy of the calculated concentration changes (Araki and Nashimoto 1989).

6.2.4 Absorption Coefficients

The absorption coefficients of HbO_2 and Hb have been obtained from in vitro studies of purified solutions. Those of cytochrome aa_3 have been obtained from in vivo studies on fluorocarbon exchange-transfused rats because it has been suggested that the in vivo and in vitro spectra of cytochrome aa_3 may differ (Jobsis et. al. 1988). Using a fluorocarbon blood substitute, it is possible to render an experimental animal virtually haemoglobin-free, while maintaining normal oxygenation and perfusion. By comparing the optical spectra obtained from the brain before and after death, a difference spectrum (oxygenated-reduced) of the cytochrome is obtained. The absorption coefficients can then be employed in the development of algorithms for use on human tissue (Wray et al. 1988).

6.2.5 Estimation of Pathlength

Quantification of NIRS data requires knowledge of the average pathlength of the photons traversing the tissue. Due to multiple scattering, this pathlength is considerably longer than the interoptode distance (the distance between the transmitting and receiving fibres). For quantification, it is therefore necessary to estimate B, the pathlength factor in the modified Beer-Lambert relationship (Eq. 6.3). Three techniques have been employed to determine this pathlength factor in brain tissue.

Firstly, use has been made of the fact that water has a broad absorption peak at 950–1050 nm. If the attenuation of light at these wavelengths is measured, the apparent concentration of water in the tissues can be calculated. Dividing this value by the known tissue water concentration allows the factor B to be derived. Using this method in the rat head, a value for B of 4.3 ± 0.4 was obtained (Wray et al. 1988).

An alternative approach is to measure the time of flight of an ultrashort pulse of infrared light as it traverses the head. The pathlength (d) can be calculated from the time of flight (t) by the equation:

$$d = c \times t/n \qquad (6.4)$$

where c is the velocity of light in a vacuum and n is the refractive index of the tissue (Bolin et al. 1989). Using picosecond pulse of light from a dye laser and a device for measuring extremely short intervals, called a streak camera, the time of flight of photons across the head of experimental animals both pre- and post-mortem have been measured and the value for B calculated (Delpy et al. 1988). In a post-mortem study of six preterm infants a mean value for B of 4.4 ± 0.3 was obtained (Wyatt et al. 1990a). A subsequent study in ten term and preterm infants with varying geometrical arrangements of the optodes gave a value of 3.9 ± 0.6 (van der Zee et al. 1991). For comparison, values for B in the adult head were 5.9 ± 0.4. The pathlength factor B changes very little despite extreme changes in physiological state and before and after death (Delpy et al. 1988). It can thus be assumed that the pathlength across the infant head will remain constant (to within 5%) during clinical studies despite any observed changes in brain oxygenation and perfusion. It might be anticipated that B would change significantly with gestational age because of changes in brain morphology such as myelination (Svaasand and Ellingsen 1983). In practice, the effects of gestational age appear to be less than the current standard deviation of the pathlength measurement. It is also of interest that values for B appear to be virtually identical for different geometrical arrangements between the transmitting and receiving fibres, provided that the interoptode spacing is greater than 2.5 cm (van der Zee et al. 1991). Thus quantification of spectroscopy data is possible with the fibres positioned at varying angles to each other on the head, provided that the interoptode spacing is measured accurately. Unfortunately, because of technical limiations it is not yet possible to measure the time of flight by this method in each patient at the bedside. Values for B obtained in previous studies can, however, be used to allow quantification of spectroscopy data with a reasonable degree of accuracy.

A third approach to the quantification of spectroscopy data has recently been developed (Lakowicz and Berndt 1990). The incident light is modulated by an ultra high-frequency sine wave. The phase difference between the incident and received light can then be measured using a phase detector and converted into pathlength directly. This technique may enable both optical density and pathlength to be determined simultaneously and continuously at the bedside and may therefore lead to further improvements in the accuracy of NIRS data.

6.2.6 The Apparatus

A number of manufacturers have produced prototype apparatus for NIRS. They are all based on a broadly similar pattern (6.2). The details of prototype apparatus designed and built in the Department of Medical Physics, University College, London have been published previously (Cope and Delpy 1988). We are currently employing a commercial version of this prototype (NIR1000, Hamamatsu Photonics KK). In this instrument, infrared light at six different wavelengths is generated by semiconduc-

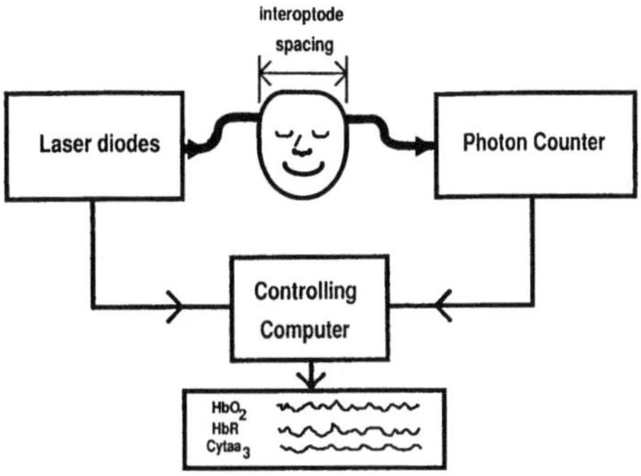

Fig. 6.2. Simplified outline of near infrared spectroscopy apparatus

tor devices known as laser diodes. The light passes down a flexible fibre optic bundle (5 mm diameter) whose end (the optode) is sited on the scalp. An identical fibre optic bundle is placed a distance of 4–8 cm away from the transmitting optode. This receiving fibre bundle conveys light to a sensitive photon detector. In the NIR1000, this is a photomultiplier tube, but in other instruments a photodiode detector is sometimes used.

In preterm infants it is usually possible to place the optodes on opposite sides of the head thus allowing transillumination of the whole brain. To provide a constant anatomical landmark we have chosen a site midway between the anterior fontanelle and the external auditory meatus. However, the exact anatomical siting of the fibres does not seem critical because the light is highly scattered within the brain. In larger infants and children the fibres are placed at an acute angle to each other, with an interoptode distance of 4–7 cm. We generally site the transmitting fibre just lateral to the anterior fontanelle and the receiving fibre overlying the temporal bone.

Changes in attenuation from an arbitrary baseline are measured at each wavelength by pulsing each laser diode rapidly in sequence. These attenuation changes are converted instantaneously into changes in [HbO_2], [Hb] and [Cyt aa_3] in mmol $\times$ l^{-1} using the previously derived algorithm. The results are displayed instantaneously and recorded on computer disk for subsequent further analysis. In the six wavelength instrument, a linear least squares algorithm is employed which also calculates a "fit error" signal that indicates the accuracy with which the derived parameters match the measured data.

The optodes are secured on the scalp using double-sided adhesive rings and flexible strapping material (Coban, 3M Ltd). Good optical coupling can be ensured by using a small amount of ultrasound contact jelly on the optode. It is not necessary to shave the scalp prior to application of the optodes, though fixation and immobilisation of the optodes is obviously more difficult if the hair is thick. The distance between the two optodes needs to be measured as accurately as possible. This is currently done using mechanical callipers. Inaccuracy in this measurement is the major source of error in the quantification of NIRS data. It is important to minimise the movement between the two optodes as this may lead to artefactual changes in the infrared indices. A change in interoptode spacing of as little as 1 mm may produce a large artefactual change in calculated chromophore concentration. Movement artefact is thus an important source of error in NIRS and every attempt must be made to minimise changes in interoptode spacing. In the future, when continuous measurement of optical pathlength at the bedside becomes feasible, this problem should be largely eliminated.

A small signal is obtained from extracerebral tissue such as scalp and skull. In the infant we estimate that less than 10% of the total signal is derived from extracerebral tissue (Wyatt et al. 1990 b). This proportion may be larger in older children and adults because of the increased thickness of the skull and scalp, but few data are currently available.

6.2.7 Safety of NIRS

In the Hamamatsu NIR1000, the average power density of light from the transmitting fibre is approximately 130 W × m^{-2}, equivalent to the output from a bright battery torch beam such as an auroscope. This value is over one order of magnitude below international safety standards for skin (IEC 825). (For comparison, the power density of tropical sunlight may exceed 10000 W × m^{-2}.) In addition, the power density within the head falls off at approximately one order of magnitude for each centimetre from the transmitting optode. Due to the geometry of the light beam as it emerges from the optodes, the power levels are also less than the international safety limits for eye exposure for both "intrabeam" and "extended source" viewing. There is therefore no risk of injury even if the transmitting fibre is accidentally placed over the orbit.

6.3 Cerebral Monitoring in Neonates

The first observations obtained by NIRS in newborn infants were published in 1985 by Brazy and her colleagues (Brazy et al. 1985) and subsequently by Ferrari et al. (1986) but quantitation of the data was not possible at that time. Since 1985 we have performed studies in over 150 newborn infants admitted to the neonatal intensive care unit at University College Hospital, London. Continuous quantification of changes in cerebral haemoglobin oxygenation and total haemoglobin concentration can be obtained. In addition, a number of important indices of cerebral haemodynamics may be derived, including cerebral blood flow (CBF), cerebral oxygen delivery (COD), cerebral blood volume (CBV) and the response to changing arterial carbon dioxide tension.

6.3.1 Continuous Observation of Changes from an Arbitrary Baseline

Continuous observation of fluctuations in cerebral oxygenation and blood volume is possible. Changes in cerebral haemoglobin oxygenation may be observed from the difference between the two haemoglobin concentrations ($[HbO_2]$–[Hb]). Alterations in the total cerebral haemoglobin concentration [TCHb] are calculated from the sum of the haemoglobin concentrations ($[HbO_2]+[Hb]$). Changes in [TCHb] in mmol × l^{-1} may be converted to changes in CBV in ml × 100 g^{-1} (see Eq. 6.9 below). With the Hamamatsu NIR1000, chromophore concentrations may be calculated every second, but unless very rapid changes are anticipated it is often preferable to average the data over a 5–30 s period, thus reducing random fluctuations in photon detection and providing an improved signal-to-noise ratio.

6.3.2 Cerebral Blood Flow

Global CBF is measured by employing a modification of the Fick principle, which states that the rate of accumulation of a tracer in an organ is equal to the difference between the rate of arrival and rate of departure of the tracer. If a tracer is rapidly introduced into the arterial supply of the brain, the amount that has accumulated in the brain may be measured later at time *t*. If this time is less than the transit time through the brain, no tracer will have appeared in the venous system. Thus CBF can be determined from the ratio of the tracer accumulated at time *t* to the quantity of tracer introduced. Previous workers have employed Cardio-Green as a near infrared absorbing tracer to give a nonquantitative measure of changes in CBF in experimental animals (Colacino et al. 1981). More recently we have used HbO_2 itself as an endogenous intravascular tracer for studies in newborn infants (Edwards et al. 1988).

A sudden increase in arterial saturation (SaO_2) over a few seconds is induced by a sharp but transient increase in inspired oxygen concentration. This causes an additional bolus of HbO_2 (the tracer) to enter the arterial supply. The quantity of tracer entering the cerebral circulation is estimated from the SaO_2 measured by a pulse oximeter on the ear. The increase from baseline in cerebral [HbO_2] is quantified by NIRS (Fig. 6.3). The cerebral haemoglobin flow (CHF) in mmol $\times$ 100 $g^{-1} \times min^{-1}$ can then be calculated from the expression:

$$CHF = k \times \Delta[HbO_2] / \int (\Delta SaO_2)\,dt \quad (6.5)$$

where k is a constant reflecting the brain density and ΔSaO_2 is the fractional change in arterial saturation. CBF can then be obtained from the relationship:

$$CBF = CHF/H \quad (6.6)$$

where H is the large vessel haemoglobin concentration (in mmol $\times l^{-1}$) measured from a peripheral blood sample. In this calculation, the effects of dissolved oxygen have been ignored since dissolved oxygen represents less than 1.5% of the total carried in the arterial blood.

Preliminary validation of this technique for blood flow measurement has been obtained from studies of the adult forearm comparing NIRS with venous occlusion plethysmography (Edwards et al. 1989). The results showed a close correspondence. Studies in sick newborn infants to compare NIRS with other methods for CBF measurement, such as xenon-133, are currently in progress.

NIRS has obvious advantages as a practical tool for CBF measurement in newborn infants. No ionising radiation is employed and measurements can be obtained at the bedside. Provided that an appropriate rapid change in SaO_2 can be induced, estimations of CBF can be performed repeatedly without risk and with minimum interference to the infant. With existing apparatus a change in SaO_2 of 5%–10% over about 5 s is required for a satisfactory measurement. Although this is both feasible and safe in many infants undergoing intensive care, it may not be possible in the sickest infants. With future improvements in sensitivity it may become feasible to obtain CBF measurements with smaller fluctuations in SaO_2. At present there are technical difficulties with the accurate measurement of SaO_2 by pulse oximetry. All commercially available pulse oximeters average their measurements over several seconds in order to increase accuracy and to minimise fluctuations in the readout of SaO_2. For CBF determination by NIRS it is necessary to modify the pulse oximeter to give "beat-to-beat" measurements with a consequent degradation in accuracy. In the future, the development of pulse oximeters specifically designed to measure small and rapid changes in SaO_2 may lead to a significant improvement in the accuracy and feasibility of the technique.

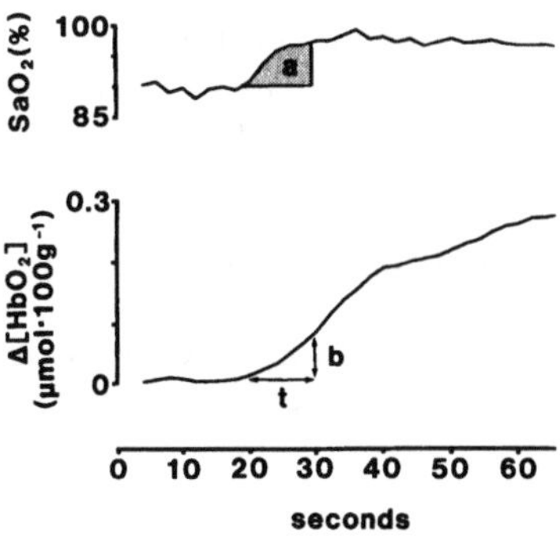

Fig. 6.3. Determination of CBF in a 26 week gestation infant with hyaline membrane disease. *Upper trace*, SaO_2 obtained from a pulse oximeter; lower trace, change in cerebral [HbO_2]. (Reprinted from Edwards et al. 1988)

6.3.3 Cerebral Oxygen Delivery

COD in ml $\times$ 100 $g^{-1} \times min^{-1}$ is obtained from the CHF using the relationship:

$$COD = k \times SaO_2 \times CHF \quad (6.7)$$

where k is a constant reflecting the quantity of oxygen in millilitres carried by each millimole of haemoglobin.

6.3.4 Cerebral Blood Volume

Absolute quantification of CBV is obtained by observing the effect on cerebral $[HbO_2]$ of a small gradual change in SaO_2 of 5%–10% over about 5 min within the range 80%–95%. The theoretical background and methodology is explained elsewhere (Wyatt et al. 1990b). An alteration in inspired oxygen concentration of about 20% is usually sufficient to induce the desired gradual change in SaO_2. This may be measured directly by a pulse oximeter or calculated from transcutaneous oxygen tension calibrated against arterial PO_2. If it is assumed that CBF, CBV and cerebral oxygen extraction remain constant during this small and gradual change in SaO_2 then the [TCHb] in mmol $\times$ l^{-1} can be calculated from the relationship:

$$[\mathrm{TCHb}] = (\Delta[\mathrm{HbO_2}] - \Delta[\mathrm{Hb}])/(2 \times \Delta \mathrm{SaO_2}) \quad (6.8)$$

where ΔSaO_2 is the fractional change in arterial saturation.

CBV in ml $\times$ 100 g^{-1} can be calculated from [TCHb] from the formula:

$$\mathrm{CBV} = [\mathrm{TCHb}] \times R \times D/10 \times H \quad (6.9)$$

where R is the cerebral : large vessel haematocrit ratio, D is the brain density in gm $\times$ ml^{-1} and H is the large vessel haemoglobin concentration in mmol $\times$ l^{-1}. Figures 6.4 and 6.5 show typical data obtained from a slow induced change in SaO_2 in a preterm infant undergoing intensive care.

CBV may be quantified at the beginning of a period of cerebral monitoring by NIRS by the method described above. This allows the total haemoglobin signal ($[HbO_2]$+[Hb]) to be calibrated giving continuous absolute quantification of CBV for the whole period of observation.

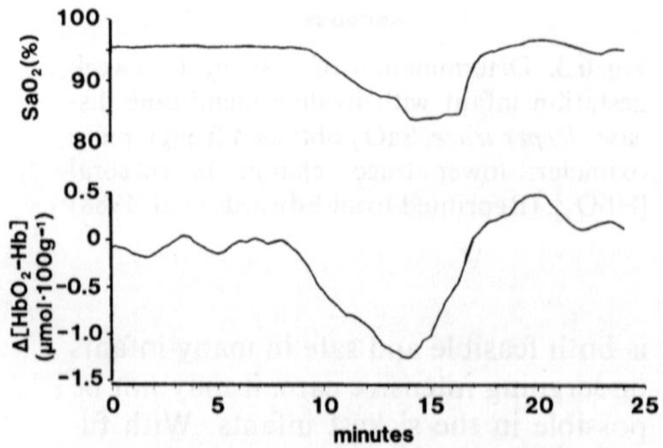

Fig. 6.4. Determination of CBV in a term infant with meconium aspiration syndrome. *Upper trace*, SaO_2 calculated from trancutaneous PO_2; lower trace, alterations in cerebral haemoglobin oxygenation. A small transient reduction in inspired oxygen concentration was induced at 9 min. (Reprinted from Wyatt et al. 1990b)

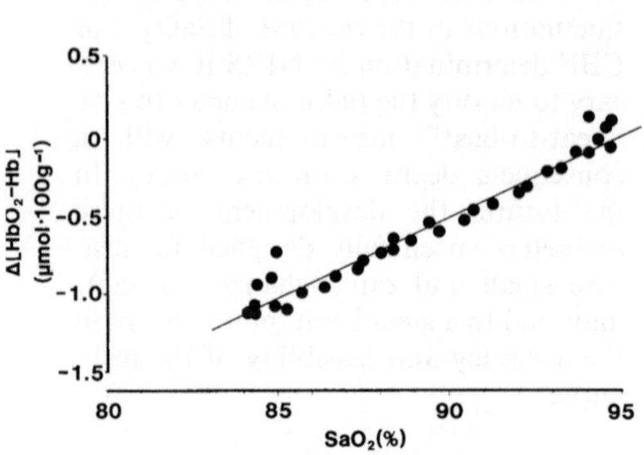

Fig. 6.5. Alteration in cerebral haemoglobin oxygenation plotted against SaO_2 with regression line. Same infant and observations as Fig. 6.4. Observations from 9 to 18 min are displayed. Each point represents data averaged over a 15 s collection period. $[HbO_2\text{-}Hb]$ plotted against SaO_2. (Reprinted from Wyatt et al. 1990b)

6.3.5 CBV Response to $PaCO_2$

The cerebral blood volume response (CBVR) to changes in arterial carbon dioxide tension ($PaCO_2$) may also be readily determined by NIRS (Wyatt et al. 1990; Pryds et al. 1990). A small change in $PaCO_2$ of 0.5–1 kPa is induced over

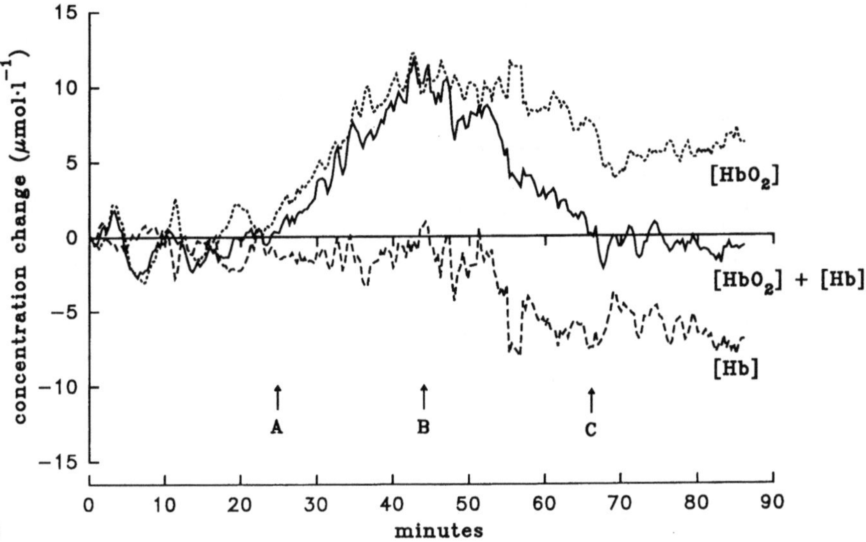

6.6

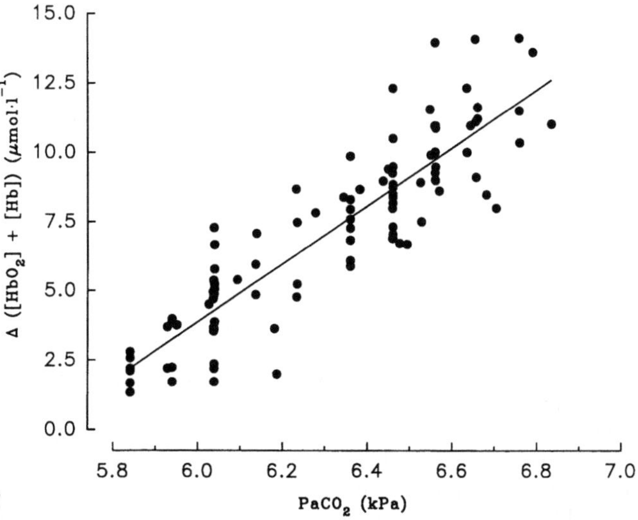

6.7

Fig. 6.6. Determination of CBVR in a term infant with diaphragmatic hernia. Changes in $[HbO_2]$, [Hb] and $[HbO_2]+[Hb]$ during a transient alteration in $PaCO_2$. The $PaCO_2$ was 5.8 kPa at *A* and rose to 6.8 kPa at *B*, returning to 5.9 kPa at *C*. (Reprinted from Wyatt et al., 1991)

Fig. 6.7. Relation between changes in $[HbO_2]$ $+[Hb]$ and $PaCO_2$ together with regression line in the same infant as Fig. 6.6. (Reprinted from Wyatt et al. 1991)

5–10 min by a change in ventilator rate or by adding a few percent of carbon dioxide to the inspired air. Changes in $PaCO_2$ may be observed by a transcutaneous electrode calibrated against arterial PCO_2, or, in infants with normal lungs, by continuous measurement of end tidal carbon dioxide concentration. Changes in [TCHb] during the alteration in $PaCO_2$ are calculated from the relationship:

$$\Delta[\mathrm{TCHb}] = \Delta[\mathrm{HbO_2}] + \Delta[\mathrm{Hb}] \quad (6.10)$$

Figure 6.6 illustrates a typical response to a small induced change in $PaCO_2$ in a term infant undergoing mechanical ventilation. The relationship between [TCHb] and $PaCO_2$ is determined and a linear regression line is then derived (Fig. 6.7). The change in CBV is calculated from [TCHb] using Eq. (6.9) above, allowing determination of CBVR in ml $\times 100\ g^{-1} \times kPa^{-1}$.

6.4 Results in Newborn Infants

6.4.1 CBF and Oxygen Delivery

At this time, few data on CBF in newborn infants with normal brains have been obtained. Preliminary studies in a heterogeneous group of newborn infants undergoing intensive care have given values for CBF of 6–30 ml $\times 100\ g^{-1} \times min^{-1}$. These results are broadly comparable with those obtained in similar infants using the xenon-133 method (Greisen and Trojaborg 1987).

6.4.2 Cerebral Blood Volume

NIRS was employed to measure CBV in 12 infants who were undergoing intensive care but who were thought to have normal brains (Wyatt et al. 1990b). Mean CBV was 2.2 ± 0.4 ml $\times 100\ g^{-1}$. There was no evidence of a systematic change in CBV with increasing gestational age. In a further ten infants who had evidence of brain injury (mostly hypoxic-ischaemic), the mean CBV was significantly elevated at 3.0 ± 1.0 ml $\times 100\ g^{-1}$. These preliminary results suggest that cerebral vasodilatation leading to elevation of global CBV is a frequent occurrence following hypoxic-ischaemic brain injury. Although intraventricular haemorrhage is common in preterm infants, the presence of blood clot within the ventricle would not be expected to cause an elevation in the CBV calculated by this technique. This is because intraventricular blood is not be involved in oxygen exchange with cerebral tissue and it would therefore be effectively "invisible" during a small induced change in SaO_2.

6.4.3 CBV Response to Changing $PaCO_2$

Observations in 14 preterm and term infants undergoing intensive care but with apprently normal brains gave values for CBVR that ranged from 0.1 to 0.7 ml $\times 100\ g^{-1} \times kPa^{-1}$ (Wyatt et al. 1991). A close linear correlation between CBVR and gestational age was observed with a marked increase in the cerebrovascular response to changing $PaCO_2$ with increasing maturity (Fig. 6.8). The values obtained for CBVR in term infants were similar to those obtained previously in adult volunteers using radiolabelled erythrocytes.

In seven infants with evidence of brain injury (mainly hypoxic-ischaemic) CBVR was significantly reduced compared with normal infants. The most pronounced reductions in CBVR were observed in infants with severe birth asphyxia, with some infants showing complete abolition of response to changing $PaCO_2$ (Wyatt et al. 1988). We have consistently observed abnormalities of the cerebral circulation after severe birth asphyxia, with elevation of CBV and attenuation or abolition of CBVR. Other investigators, employing alternative techniques, have found elevation of CBF and

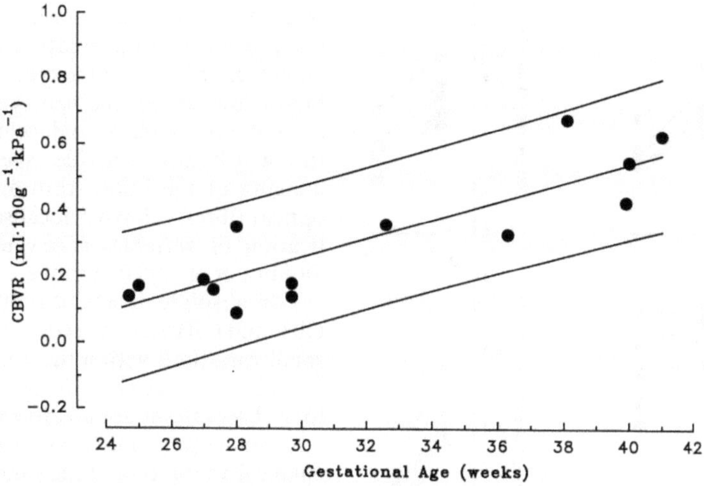

Fig. 6.8. CBVR in ml · 100 g^{-1} · kPa^{-1} plotted against gestational age in infants with apparently normal brains. (Reprinted from Wyatt et al. 1991)

blood flow velocity in term infants with birth asphyxia. All this evidence is consistent with the presence of marked vasodilatation and vasoparalysis of the cerebral circulation following an acute hypoxic-ischaemic insult in term infants. The findings of an elevated CBV and reduced CBVR in infants with suspected hypoxic-ischaemic injury may be predictive of a poor outcome, although this hypothesis is not yet substantiated. In a small number of infants who have been studied both by NIRS and phosphorus MRS, these haemodynamic abnormalities have been observed immediately after birth and prior to the development of the delayed or "secondary" energy failure, which is observed more than 24 h after birth (Wyatt et al. 1989) (Fig. 6.9). In the future, NIRS may be employed to identify those infants in whom the prognosis is particularly poor and in whom novel cerebroprotective agents might be tested by controlled trials.

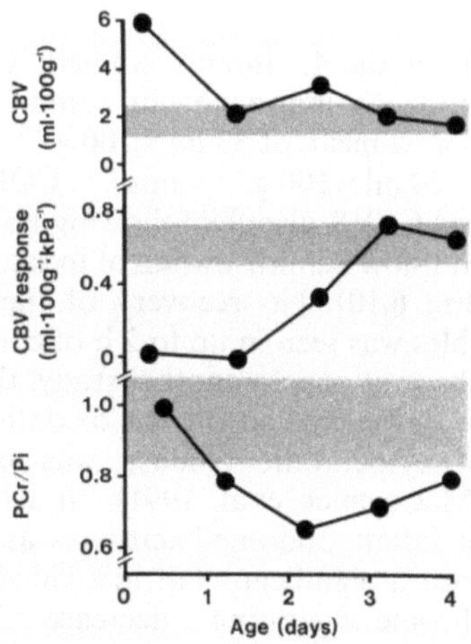

Fig. 6.9. CVB, CBVR and phosphocreatine/inorganic phosphate ratio (PCr/Pi) in an infant with severe birth asphyxia born at 36 weeks gestation who developed cerebral atrophy and died and age 7 weeks. *Hatched areas* represent data from control infants. (Reprinted from Wyatt et al. 1989)

6.4.4 Indomethacin Administration

The effect on the brain of indomethacin, administered for treatment of a patent ductus arteriosus, has been recently studied by NIRS (Edwards et al. 1990). In

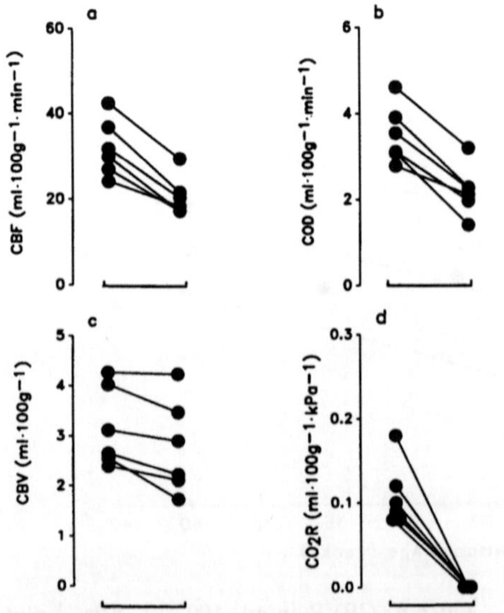

Fig. 6.10. Effect of a slow infusion of indomethacin on cerebral blood flow (CFB), oxygen delivery (COD), blood volume (CBV) and response to changing $PaCO_2$ (CO_2R) in six preterm infants with patent ductus arteriosus. (Reprinted from Edwards et al. 1990)

all of the 13 infants studied, CBF fell following indomethacin administration, from a mean of 33 $ml \times 100\ g^{-1} \times min^{-1}$ to 20 $ml \times 100\ g^{-1} \times min^{-1}$. COD, CBV and CBVR also fell following both rapid and slow administration of indomethacin (Fig. 6.10). No recovery of these variables was seen in up to 2 h of continuing observations. In another study, the effect of indomethacin on the oxidation state of cytochrome oxidase was observed (McCormick et al. 1991). In a minority of infants indomethacin was associated with a significant fall in oxidised cytochrome suggesting a decrease of oxygen availability at a mitochondrial level.

6.5 Limitations of NIRS

Since infrared light is highly scattered within the brain, existing techniques for NIRS provide information on global cerebral oxygenation and haemodynamics. Little or no information on the regional distribution of oxygenation and blood flow can be obtained. Attempts are currently being made to develop apparatus which will provide spectroscopic imaging of the brain from an array of optical fibres, allowing localised quantification of variables (Jarry et al. 1984; Tamura et al. 1987; Arridge et al. 1990).

For absolute quantification of CBF, CBV and CBVR, it is necessary to induce small variations within the normal range in SaO_2 and $PaCO_2$. Although satisfactory observations are possible in most infants undergoing intensive care with mechanical ventilation, it may not be possible to perform these manoeuvres in the most critically ill infants. Infants who are breathing spontaneously in air may require the administration of modified gas mixtures by mask to obtain the necessary variations in SaO_2 and $PaCO_2$.

6.6 Prognostic Value of Data Obtained by NIRS

NIRS has been introduced only recently; thus, little information is available on the prognostic significance of the haemodynamic data that has been obtained. It is likely that "critical" values of CBF and COD will be defined in newborn infants of different gestational ages. This will allow detection of those infants in whom COD is critically impaired leading to a poor outcome. Characteristic haemodynamic abnormalities have also been observed following perinatal asphyxia (see above), and it is likely that these abnormalities are predictive of long-term neurodevelopmental impairment or death.

6.7 Conclusion

NIRS has many advantages as a technique for providing quantitative noninvasive information about cerebral oxygenation and haemodynamics. No ionising radiation is employed, and repeated measurements can be made safely. Continuous recording of changes in oxygenation and haemodynamics can be carried out for long periods. The apparatus is portable and studies can be performed in the intensive care unit without interference with normal medical and nursing procedures. No regional information is yet available with NIRS but future developments may allow spectroscopic imaging of the head.

Acknowledgements. The authors wish to thank Prof Osmund Reynolds, Dr Mark Cope, Dr David Edwards, Dr David McCormick, Ms Anna Potter, Dr Simon Roth, Mr Peter Van Der Zee and the staff of the Neonatal Unit, UCH. This work has been supported by the Medical Research Council, the Wellcome Trust, the Wolfson Foundation and Hamamatsu Photonics KK.

References

Araki R, Nashimoto I (1989) Multicomponent analysis of near infrared spectra of anaesthetised rat head: (ii) Quantitative multivariate analysis of haemoglobin and cytochrome oxidase by non-negative least squares method. Adv Exp Med Biol 248:11–20

Arridge SR, van der Zee P, Delpy DT, Cope M (1990) Aspects of clinical infrared absorption imaging. In: Todd-Pokropek A, Viergever MA (eds) The formation, handling and evaluation of medical images. Springer, Berlin Heidelberg New York, pp 407–418

Bolin FP, Preuss LE, Taylor RC, Ference RJ (1989) Refractive index of some mammalian tissues using a fibre optic cladding method. Appl Optics 28:2297–2303

Boulnois JL (1986) Photophysical processes in recent medical laser developments: a review. Lasers Med Sci 1:47–66

Brazy JE, Lewis DV, Mitnick MH, Jobsis FF (1985) Noninvasive monitoring of cerebral oxygenation in preterm infants: preliminary observations. Pediatrics 75:217–225

Brinkman R, Zijlstra WG, Koopmans RK (1950) A method for continuous observation of percentage oxygen saturation in patients. Arch Chir Neerl 1:333–344

Colacino JM, Grubb B, Jobsis FF (1981) Infrared technique for cerebral blood flow: comparison with 133 Xenon clearance. Neurol Res (1):17–31

Cope M, Delpy DT (1988) A system for long term measurement of cerebral blood and tissue oxygenation in newborn infants by near-infrared transillumination. Med Biol Eng Comput 26:289–294

Cope M, Delpy DT, Reynolds EOR, Wray S, Wyatt J, van der Zee P (1988) Methods of quantitating near infrared spectroscopy data. Adv Exp Med Biol 222:183–189

Delpy DT, Cope M, van der Zee P, Arridge S, Wray S, Wyatt JS (1988) Estimation of optical pathlength through tissue from direct time of flight measurement. Phys Med Biol 33:1433–1442

Edwards AD, Wyatt JS, Richardson EC, Delpy DT, Cope M, Reynolds EOR (1988) Cotside measurement of cerebral blood flow in ill newborn infants by near infrared spectroscopy. Lancet ii:701–702

Edwards AD, Reynolds EOR, Richardson CE, Wyatt JS (1989) Estimation of blood flow in man using near infrared spectroscopy. J Physiol (Lond) 410:50P

Edwards AD, Wyatt JS, Richardson CE, Potter A, Cope M, Delpy DT, Reynolds EOR (1990) Effects of indomethacin on cerebral haemodynamics and oxygen delivery investigated by near infrared spectroscopy in very preterm infants. Lancet i:1491–1495

Ferrari M, de Marchis C, Giannini I, di Nicola A, Agostino R, Nodari S, Bucci G (1986) Cerebral blood volume and haemoglobin oxygen saturation monitoring in neonatal brain by near IR spectroscopy. Adv Exp Med Biol 200:203–212

Greisen G, Trojaborg W (1987) Cerebral blood flow, $PaCO_2$ changes and visual evoked potentials in mechanically ventilated preterm infants. Acta Paediatr Scand 76:394–400

Jarry G, Ghesquire S, Maarek JM, Debray S, Bui-Mong-Hung, Laurent D (1984) Imaging mammalian tissues and organs using laser collimated transillumination. J Biomed Eng 6:70–74

Jobsis FF (1977) Noninvasive infrared monitoring of cerebral and myocardial sufficiency and circulatory parameters. Science 198:1264–1267

Jobsis FF, Piantadosi CA, Sylvia AL, Lucas SK, Keizer HH (1988) Near infrared monitoring of cerebral oxygen sufficiency. Neurol Res 10:7–17

Lakowicz JR, Berndt K (1990) Frequency domain measurements of photon migration in tissue. Chem Phys Lett 166:246–252

Matthes K (1935) Untersuchungen über die Sauerstoffsättigungen des menschlichen Arterienblutes. Arch Exp Pathol Pharmac 179:698–711

McCormick DC, Edwards AD, Wyatt JS, Potter A, Cope M, Delpy DT, Reynolds EOR (1991) The effect of indomethacin on cerebral oxidised cytochrome aa_3 concentration in preterm infants (abstr). Pediatr Res (in press)

Merrick E (1975) A multi-wavelength ear oximeter. Proc BIOCAPT 75(2):185–190

Millikan GA (1942) The oximeter, an instrument for measuring continuously oxygen saturation of arterial blood in man. Rev Sci Instrum 13:434–444

Pryds O, Greisen G, Skov LL, Friis-Hansen B (1990) Carbon dioxide related changes in cerebral blood volume and cerebral blood flow in mechanically ventilated preterm neonates. Comparison of near infrared spectrophotometry and 133 Xenon clearance. Pediatr Res 27:445–449

Svaasand LO, Ellingsen R (1983) Optical properties of human brain. Photochem Photobiol 38(3):293–299

Tamura M, Nomura Y, Hazeki O (1987) Laser tissue spectroscopy – near infrared CT. Rev Laser Eng 15(8):74–82

van der Zee P, Cope M, Arridge SR, Essenpreis M, Potter LA, Edwards AD, Wyatt JS, McCormick DC, Roth SC, Reynolds EOR, Delpy DT (1991) Experimentally measured optical pathlength for the adult head, calf and forearm, and the head of the newborn infant as a function of interoptode spacing. Adv Exp Med Biol (in press)

Wray S, Cope M, Delpy DT, Wyatt JS, Reynolds EOR (1988) Characterization of the near infrared absorption spectra of cytochrome aa_3 and haemoglobin for the non-invasive monitoring of cerebral oxygenation. Biochim Biophys Acta 933:184–192

Wyatt JS, Cope M, Delpy DT, Wray S, Richardson CE, Reynolds EOR (1988) Responses of cerebral vasculature to changes in arterial carbon dioxide tension measured by near infrared spectroscopy in newborn infants (abstr). Pediatr Res 22:230

Wyatt JS, Edwards AD, Azzopardi D, Reynolds EOR (1989) Magnetic resonance and near infrared spectroscopy of perinatal hypoxic-ischaemic brain injury. Arch Dis Child 64:953–963

Wyatt JS, Cope M, Delpy DT, Van der Zee P, Arridge S, Edwards AD, Reynolds EOR (1990a) Measurement of optical pathlength for cerebral near infrared spectroscopy in newborn infants. Dev Neurosci 12:140–144

Wyatt JS, Cope M, Delpy DT, Richardson CE, Edwards AD, Wray S, Reynolds EOR, (1990b) Quantitation of cerebral blood volume in newborn human infants by near infrared spectroscopy. J Appl Physiol 68:1086–1091

Wyatt JS, Edwards AD, McCormick DC, Cope M, Delpy DT, Reynolds EOR (1991) Response of cerebral blood volume to changes in arterial carbon dioxide tension in preterm and term infants. Pediatr Res 29: 553–557

7 Single Photon Emission Computed Tomography of the Brain Perfusion in Neonates

J. HADDAD, A. CONSTANTINESCO, and B. BRUNOT

CONTENTS

7.1 Introduction

In the neonatal period, neurologic morbidity is a significant problem and contributes to an abnormal development outcome. Detecting cerebral disorders early in the neonatal period by means of clinical examination, electrophysiological measurements and conventional brain imaging, such as US, MRI and CT, scan, is helpful. Unfortunately, it seems to be insufficient since some infants show more severe cerebral impairment than expected despite these neonatal investigations. In order to address this issue, another approach to evaluate brain disorders has been developed, measuring functional and metabolic activities of the CNS.

In the last few years, increasing interest has been focussed on techniques using radionuclides to measure cerebral blood flow (CBF). Among them, single photon emission computed tomography (SPECT) is far less expensive and not as complicated as the others. Moreover, it has proven to be useful for evaluating cerebral perfusion (CP) or regional cerebral blood flow (rCBF) in adults and children (Podreka et al. 1987; Denays et al. 1989; Cordes et al. 1990). In neonates few data are available on this relatively new technique (Schober et al. 1987; Tzourio et al. 1988; Denays et al. 1989). In this paper we will give an overview of the use of cerebral perfusion by SPECT in neonates, based on reports in the literature and our own experience. Today, in our institution, 22 neonates have been evaluated by this method. Our conclusions must nonetheless be considered preliminary.

7.2 Principles of Brain Perfusion Imaging by SPECT

SPECT uses a rotating gamma camera for reconstructing cross-sectional images of radiotracer distribution in organs.

7.2.1 Radiotracers

A number of radiotracers have been developed that cross the blood-brain barrier, distribute within the brain proportional to rCBF and remain fixed for several hours. Single photon lipophilic cerebral perfusion tracers, such as iodine-123 iodoamphetamine (IMP) and technetium

99m hexamethyl-propylenamineoxime (HMPAO), are currently used with safety in newborns. According to Denays et al. (1989), the dose injected should be 0.5 mCi of IMP and 3 mCi of HMPAO. Xenon-133 was also used (Tzourio et al. 1988) to measure rCBF during cerebral maturation.

7.2.2 Methods

The intracerebral distribution of the radiotracer is measured with a rotating gamma camera. The camera, equipped with a low-energy high-resolution collimator, rotates step by step or continuously through 180° or 360° and as close as possible to the head of the patient. Some 30–60 projections are currently obtained within 20–30 min in a 64 × 64 matrix. After optimal spatial prefiltering, the images are reconstructed by filtered back-projection into axial (parallel to the orbitomeatal line), coronal and sagittal slices with a thickness ranging from 5 to 10 mm.

In our institution, for HMPAO-SPECT, we use a Phillips rectangular gamma camera equipped with a low-energy high-resolution collimator connected to a Medasys A3 processing system. The injected activity is 3 mCi. The color scale used to evaluate cerebral perfusion progresses from dark blue (hypoperfusion) to bright white (high perfusion).

7.2.3 Patient Handling

For SPECT examination, the following conditions are required:

1. An intravenous line inserted in an upper or lower limb of the neonate 2 h before the examination.

2. Since HMPAO-SPECT will depict instantaneously the distribution of the radiotracer at the moment of the injection, the radiotracer must be injected in a quiet environment to avoid disturbance of CBF.

3. Absolute immobility of the neonate is required during data acquisition in order to avoid movement artefacts. In prematures the examination often occurs after feeding. In neonates and early infancy, sedation is used. Chloral hydrate is given via a nasogastric tube (50 mg/kg). However, it is important to stress that sedation must be performed after injection of the radiotracer in order to avoid disturbance of CBF by any drug.

4. The infant is brought to the SPECT facilities and placed in a specially designed cot. The infant must be supine, the head in the field of view of the gamma camera, and positioned with the head axis corresponding to the axis of rotation. Beside hearing, touching and seeing the infants, surveillance is maintained by an ECG.

7.2.4 Interpretation

Interpreting scans drawn from IMP or HMPAO-SPECT studies is mainly qualitative. Visual evaluation of cerebral perfusion by means of a gray to white scale or color scales is used. Regional CP is studied in each frontal, parietal, temporal and occipital lobe and corresponding cortex and in basal ganglia, brain stem and cerebellum. Side to side differences in brain isotope uptake are obtained by visual estimation and by calculation of the left to right percentage in a region of interest (ROI) larger than 2 × FWHM (full width at half maximum) of the spatial resolution of the detector. Side to side differences above 12% are defined as abnormal based upon previous data in healthy subjects (Cordes et al. 1990).

Quantitative evaluation of IMP or HMPAO-SPECT scans are difficult. However counts per pixel of the individual ROIs allows one to determine a regional index (RI) and a perfusion index (PI) (Cordes et al. 1990). RI is the counts per pixel on the right divided by the counts per pixel on the left. PI is the ROI mean counts per pixel divided by the mean of the counts per pixel of the whole brain.

The RI evaluates the distribution of the perfusion between the two hemisphere sides and PI indicates an increase or a decrease in perfusion as compared with the mean.

7.3 Neonatal Applications

7.3.1 Normal Results

The pattern of HMPAO-SPECT and IMP-SPECT images in the neonatal period is well defined (Denays et al. 1989; Rubinstein et al. 1989).

In prematures, prominent perfusion is seen mainly in the thalami and brain stem. With progression of gestational age (GA), cerebral perfusion gradually increases in the cerebellum, the striatum, the parietal white matter and parietal cortex. At term, low activity is seen in the occipital region, most markedly in the frontal area (Fig. 7.1).

The HMPAO-SPECT data described above are in general agreement with cerebral functional activity as detected by PET with 2-deoxy-2[18-F]-fluoro-D-Glucose (DFG) (Chugani et al. 1986, 1987). Indeed, we have found that patterns of local cerebral metabolic rates for glucose in the neonatal period, as revealed by PET scan, were similar to rCBF detected by HMPAO-SPECT (Fig. 7.1). Moreover, a good correlation using quantitative data was found by Tzourio et al. (1988) when comparing the rCBF measured by ^{133}Xe-SPECT and the data of DFG distribution during cerebral maturation as determined by Chugani et al. 1986.

We have also noted that there is a good correlation between myelination as depicted by MRI in the neonatal period (Dietrich 1990) and rCBF detected by HMPAO-SPECT. Myelin deposition occurs in regions of maximum cerebral functional activity. The progression of myelination observed by MRI is similar to the increase of rCBF measured by HMPAO-SPECT (cephalad progression).

SPECT data are congruous with neonatal behavior. Intrinsic brain stem reflexes (Moro, root and grasp reflexes) are prominent in neonates and correlate with the high CP of the brain stem. Nonpurposeful limb movements, mediated by an imbalance between basal ganglia and cerebral cortex, are well correlated with the ratio of CP between basal ganglia and cerebral cortex. Sensorimotor cortex (parietal cortex) is the most highly perfused area in the neonatal period, which is in agreement with the motor and sensorial capacities of the newborn. From these findings, we emphasize that HMPAO-SPECT can be a useful indicator of brain maturation in the neonatal period.

7.3.2 HMPAO-SPECT and Brain Disorders in Neonates

7.3.2.1 Perinatal Asphyxia

Perinatal asphyxia is the initiating event in most neurologic sequelae in both prematures and full-term infants. It is well known that asphyxia induces an impairement in the autoregulation of CBF and leads to ischemic or hemorrhagic lesions. US is currently used to diagnose and follow these cerebral injuries. Despite its broad application, the sensitivity and specificity of this technique remains questionable (see Chap. 2 in this book). Relatively little data are available on HMPAO-SPECT studies and asphyxia in neonates. The following data are collected from the literature and from our own experience using SPECT to monitor perinatal asphyxia.

7.3.2.2 Perinatal Asphyxia in Prematures

In prematures, *periventricular-intraventricular hemorrhages* (PV-IVH) are the

7.1

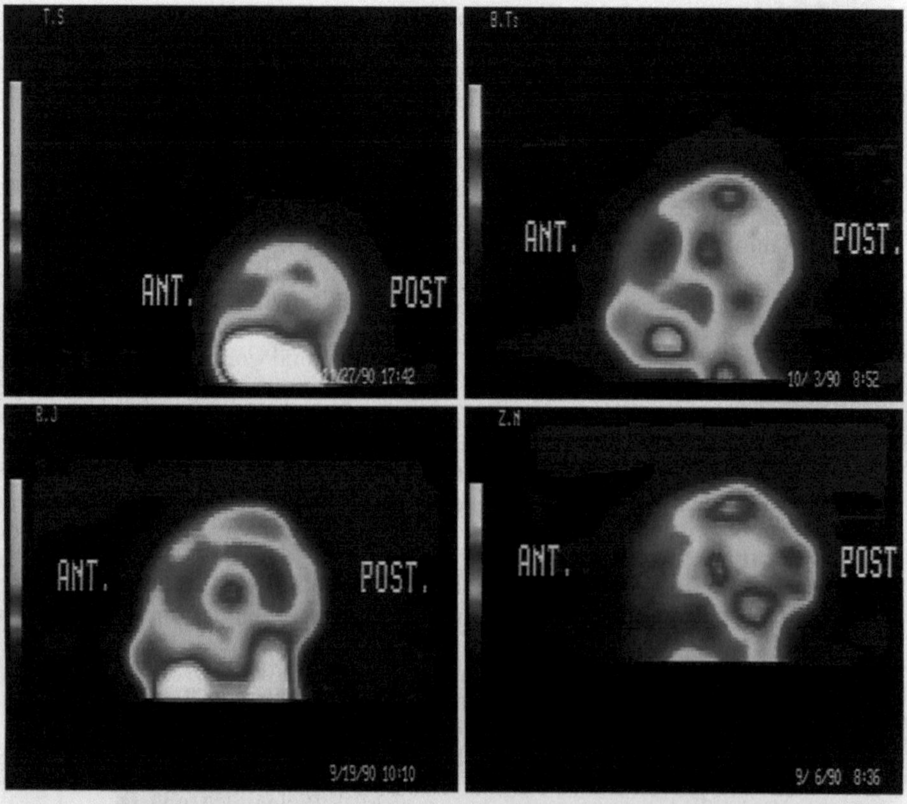

7.2

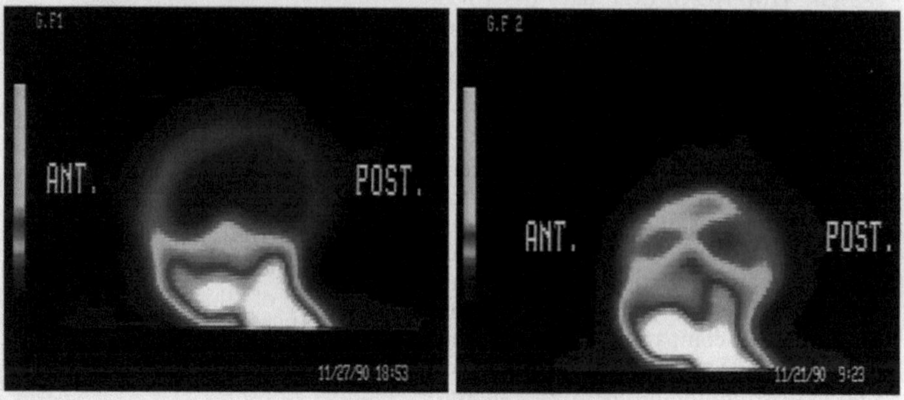

Fig. 7.1. Patterns of rCBF displayed by HMPAO-SPECT at 32 weeks (*upper left*), 40 weeks (*upper right*), 44 weeks (*bottom left*) and 46 weeks (*bottom right*) postconceptional age; 8 mm slice thickness, sagittal views. Note progression of perfusion from basal ganglia to cerebellum to parietal lobes, then to occipital lobes. Frontal lobes are poorly perfused

Fig. 7.2. Premature of 31 weeks gestational age suffering from intraventricular hemorrhage with acute hydrocephalus (as diagnosed by conventional brain imaging); HMPAO-SPECT; 8 mm slice thickness, sagittal cross-section before ventriculoperitoneal shunt (*left*). Note the low cerebral perfusion over all areas of the brain before treatment and reappearance of cerebral perfusion after treatment (*right*)

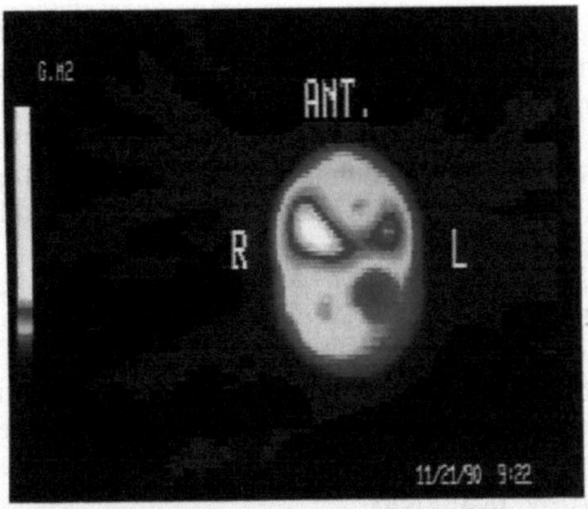

7.3

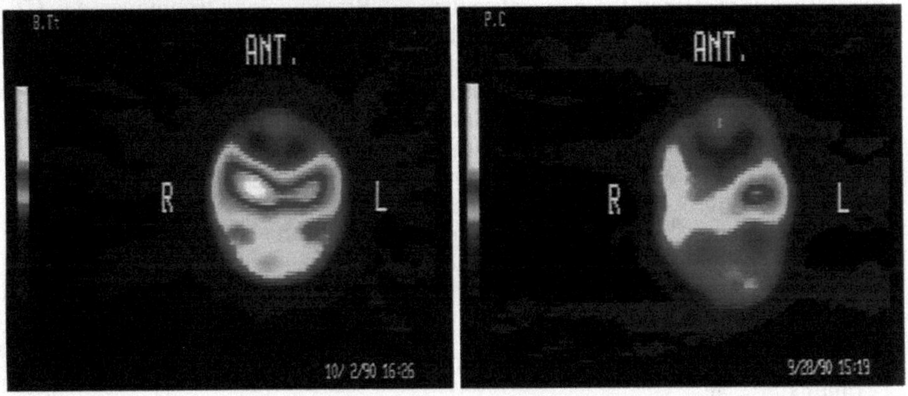

7.4

Fig. 7.3. Premature of 38 weeks postconceptional age. Left intraventricular hemorrhage with left parietal involvement (diagnosed by conventional brain imaging); 8 mm slice thickness, transverse cross-section; HMPAO-SPECT. Low perfused area on the left parietal area reaching the cortex

Fig. 7.4. HMPAO-SPECT; 8 mm slice thickness, transverse cross-section obtained from two full-term infants: normal full-term infant (*left*) and full term infant suffering of bilateral cerebral leucomalacia located at the frontal lobe (*right*) (as diagnosed by conventional brain imaging). Note low perfusion in both frontal and parietal lobes and ventricular size when compared to normal

most often encountered. They are classified into grades 1, 2 or 3 (see Chap. 2, Sect. 2.6) and are often complicated by hydrocephalus and parenchymal involvement.

Although HMPAO-SPECT may not have any further benefit, compared to US, in the recognition of PV-IVH, it has been useful in the evaluation of complications; the effect of hydrocephalus on cerebral perfusion is well displayed by HMPAO-SPECT (Fig. 7.2). Excessive ventricular dilatation leads to a disturbance of rCBF marked by hypoperfusion. HMPAO-SPECT data, acquired after ventriculo-peritoneal shunt, show a reappearence of rCBF. We can state that HMPAO-SPECT is a useful monitor of CNS complications brought on by hydrocephalus and thus leads to rational patient management.

Parenchymal involvement associated with PV-IVH refers to hemorrhagic infarction or hemorrhagic leucomalacia. In the pathogenesis of both, ischemia is the most important event leading to an impairment in behavioral outcome. Parenchymal involvement is readily identified by US and located in the periventricular areas. However the importance of the ischemic damage seems to be underestimated by US, CT or MRI. HMPAO-SPECT shows (Fig. 7.3) a marked hypoperfusion reaching the cortical areas in a premature baby suffering from PV-IVH with parenchymal involvement. Thus the extent of the defect is often greater on HMPAO-SPECT than on other brain imaging methods.

Cerebral leucomalacia refers to necrosis of white matter in the periventricular areas and in some patients, subcortically (see Chap. 2, Sect. 2.5.4). This ischemic injury is well displayed by conventional brain imaging but, as emphasized above, the ischemic damage seems to be underestimated. HMPAO-SPECT is more informative (Fig. 7.4). It identifies a hypoperfused area more significant than that shown by imaging techniques such as US or MRI.

7.3.2.3 Perinatal Asphyxia in Full-Term Infants

It is well known that the usual methods of brain imaging are of limited value in the acute phase of severe birth asphyxia. CR, MRI or US findings remain normal for some time after onset of symptoms, while HMPAO-SPECT documents the changes in cerebral perfusion that are present at the onset (Figs. 7.5 and 7.6). Anomalies of rCBF can be noted in cortical, subcortical, thalamic or cerebellar regions, depending on the severity of perinatal asphyxia. Generally, basal ganglia and brain stem remain highly perfused, whereas cortical and subcortical regions are less perfused (Figs. 7.5 and 7.6).

7.3.2.4 Other Brain Disorders in the Neonate

The clinical course of *CNS infections* can be altered by several complications such as ventriculitis, hydrocephalus, abscess or subdural effusion. The usual forms of brain imaging are useful in assessing such anomalies. Therefore, HMPAO-SPECT seems to be more useful only in evaluating rCBF in patients with hydrocephalus, as mentioned above.

White matter diseases are well displayed by MRI. To our knowledge no HMPAO-SPECT data are available for this pathology. However, as myelination is altered in such diseases, one expects that rCBF would be abnormal in subcortical areas.

Brain imaging techniques, e.g. CT, US and MRI, seem to provide better information regarding congenital malformations and tumors. HMPAO-SPECT constitutes an additional source of information but is not imperative.

7.3.3 Limits of the Method

Cerebral perfusion SPECT examination, as with other imaging techniques (CT and MRI), is carried out of the neonatal unit. Therefore, removal of critically ill neonates remains questionable, unless information expected from SPECT is of major interest with respect to withdrawal of the intensive care or birth asphyxia, for example.

Absolute immobility is required to perform SPECT. Chloral hydrate is often used to sedate the infant. It is widely used in MRI examinations, and no side effects have, as yet,been noted when the sedative is correctly used. However, it needs careful attention and surveillance of vital parameters.

To perform SPECT examination, one ought to be cautious that the injection of the radiotracer must be done in the absence of any stimuli or drug effects.

Consent from parents is important to obtain since radionuclide tracer is used. It should also be noted that, for image quality reasons, the administered activity is approximately three times greater, normalized to weight, than that usually

7.5

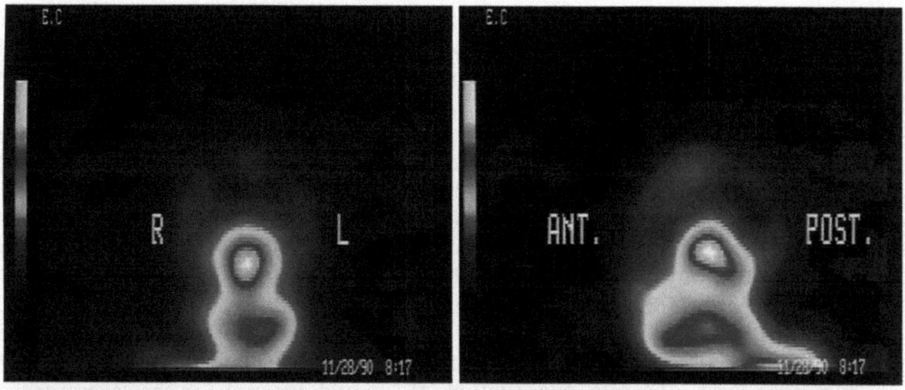

7.6

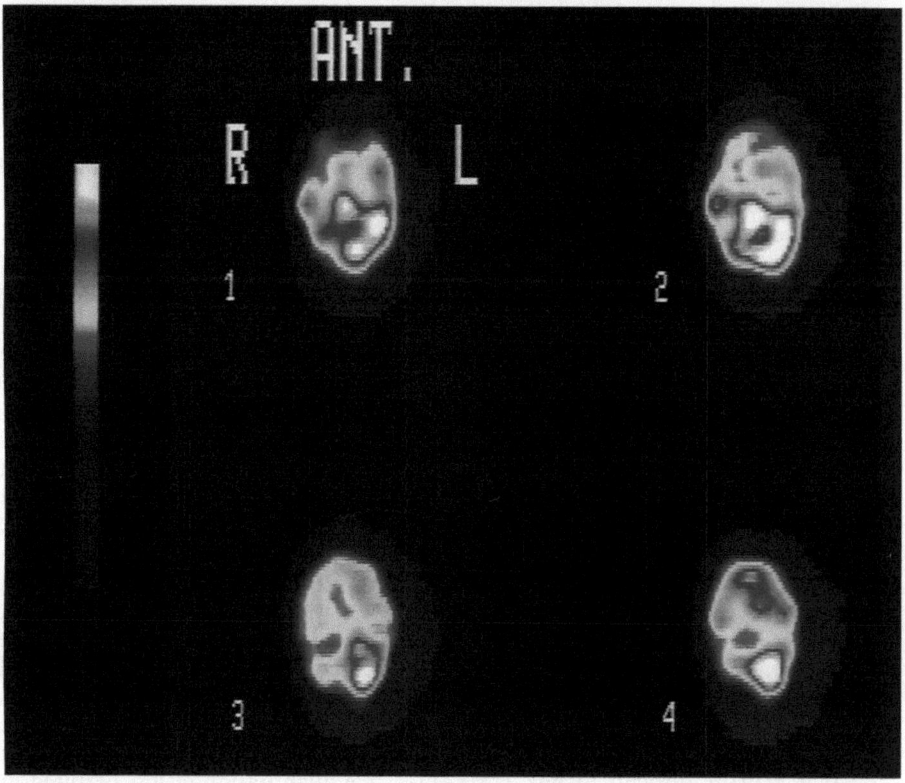

Fig. 7.5. HMPAO-SPECT; 8 mm slice thickness. Frontal cross-section (*left*), sagittal cross-section (*right*) showing an anoxic-ischemic brain injury in a full-term baby (conventional brain imaging diagnosis: intraventricular hemorrhage only). Note very low perfusion in cerebellum, cortical and subcortical regions. Only brain stem and basal ganglia centers are perfused. Outcome: died

Fig. 7.6. HMPAO-SPECT; 8 mm slice thickness, 4 contiguous transverses cross-section images from base to vertex in a 37 weeks gestational age infant suffering from birth asphyxia (normal as diagnosed by conventional brain imaging). Note low cerebral perfusion in temporal, parietal, frontal and occipital lobes. Only basal ganglia, brain stem and the cerebellum seem to be spared. Outcome: died given to an adult patient. The absorbed dose is therefore about twice that of an adult patient, as reported by Denays et al. (1989).

HMPAO-SPECT data will show, instantaneously, distribution of the radiotracer in the CNS. Thus, it will report only about the blood flow of the CNS at the moment of injection. It does not allow one to study the evaluation of rCBF over the period following tracer administration.

Difficulties can arise in interpreting images. First, absolute quantitation of tracer uptake by the brain is not actually realistic. Second, relative analysis after defining RI and PI, based on ROI, is possible, knowing that qualitative evaluation requires at least two interpretations from persons unaware of the pathology. Moreover, some cerebral regions, such as the frontal lobes, are poorly perfused. Thus, damage occurring in such regions is difficult to assess. It is also difficult to distinguish between the lenticular nuclei, striatum and thalami since the head circumference of newborns is small, leading to a poor spatial resolution in the 64 × 64 pixels reconstructed images.

Absence of healthy newborn controls, for ethical reasons, constitutes a limitation. However, normal findings could be drawn from infants who are neurologically normal at follow-up.

7.4 Prognosis Based on HMPAO-SPECT in the Neonatal Period

It is actually difficult to link HMPAO-SPECT data in the neonatal period to a prognosis since no long-term clinical follow-up data are available. However, it seems important to predict neurodevelopmental outcome in order to adopt, in severely ill neonates, a rational management scheme. Thus, HMPAO-SPECT data must be integrated with other data drawn from clinical examination, conventional brain imaging techniques, Doppler and other CNS investigations. HMPAO-SPECT can be helpful in situations in which brain imaging seems to be normal (birth asphyxia). Disturbance of rCBF, displayed by HMPAO-SPECT, seems to be related to an abnormal functional activity in the affected area. In some instances the defect shown by HMPAO-SPECT is often greater than that exhibited by US, CT or MRI. One should emphasize that the extent of the defect displayed by HMPAO-SPECT could account for the severe neurologic delay in infants whose prognosis, when based on other forms of brain imaging, was less obvious.

7.5 Conclusions and Perspectives

Cerebral perfusion imaging in neonates appears to be interesting in evaluating brain injuries, especially those induced by perinatal asphyxia. It constitutes a functional approach to studying the CNS. Combined with conventional brain imaging (US, CT and MRI), it will be helpful in providing a better diagnosis of the injury and its extent. Prognosis based only on this technique is hazardous, due to the various limits of the method. More data are needed to know to what extent this technique will be helpful in monitoring the neonatal period. The future is promising. Emphasis must be placed on reducing the limits of the method and especially on providing a better quantitative evaluation. Tridimensional images will soon be available leading to a possible quantitation of low perfused injured cerebral volumes. We hope that by ameliorating this technique and initiating more investigations, HMPAO-SPECT will be more useful and desireable for the clinician.

References

Cordes M, Christe W, Henkes H, Delavier U, Eichstadt H, Schorner W, Langer R, Felix R (1990) Focal epilepsies: HMPAO-SPECT compared with CT, MR and EEG. J Comput Assisted Tomogr 14:402–409

Chugani H, Phelps M (1986) Maturation changes in cerebral function in infants determined by 18-FDG positron emission tomography. Science 231:840–843

Chugani H, Phelps M, Mazziota J (1987) Positron emission tomography study of human brain functional development. Ann Neurol 22:487–497

Denays R, Tondeur M, Foulon M, Verstraeten F, Ham H, Piepz A, Noel P (1989) Regional brain blood flow in congenital dysphasia. Studies with technetium-99m HMPAO-SPECT. J Nucl Med 30:1825–1829

Denays R, Van Pachterbeke TV, Tondeur M, Spehl M, Toppet V, Ham H, Piepz A, Rubinstein M, Noel P, Haumont D (1989) Brain single photon emission computed tomography in neonates. J Nucl Med 30:1338–1341

Dietrich R (1990) Magnetic resonance imaging of normal brain maturation. Semin Perinatol 14:201–211

Podreka I, Suess E, Goldenberg G, Steiner M, Brucke T, Muller C, Lang N, Neirinckx RD, Deecke L (1987) Initial experience with Tc99m HMPAO brain SPECT. J Nucl Med 28:1657–1666

Rubinstein M, Denays R, Ham H, Piepz A, Van Pachterbeke T, Haumont D, Noel P (1989) Functional imaging of brain maturation in humans using iodine 123 iodoamphetamine and SPECT. J Nucl Med 30:1982–1985

Schober O, Galaske R, Heyer R (1987) Determination of brain death with 123-I-IMP and 99m-Tc-HMPAO. Neurosurg Rev 10:19–22

Tzourio N, Chiron C, Raynaud C, Dulac O, Zilbovicius M, Mazoyer B, Bourguignon M, Syrota A (1988) Etude de la maturation cerebrale du nourrisson a l'aide du SPECT et du xenon 133. J Med Nucl Biophys 12(4):133

8 Positron Emission Tomography in the Study of Neonatal Brain *

D. I. ALTMAN and J. J. VOLPE

CONTENTS

8.1 Introduction

Emission tomography is a technique that produces an image of the distribution of a previously administered radionuclide in any desired organ of the body, e.g., the head. Positron emission tomography (PET) takes advantage of the unique properties of annihilation radiation that is generated when positrons are absorbed in matter to provide an image that is a highly accurate representative of that radionuclide at a selected plane through the organ. PET has been used in humans to measure cerebral blood flow (CBF), blood volume, cerebral metabolism of glucose and oxygen, acid-base balance, receptor pharmacology and neurotransmitter metabolism. The application of PET to study cerebral physiology and neurologic disease in newborn infants is in its formative stage and has been restricted primarily to measurements of CBF and cerebral glucose metabolism. In this chapter we review and discuss aspects of PET that are pertinent to its application in newborn infants. We begin with a discussion of technological and methodologic considerations of PET with special reference to newborn infants. We then present clinical and research observations that have been made in the past few years.

8.2 Basic Principles of PET

The application of PET to the study of cerebral physiology and neurologic disease requires: (a) a positron emission tomography to measure accurately the administered radioactivity in vivo, (b) a cyclotron or linear accelerator to generate the positron-emitting radionuclides, and (c) mathematical models of radiotracer kinetics that relate tissue radioactivity measured by PET to a quantitative value, e.g., CBF (Powers and Raichle 1985; Raichle 1983).

* This review has been published in identical form in *Clinics of Perinatology*.

8.2.1 The Positron Emission Tomograph

PET is based on the in vivo detection of the two high-energy gamma photons (511 keV) that are generated from the annihilation of positrons in matter (Fig. 8.1). These photons are emitted at 180° to each other and their detection is based on the use of electronic coincidence circuits, i.e., two external radiation detectors are connected in coincidence to record an event in the tissue between them only when two annihilation photons arrive virtually simultaneously (Phelps et. al. 1975). In a modern tomograph, detectors are arranged about the head in a circular fashion and the tomograph consists of multiple rings that allow simultaneous measurement of radioactivity of multiple transverse slices. The information recorded by the detectors is analyzed by a technique called filtered-back projection to reconstruct an image which is an accurate quantitative representation of regional tissue radioactivity. The performance characteristics and other technical details of tomo-

Fig. 8.1. Basic principle of positron emission tomography (PET). Isotopes utilized decay by emission of a positron (B+) which travels a few millimeters before colliding with an electron (B−) producing an annihilation event. Latter event results in emission of two high-energy photons, which travel at approximately 180° from each other and are detected by radiation detectors linked in coincidence circuits. (From Raichle 1983)

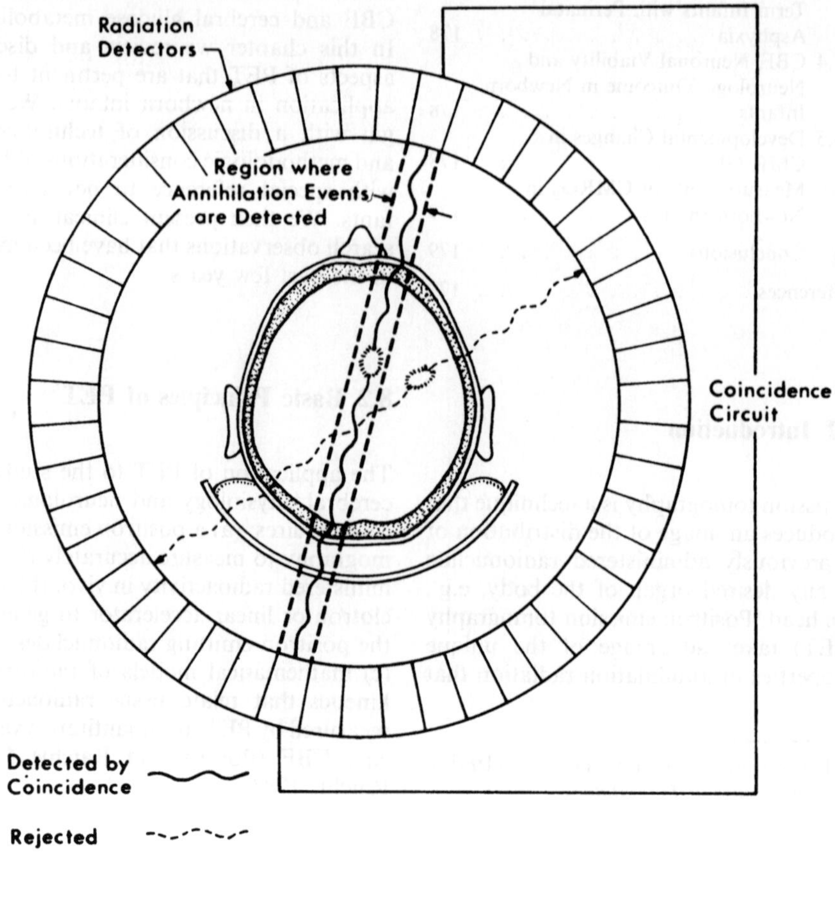

graphic design are described in a number of general reviews and will not be discussed here (Hoffman and Phelps 1986; Ter-Pogossian 1977). However, two aspects of PET, i.e., spatial resolution and photon attenuation, that are especially important to studies of newborn infants require further discussion.

8.2.1.1 Spatial Resolution

In the PET image, radioactivity from a given region is redistributed or "smeared" over a larger area. This spatial distribution is based on the spatial distribution of measured radioactivity produced by a single point of radioactivity, often called a line-spread function. The resolution of a PET system is defined as the width of this distribution at one-half of the maximum counting rate, i.e., full width at half maximum, abbreviated FWHM. The FWHM is a description of the degree of smearing or redistribution of radioactivity in the reconstructed image and is not a measure of the smallest object that can be measured accurately. As a result of this redistribution, a given region in the reconstructed PET image contains only a portion of the radioactivity actually emitted from that region in the original structure. The remainder of the radioactivity has been redistributed into surrounding areas of the image. Similarly radioactivity from the surrounding regions has been redistributed into the region of interest. Thus, the regional radioactivity measurement made by the PET represents not only the contribution of the radioactivity actually within that region but also a contribution from radioactivity in surrounding regions (Hoffman et al. 1979; Mazziotta et al. 1981; Powers and Raichle 1985). This effect is known as partial volume averaging. Thus, it is impossible to sample pure cortical gray and subcortical white matter because of their small size. In addition, any region that is close to the surface of the brain or to the ventricles will include recording of activity from the cerebrospinal fluid. Inclusion of this physiologically "inactive" fluid will lead to underestimation of the regional measurement for contiguous brain regions (Herscovitch et al. 1986).

8.2.1.2 Photon Attenuation

Only a fraction of the photons emitted from the radioactive source in the sampled region reach the external detectors, since some are absorbed by the tissue. In order to correct for the absorption of photons, a correction factor is derived as follows. Prior to performing an individual scan, an external positron-emitting source is placed within the detector field and the number of coincidences for each detector is recorded. The infant's head is then placed in the detector field (with the external source still in position) and the number of coincidences that each detector now registers is recorded. The difference in recorded coincidences is due to absorption of the photons by the infant's head, i.e., there was attenuation of the emitted photons as they passed through the infant's head. The attenuation fraction can then be calculated and used to correct data for the subsequent emission scans. Failure to correct for attenuation will underestimate the radioactivity present in the sampled tissue and result in an erroneously low value. Moreover, utilization of an adult value for attenuation correction in infants will produce spurious data, because the degree of attenuation produced by the newborn infant's smaller brain volume and thinner skull will be less than in adults. Finally, individual attenuation corrections should be performed in all infants to correct for small individual differences in photon attenuation among infants.

8.2.2 Radiotracers

The second requirement to study cerebral physiology with PET is a radiotracer that contains a positron-emitting radionuclide (Fowler and Wolf 1986). Certain elements (such as ^{15}O, ^{11}C, ^{13}N) decay by positron emission and can be generated and incorporated into biological molecules, e.g., $H_2{}^{15}O$. In other cases, when incorporation of these radionuclides into a biological molecule is not possible, another positron emitter such as ^{18}F can be generated and incorporated into chemically analogous molecules, e.g., ^{18}F-labelled deoxyglucose. Most of these radionuclides have short half-lives, ranging from 123 s for ^{15}O, to 20 min for ^{11}C or 110 min for ^{18}F. This short half-life allows relatively large amounts of radioactivity to be administered to the infant, while minimizing the absorbed radiation. Since radiation decay is rapid, especially for ^{15}O, sequential scanning is possible. The major disadvantage to these radioisotopes is that they must be prepared by a facility in the same institution or shipped only short distances. Since they are produced primarily by a cyclotron or linear acceleration, the ability to perform PET measurements depends on availability of these costly systems.

8.2.3 Mathematical Models

The third requirement for PET is a mathematical model that quantitatively relates tissue concentration of the radiotracer to the physiologic variable under study. These models must take into account a variety of factors, including delivery of tracer to the tissue, uptake and metabolism of the tracer in the tissue, egress of tracer and metabolites from the tissue and recirculation of metabolized and unmetabolized tracer. The model must be practical in its applicability and allow safe amounts of radioactivity to be administered. Finally, the assumptions in the models should be validated in normal subjects and under the pathologic conditions to be studied. We review next the methods to measure CBF cerebral blood volume (CBV), cerebral glucose metabolism (CMR-Glc) and cerebral oxygen metabolism ($CMRO_2$).

8.2.3.1 Cerebral Blood Flow

The method employed to measure CBF in infants with PET is based on the classic tissue autoradiographic technique described initially by Kety (1960) and Landau et al. (1955). This method, described in detail elsewhere, is reviewed briefly here (Altman et al. 1988; Herscovitch et al. 1983; Raichle et al. 1983). The method utilizes a hand-held injection of $H_2{}^{15}O$ in a peripheral vein over 5 s, followed by a 40 s emission scan. Quantification of absolute values of CBF requires a simultaneous arterial time-activity curve which is obtained by rapid arterial sampling from a peripheral artery. The arterial curve, generated from samples obtained either from a peripheral artery (radial, tibial), or from the descending aorta (via an umbilical arterial catheter), is assumed to be the same as that for the cerebral arteries. Any difference in the systemic and cerebral curves will lead to errors in the calculated CBF. The difference in arrival time of the radioactive bolus in the arterial curve and the head can be compensated for by defining the arrival time of the radioactive bolus in the head and in the arterial curve and then shifting the arterial curve accordingly.

Although water is a highly desirable tracer for the measurement of CBF because of its nearly free diffusibility, even the use of water is subject to some error. First, the blood-brain barrier is not completely permeable to water (Eichling et al. 1974). At high flow, water is incompletely extracted and consequently blood flow is underestimated (Herscovitch et al. 1987). Fortunately, in newborn infants, quantitative CBF is relatively low and the permeability of water does not result in a significant error in the calculation of CBF. Another possible cause of error in the use of water as tracer is the estimation of the partition coefficient of water in brain. This coefficient is affected by changes in the water content of brain and blood. The newborn brain contains relatively greater amounts of water than does adult brain, and hence, the value of the partition coefficient is different from the adult value. Therefore, an age-appropriate value is used in the calculation of CBF in the newborn (Herscovitch and Raichle 1985). In addition, the partition coefficient of water in injured brain could be different from the coefficient in normal brain. Nevertheless, experiments on neonatal animals suggest that the brain water content changes little with ischemia, e.g., by no more than approximately 3% (Rice et al. 1981). In general, large changes in the value of the partition coefficient are required to exert an appreciable effect on calculated CBF, because the mathematical algorithm used to calculate CBF is relatively insensitive to changes in the coefficient.

8.2.3.2 Cerebral Blood Volume

Measurement of CBV in newborn infants is performed following hand ventilation of air containing trace amounts of ^{15}O-labelled carbon monoxide via an endotracheal tube into the infant's lungs (Martin et al. 1987). The $C^{15}O$ combines with hemoglobin to form carboxyhemoglobin, which serves as a red blood cell, i.e., intravascular, tracer. Following a 2 min period of equilibration, a 5 min emission scan is performed. CBV is calculated by measuring the radioactivity in a peripheral blood sample and correcting for the difference in cerebral hematocrit and peripheral large vessel hematocrit and for the difference in density of blood and brain. The primary source of error in the measurement of CBV with this method arises from the application of a single average value for the ratio of cerebral tissue hematocrit to large vessel hematocrit. Recent evidence suggests that there is local variation in this ratio in adults, and the value for newborn infants is not known (Lammertsma et al. 1984; Sakai et al. 1985). Although small errors in the absolute CBV values may be obtained by this method, CBV data can be used to correct for intravascular radiotracer in other models (see below, $CMRO_2$).

8.2.3.3 Cerebral Glucose Metabolism

CMR-Glc in newborn infants has been measured by a modification for PET of the deoxyglucose (DG) method, detailed initially by Sokoloff and colleagues (Sokoloff et al. 1977). This method is based on the behavior of the glucose analogue DG, which is transported into brain, phosphorylated in a manner similar to glucose, but not metabolized further. Glucose metabolic rate is calculated in terms of three rate constants (RC) that describe influx, phosphorylation and efflux of DG and an isotope effect correction factor or lumped constant (LC). The LC itself is composed of six constants that describe the ratios of uptake and phosphorylation of glucose and DG, the dephosphorylation of glucose and the ratio of distribution space of DG in the tissue to that of glucose. The DG method has been applied to PET using ^{18}F-labelled DG as the radiotracer (Huang et al. 1980; Phelps et al. 1979; Reivich et al. 1979). A single, usually 5 min, PET scan is performed 45 min after injection of the radiotracer and average adult values of the RC and LC are used to calculate quantitative glucose metabolism. This approach may be subject to error since in normal newborn infants the values of the RC and LC may differ greatly from normal adult values. Furthermore, the value of these constants may vary markedly in ischemic and infarcted tissue, particularly when tissue glucose demand exceeds glucose supply (Crane et al. 1981; Gjedde et al. 1985; Hawkins et al. 1981; Nerdergaard et al. 1986). Unless these constants are measured in individual patients and in disease situations, large errors in calculated glucose metabolism can occur. Unfortunately, these measurements are difficult to perform, require significant blood volumes to be drawn from the infant and are time-consuming.

8.2.3.4 Cerebral Oxygen Metabolism

$CMRO_2$ has been measured by two methods, the steady state $[^{15}O]CO_2$ method and the bolus inhalation $[^{15}O]O_2$ method (Frackowiak et al. 1980; Mintun et al. 1984; Videen et al. 1987). Only the latter method has been adapted for newborn infants. Cerebral oxyen extraction fraction (OEF) and $CMRO_2$ are calculated following hand ventilation of air containing trace amounts of $[^{15}O]O_2$ into the infant's lungs via an endotracheal tube. Data from separately performed parallel CBF and CBV studies (see above) and from an accurate simultaneous measurement of arterial oxygen content are required to calculate OEF and $CMRO_2$. Calculated $CMRO_2$ by this method is subject to any errors in the measurements of CBF or CBV. Furthermore, when $CMRO_2$ is low, the effect of these errors on calculated $CMRO_2$ can be magnified considerably.

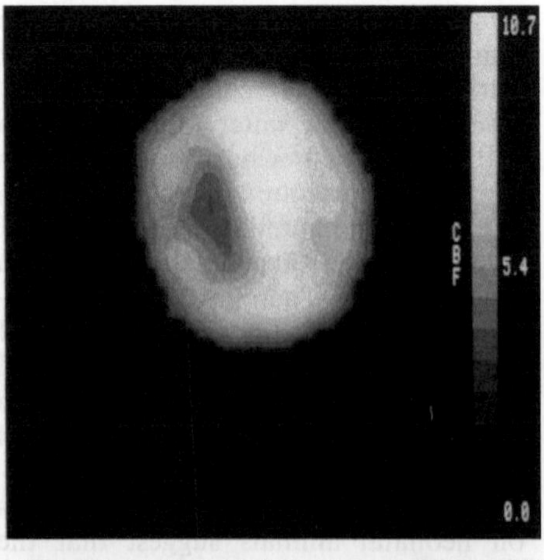

Fig. 8.2. Positron emission tomography (PET) scan in a premature infant with intraventricular hemorrhage and hemorrhagic parenchymal infarct in the left cerebral hemisphere. Scans represent horizontal section with right side of brain to readers right. The scale is a linear representation of cerebral blood flow (CBF). Extensive impairment of CBF in the hemisphere containing the intracerebral blood is apparent

8.3 PET Studies in Newborn Infants

8.3.1 PET Measurements of CBF in Newborn Infants with Intraventricular Hemorrhage

A single study reported the use of PET to measure CBF in premature infants with intraventricular hemorrhage (IVH) (Volpe et al. 1983). CBF was measured in six infants, 1–15 days after cranial ultrasonography had documented IVH associated with a unilateral parenchymal echodensity indicative of hemorrhagic parenchymal infarction. Analysis of the CBF images revealed the expected markedly reduced blood flow in the region of the parenchymal echodensity (Fig. 8.2). However, blood flow was apparently reduced also in the affected hemisphere in areas distant to and not involved by the hemorrhage. Neuropathologic studies in these infants revealed hemorrhagic infarction in the region of the parenchymal echodensity and nonhemorrhagic infarction in the periventricular regions distant to the hemorrhagic infarction and apparently corresponding to the areas of reduced blood flow. This finding suggests that the hemorrhagic parenchymal infarct is part of a larger lesion that presumably is ischemic in its basic nature. However, because injured tissue from any cause will result in reduced local blood flow, the data do not prove that the cause of the injured periventricular white matter was prior reduction in CBF due to arterial hypotension

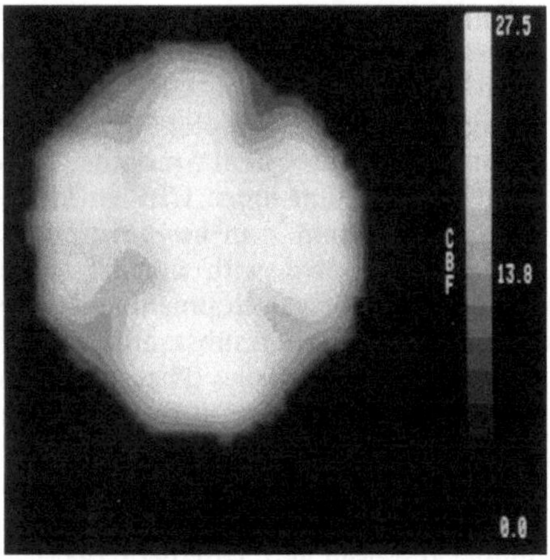

Fig. 8.3. Positron emission tomography (PET) scan in a term infant with hypoxic-ischemic encephalopathy. Reduction in CBF in the parasagittal regions is apparent

or increased intracranial venous pressure. Moreover, other explanations for the apparent wide area of decreased blood flow need to be considered. For example, it is necessary to consider the effect of partial volume averaging, discussed above, which can be appreciable in the premature infant. This problem may be aggravated if there is ventriculomegaly, a frequent feature in infants with IVH and parenchymal infarction (Guzetta et al. 1986). In addition, destruction of afferent and efferent fiber pathways by a cerebral lesion may cause reductions in both CBF and metabolism in regions which show no structural abnormality, such as in the cortex overlying purely subcortical lesions (Metter et al. 1985; Videen et al. 1987).

This single report indicates that abnormalities of CBF are apparent in infants with IVH and parenchymal infarction. Further studies are needed in premature infants at high risk for the development of IVH and the parenchymal lesion prior to the development of the lesions to determine if there is reduced CBF and evidence of hemodynamic compromise prior to the development of the parenchymal infarction.

8.3.2 Measurement of CBF in Term Infants with Perinatal Asphyxia

A single study reports measurements of CBF in 17 asphyxiated newborn infants performed during the acute phases of their illness (Volpe et al. 1985). Quantitative CBF values were not obtained in all infants. An apparently unifying abnormal pattern of CBF was observed in these infants, i.e., a relative decrease in CBF to parasagittal regions of the cerebrum, more marked posteriorly than anteriorly (Fig. 8.3). In infants who subsequently developed normally, the ratio of parasagittal CBF to the highest CBF recorded in the sylvian region was 0.78. In infants who suffered permanent neurologic deficits, the ratio was 0.60, approximately 20% lower. Support for cerebral injury in the watershed regions of the brain of these asphyxiated infants was provided by the finding of abnormal technetium uptake in this region on brain scan in three infants and postmortem evidence of parasagittal ischemic cortical and white matter injury in the single autopsied patient. This patient also had evidence of diffuse cerebral and brain stem neuronal injury, indicating the difficulty in correlating the PET findings to a single pathologic entity. Since quantitative CBV values were not obtained in all infants, the biological significance of this apparent reduction in CBF remains to be determined conclusively. Recently, we and others have found that the CBF requirement for brain viability in newborn infants is lower than in adults (see below). Whether CBF in the parasagittal regions was below these ischemic thresholds remains to be determined. As discussed above, it may not be possible to resolve this question until the resolution of modern tomographs improves, since it is not possible to measure accurately CBF in these discrete regions.

8.3.3 Measurement of DG Uptake in Term Infants with Perinatal Asphyxia

Various patterns of DG uptake have been reported in 13 infants with perinatal asphyxia and newborn seizures (Doyle et al. 1983; Thorp et al. 1988). Quantitative values for CMR-Glc were not calculated. The patterns of DG uptake observed included no focal abnormality, focal increase or decrease uptake of DG and loss of metabolic definition (all regions containing approximately equal amounts of radiotracer). While these studies demonstrate the technical feasibility of performing PET studies on such newborn infants, the biological significance of these findings remain to be determined conclusively. However, they do stress the heterogeneity of the clinical and neuropathologic characteristics of infants with perinatal asphyxia.

8.3.4 CBF, Neuronal Viability and Neurologic Outcome in Newborn Infants

Measurements of CBF in adults with cerebrovascular disease have demonstrated that CBF values below 10 ml 100 g^{-1} min^{-1} occur only in infarcted brain (Powers et al. 1985). In experimental animals, the ischemic threshold for electrocerebral silence is approximately 16–20 ml 100 g^{-1} min^{-1}, and the threshold for neuronal death is approximately 10 ml 100 g^{-1} min^{-1} (Astrup 1982). Recently, we reported our observations of CBF in 16 preterm and 14 term infants with a variety of neurologic conditions and correlated these values of CBF measured in the newborn period with neurologic and cognitive outcome (Altman et al. 1988). Two major findings were apparent. The first finding was that the CBF requirement for brain viability in newborn infants is lower than in adults. Three preterm infants with mean hemispheric CBF of 4.9, 5.2, and 9.3 ml 100 g^{-1} min^{-1} had normal neurologic examinations and cognitive scores at follow-up of 6–18 months. One term infant with mean hemispheric CBF of 9.0 ml 100 g^{-1} min^{-1} was developing normally when he died of sepsis at 5 months. These data indicate that mean CBF as low as 5 ml 100 g^{-1} min^{-1} in newborn infants can be associated with normal subsequent neurologic development and therefore preservation of a substantial proportion of cerebral tissue. These data are consistent with observations of other investigators who have documented intact visual evoked responses in preterm infants with CBF below 10 ml 100 g^{-1} min^{-1} (Greisen and Trojaberg 1987).

The second finding of the report was that the absolute value of CBF measured during the newborn period did not predict subsequent neurologic outcome. Thus, there was no statistically significant relationship between newborn CBF values and the degree of neurologic and cognitive deficits. This finding was not totally unexpected, since, in the acute period after brain injury, normal mechanisms of CBF regulation are impaired. Thus, CBF is often normal or elevated in a damaged tissue with a reduced metabolic rate (Powers and Raichle 1985; Obrist et al. 1984).

8.3.5 Developmental Changes in CMR-Glc

Chugani et al. (1987; Chugani and Phelps 1986) have reported striking changes in CMR-Glc during brain development from the newborn period through infancy and childhood. Of note for this review, they have measured CMR-Glc in a few newborn infants who suffered newborn seizures but who were subsequently normal at follow-up. Reduced CMR-Glc was found in these infants, with values approximately 60% of adult values. CMR-Glc appeared highest in the sensorimotor cortex, thalamus and brain stem, and relatively lower values were found in frontal areas and in striatal regions.

These findings are consistent with developmental changes in CBF, CMR-Glc and enzyme activity levels in a number of animal species (Abrams et al. 1984; Booth et al. 1980; Himwich and Fazekas 1941; Nehlig et al. 1988; Patel et al. 1975; Tyler and van Harreveld 1942).

8.3.6 Measurements of $CMRO_2$ in Newborn Infants

Preliminary measurements of $CMRO_2$, CBV and OEF have been reported in abstract form in five preterm and four term infants (Altman et al. 1989). In the term infants the range of $CMRO_2$ was from 0.4 to 1.3 ml 100 g^{-1} min^{-1}. These values are lower than values found in viable adult brain and suggest that the $CMRO_2$ requirement for brain viability is lower in newborn infants than in adults. In two preterm infants of gestational ages 26 and 28 weeks, who had minimal or no evidence of brain injury in the newborn period, $CMRO_2$ was very low, i.e., <0.06 ml 100 g^{-1} min^{-1}. This finding, although preliminary, suggests that cerebral energy requirements at this gestational age may be minimal and/or that they are met by nonoxidative mechanisms such as glycolysis.

8.4 Conclusions

In the preceding discussion we have reviewed the technical and methodologic aspects of PET that pertain to measurements of CBF, CBV and cerebral metabolism in newborn infants. The use of PET in the study of cerebral physiology and neurologic disease in newborn infants is still in its formative stages, but accurate measurements are possible. There are many methodologic and technical problems that need to be considered when these methods are applied to newborn infants. However, from the data presented in this review, it is apparent that PET has provided important new insights into the cerebral circulatory and metabolic changes that occur during development and with cerebral injury. Clearly, more studies, critically analyzed and correlating PET measurements with neuropathologic changes, clinical syndromes and neuroradiologic imaging features are needed. Of particular importance will be studies of infants with minimal or no brain injury who are at highest risk for developing cerebral injury.

References

Abrams RM, Ito M, Frisinger JE, et al. (1984) Local cerebral glucose utilization in fetal and neonatal sheep. Am J Physiol 246:R608–R618

Altman DI, Powers WJ, Perlman JM, et al. (1988) Cerebral blood flow requirement for brain viability in newborn infants is lower than in adults. Ann Neurol 24:218–226

Altman DI, Perlman JM, Volpe JJ, et al. (1989) Cerebral oxygen metabolism in newborn infants measured with positron emission tomography. J Cereb Blood Flow Metab 9:S25

Astrup J (1982) Energy requiring cell functions in the ischemic brain. J Neurosurg 56:482–497

Booth REG, Patel TB, Clark JB (1980) The development of enzymes of energy metabolism in the brain of a presocial (Guinea pig) and non-presocial (rat) species. J Neurochem 34:17–25

Chugani HT, Phelps ME (1986) Maturational changes in cerebral function in infants determined by ^{18}FDG positron emission tomography. Science 231:840–843

Chugani HT, Phelps ME, Mazziota JC (1987) Positron emission tomography study of human brain functional development. Ann Neurol 22:487–497

Crane PD, Pardridge WM, Braun LD, et al. (1981) The interaction of transport and metabolism on brain glucose utilization: a re-evaluation of the lumped constant. J Neurochem 36:1601–1604

Doyle LW, Nahmias C, Firnau G, et al. (1983) Regional cerebral glucose metabolism of newborn infants measured by positron

emission tomography. Dev Med Child Neurol 25:143–151
Eichling JO, Raichle ME, Grubb RL Jr, et al. (1974) Evidence of the limitations of water as a freely diffusible tracer in the brain of the rhesus monkey. Circ Res 35:358–364
Fowler JS, Wolf AP (1986) Positron emitter-labelled compounds: priorities and problems. In: Phelps ME, Mazziotta J, Shelbert H (eds) Positron emission tomography and autoradiography: principles and applications for the brain and heart. Raven, New York, pp 391–450
Frackowiak RSJ, Lenzi GL, Jones T, et al. (1980) Quantitative measurement of regional cerebral blood flow and oxygen metabolism in man using ^{15}O and positron emission tomography: theory procedure and normal values. J Comput Assist Tomogr 4:727–736
Gjedde A, Wienhard K, Heiss WD, et al. (1985) Comparative regional analysis of 2-fluorodeoxyglucose and methylglucose uptake in brain of four stroke patients with special reference to the regional estimation of the lumped constant. J Cereb Blood Flow Metab 5:163–178
Greisen G, Trojaberg W (1987) Cerebral blood flow, $paCO_2$ changes, and visual evoked potentials in mechanically ventilated, preterm infants. Acta Pediatr Scand 76:394–400
Guzzetta FF, Shackelford GD, Volpe S, et al. (1986) Periventricular intraparenchymal echodensities in the premature newborn: critical determinant of neurologic outcome. Pediatrics 78:995–1006
Hawkins R, Phelps ME, Huang SL, et al. (1981) Effect of ischemia on quantification of local cerebral glucose metabolic rate in man. J Cereb Blood Flow Metab 1:37–52
Herscovitch P, Raichle M (1985) What is the correct value for the brain-blood partition coefficient of water? J Cereb Blood Flow Metab 5:65–69
Herscovitch P, Markham J, Raichle ME (1983) Brain blood flow measured with intravenous $H_2{}^{15}O$. I. Theory and error analysis. J Nucl Med 24:782–789
Herscovitch P, Auchus AP, Gado M, et al. (1986) Correction of positron emission tomography data for cerebral atrophy. J Cereb Blood Flow Metab 6:120–124
Herscovitch P, Raichle M, Kilbourn M, et al. (1987) Positron emission tomographic measurement of cerebral blood flow and permeability-surface area product of water using ^{15}O-water and ^{11}C-butanol. J Cereb Blood Flow Metab 7:527–542
Himwich H, Fazekas J (1941) Comparative studies of the metabolism of the brain of infant and adult dogs. Am J Physiol 132:454–459
Hoffman EJ, Phelps ME (1986) Positron emission tomography: principles and quantitation. In: Phelps ME, Mazziotta J, Schelbert H (eds) Positron emission tomography and autoradiography: principles and applications for the brain and heart. Raven, New York, pp 237–286
Hoffman EJ, Huang S, Phelps ME (1979) Quantitation in positron emission tomography. I. Effect of object size. J Comput Assist Tomogr 3:299–308
Huang SC, Phelps ME, Hoffman EJ, et al. (1980) Non-invasive determination of local cerebral metabolic rate of glucose in man. Am J Physiol 238:E69–E82
Kennedy C, Grave GD, Jehle JW, et al. (1972) Changes in blood flow in the component structures of the dog brain during postnatal maturation. J Neurochem 19:2423–2433
Kety SS (1960) Measurement of local blood flow by the exchange of an inert diffusible substance. Methods Med Res 8:125–129
Lammertsma AA, Brooks DJ, Beaney RP, et al. (1984) In vivo measurement of regional cerebral hematocrit using positron emission tomography. J Cereb Blood Flow Metab 4:317–322
Landau WM, Freygang WH Jr, Rowland LP (1955) The local circulation of the living brain, values in the unanesthetized and anesthetized cat. Trans Am Neurol Assoc 80:125–129
Martin WRW, Powers WJ, Raichle ME (1987) Cerebral blood volume measured with inhaled $C^{15}O$ and positron emission tomography. J Cereb Blood Flow Metab 7:421–426
Mazziotta JC, Phelps ME, Plummer D, et al. (1981) Quantitation in positron emission computed tomography. V. Physical-anatomical effects. J Comput Assist Tomogr 5:734–743
Metter EJ, Mazziotta JC, Itabaski HH, et al. (1985) Comparison of glucose metabolism, X-ray CT, and postmortem data in a patient with multiple cerebral infarcts. Neurology (NY) 35:1695–1701
Mintun MA, Raichle ME, Martin WRW, et al. (1984) Brain oxygen utilization mea-

sured with O-15 radiotracers and positron emission tomography. J Nucl Med 25:177–187

Nehlig A, de Vasconcelos AP, Boyet S (1988) Quantitative autoradiographic measurement of local cerebral glucose utilization in freely moving rats during postnatal development. J Neurosci 8:2321–2333

Nerdergaard M, Gjedde A, Diemer NH (1986) Focal ischemia of the rat brain: autoradiographic determination of cerebral glucose utilization, glucose content, and blood flow. J Cereb Blood Flow Metab 6:414–424

Obrist WD, Langfitt TW, Jaggi JL, et al. (1984) Cerebral blood flow and metabolism in comatose patients with acute head injury. J Neurosurg 61:241–253

Patel MS, Johnson CA, Rajan R, et al. (1975) The ontogeny of ketone bodies in developing human brain: development of ketone-body-producing enzymes and ketone bodies as precursors for lipid synthesis. J Neurochem 25:905–908

Phelps ME, Hoffman EJ, Mullani NA, et al. (1975) Application of annihilation coincidence detection to transaxial reconstruction tomography. J Nucl Med 16:210–223

Phelps ME, Huang SC, Hoffman EJ, et al. (1979) Tomographic measurement of local cerebral glucose metabolic rate in humans with (F-18)2-fluro-2-deoxy-D-glucose: validation of method. Ann Neurol 6:371–388

Powers WJ, Raichle ME (1985) Positron emission tomography and its application to the study of cerebrovascular disease in man. Stroke 16:361–376

Powers WJ, Grubb RL, Darriet D, et al. (1985) Cerebral blood flow and cerebral metabolic rate of oxygen requirements for cerebral function and viability in humans. J Cereb Blood Flow Metab 5:600–608

Raichle ME (1983) Positron emission tomography. Annu Rev Neurosci 6:249–267

Raichle ME, Martin WRW, Herscovitch P, et al. (1983) Brain blood flow measured with intravenous $H_2{}^{15}O$. XI. Implementation and validation. J Nucl Med 24:790–798

Reivich M, Kuhl D, Wolf A, et al. (1979) The (^{18}F)-fluorodeoxyglucose method for the measurement of local cerebral glucose utilization in man. Circ Res 44:127–137

Rice JE, Vannucci RC, Brierly JB (1981) The influence of immaturity on hypoxic-ischemic brain injury in the rat. Ann Neurol 9:131–141

Sakai F, Nakazawa K, Tazaki Y, et al. (1985) Regional cerebral blood volume and hematocrit measured in normal human volunteers by single-photon emission computed tomography. J Cereb Blood Flow Metab 5:707–713

Sokoloff L, Reivich M, Kennedy L, et al. (1977) The [^{14}C] deoxyglucose method for the measurement of local cerebral glucose utilization: theory procedure and normal values in the conscious and anesthetized albino rat. J Neurochem 28:897–916

Thorp PS, Levin SD, Garnett ES, et al. (1988) Patterns of cerebral glucose metabolism using ^{18}FDG and positron tomography in the neurologic investigation of the full term infant. Neuropediatrics 19:146–153

Ter-Pogossian MM (1977) Basic principles of computed axial tomography. Semin Nucl Med 7:109–127

Tyler DB, van Harreveld A (1942) The respiration of the developing brain. Am J Physiol 136:600–603

Videen TO, Perlmutter JS, Herscovitch P, et al. (1987) Brain blood volume, flow, and oxygen utilization measured with ^{15}O radiotracers and positron emission tomography: revised metabolic computations. J Cereb Blood Flow Metab 7:513–516

Volpe JJ, Herscovitch P, Perlman JM (1983) Positron emission tomography in the newborn: extensive impairment of regional cerebral blood flow with intraventricular hemorrhage and hemorrhagic intracerebral involvement. Pediatrics 72:589–601

Volpe JJ, Herscovitch P, Perlman JM, et al. (1985) Positron emission tomography in the asphyxiated term newborn: parasagittal impairment of cerebral blood flow. Ann Neurol 17:287–296

Subject Index

MIX
Papier aus verantwortungsvollen Quellen
Paper from responsible sources
FSC® C105338

If you have any concerns about our products,
you can contact us on
ProductSafety@springernature.com

In case Publisher is established outside the EU,
the EU authorized representative is:
Springer Nature Customer Service Center GmbH
Europaplatz 3, 69115 Heidelberg, Germany

Printed by Libri Plureos GmbH
in Hamburg, Germany